# Sudden Cardiac Death

# Cardiovascular Clinics Series

*Not Available

# Sudden Cardiac Death

## Mark E. Josephson, M.D. | Editor

Robinette Foundation Professor of Medicine
University of Pennsylvania School of Medicine
Chief, Cardiovascular Section
Hospital of the University of Pennsylvania
Philadelphia, Pennsylvania

## CARDIOVASCULAR CLINICS
## Albert N. Brest, M.D. | Editor-in-Chief

James C. Wilson Professor of Medicine
Director, Division of Cardiology
Jefferson Medical College
Philadelphia, Pennsylvania

 F. A. DAVIS COMPANY, PHILADELPHIA

Cardiovascular Clinics, 15/3, Sudden Cardiac Death

Copyright © 1985 by F. A. Davis Company

Printed in the United States of America

NOTE: As new scientific information becomes available through basic and clinical research, recommended treatments and drug therapies undergo changes. The authors and publisher have done everything possible to make this book accurate, up-to-date, and in accord with accepted standards at the time of publication. However, the reader is advised always to check product information (package inserts) for changes and new information regarding dose and contraindications before administering any drug. Caution is especially urged when using new or infrequently ordered drugs.

**Library of Congress Cataloging in Publication Data**

Cardiovascular clinics. 1–

  Philadelphia, F. A. Davis, 1969–

    v. ill. 27 cm.

    Editor: v. 1–  A. N. Brest
    Key title: Cardiovascular clinics, ISSN 0069-0384
    1. Cardiovascular system—Diseases—Collected works. 1. Brest, Albert N., ed.
    [DNLM: W1 CA77N]
    RC681.A1C27     616.1      70-6558
    ISBN 0-8036-5098-1                                    MARC-S

Library of Congress      75[8307]

# Preface

Sudden cardiac death remains one of the most pressing, unresolved problems in Medicine today and remains the major cause of death in patients with coronary artery disease. Over the past 10 years, significant efforts have been made in an attempt to predict those patients at risk for sudden death and to develop pharmacologic and nonpharmacologic methods to prevent patients at risk from dying.

This volume provides a comprehensive review of up-to-date information concerning epidemiology, pathology and underlying mechanisms, and therapeutic interventions possible for the prevention of sudden cardiac death. Holter monitoring and electrophysiologic testing have aided greatly in our understanding of the electrophysiologic milieu that characterizes patients at risk for sudden death. In addition, pharmacologic therapy has been improved with the development of new antiarrhythmic agents as well as the use of both Holter monitoring and programmed stimulation to identify patients at risk and to develop therapeutic regimens. In addition to the pharmacologic therapy of malignant ventricular arrhythmias, the role of implantable electronic devices and surgery in managing these arrhythmias is discussed. Newer methods to predict patients at risk for sudden arrhythmic death are discussed, as well as the potential role of platelets, prostaglandins, coronary spasm, and the autonomic nervous system in the initiation of lethal arrhythmias.

I wish to thank all of the contributing authors for their detailed and well-developed discussion of these topics. I would like to acknowledge the help of the Electrophysiology Fellows and the technical staff at the University of Pennsylvania for helping to generate much of the information published in this book. Special thanks go to Ms. Maria Coscia and Angelika Boyce for assuring the completion of all the authors' manuscripts and meeting all necessary deadlines for this text.

It is my hope that this text will provide the most up-to-date review of all aspects of sudden cardiac death syndrome.

Mark E. Josephson, M.D.
Guest Editor

# Editor's Commentary

In years past, cardiac arrest had been invariably fatal. More recently, we have learned how to reverse the condition and how to prevent additional attacks, at least in some instances. Moreover, we have begun to recognize precursors of this disorder. Nonetheless, sudden cardiac death continues to be the leading cause of mortality in the United States. Clearly, therefore, we need to enlarge our understanding of this disorder. This issue of CARDIOVASCULAR CLINICS deals broadly and specifically with the pathology, electrophysiology, pathogenesis, clinical characteristics (initiating events, epidemiology, identification of risks), diagnostic approaches (signal averaging, ambulatory monitoring, programmed electrical stimulation), and management (drug, surgical approaches) of sudden death. The discussions presented in this book by leading authorities in the field suggest that we are on the threshold of firm understanding and of rational dealing with this pervasive problem. I am deeply grateful to Dr. Mark E. Josephson for his guidance in the formulation of this book, and both of us are indebted to the individual authors for their outstanding contributions.

Albert N. Brest, M.D.
Editor-in-Chief

# Contributors

Jesus M. Almendral, M.D.
*Fellow in Electrophysiology, Cardiovascular Section, Hospital of the University of Pennsylvania, Philadelphia, Pennsylvania*

Saroja Bharati, M.D.
*Clinical Professor of Pathology, Temple University Medical School, Philadelphia, Pennsylvania; Clinical Professor of Pathology, The Pennsylvania State Unviersity, The Milton S. Hershey Medical Center, Hershey, Pennsylvania; Chairperson, Department of Pathology, Deborah Heart and Lung Center, Browns Mills, New Jersey; Research Professor of Medicine, University of Illinois College of Medicine at Chicago, Chicago, Illinois*

J. Thomas Bigger, M.D.
*Professor of Medicine and Pharmacology, Division of Cardiology, Department of Medicine, Columbia University; Director, Arrhythmia Control Unit, The Columbia-Presbyterian Medical Center, New York, New York*

Alfred E. Buxton, M.D.
*Assistant Professor of Medicine; University of Pennsylvania School of Medicine; Director, Clinical Electrophysiology Laboratory, Hospital of the University of Pennsylvania, Philadelphia, Pennsylvania*

Dennis M. Cassidy, M.D.
*Fellow in Electrophysiology, Cardiovascular Section, Hospital of the University of Pennsylvania, Philadelphia, Pennsylvania*

Agustin Castellanos, M.D.
*Professor of Medicine, University of Miami School of Medicine; Director, Clinical Electrophysiology, Jackson Memorial Hospital, Miami, Florida*

James Coromilas, M.D.
*Assistant Professor of Medicine, Division of Cardiology, Department of Medicine, Columbia University; Director, Ambulatory ECG Laboratory, The Columbia-Presbyterian Medical Center, New York, New York*

John U. Doherty, M.D.
*Assistant Professor of Medicine, University of Pennsylvania School of Medicine; Director of Holter Monitoring, Hospital of the University of Pennsylvania, Philadelphia, Pennsylvania*

Carol A. Dresden, M.S.
*Research Associate, Cardiovascular Section, Hospital of the University of Pennsylvania, Philadelphia, Pennsylvania*

Daneil Estes, R.N., C.C.R.N.
*Clinical Research Assistant, Division of Cardiology, University of Miami School of Medicine, Miami, Florida*

Rita A. Falcone, M.S.
*Research Associate, Cardiovascular Section, Hospital of the University of Pennsylvania, Philadelphia, Pennsylvania*

William H. Frishman, M.D.
*Director, Department of Medicine, The Hospital of the Albert Einstein College of Medicine, Bronx, New York*

Curt D. Furberg, M.D.
*Director, Clinical Trials Branch, National Heart, Lung and Blood Institute, Bethesda, Maryland*

John S. Gelman, M.B., B.S., F.R.A.C.P.
*Fellow, Division of Cardiology, University of Florida College of Medicine, Gainesville, Florida*

Sheldon Goldberg, M.D.
*Associate Professor of Medicine, Jefferson Medical College; Director, Cardiac Catheterization Laboratory, Thomas Jefferson University Hospital, Philadelphia, Pennsylvania*

Allan M. Greenspan, M.D.
*Associate Professor of Medicine; Associate Director, Clinical Cardiac Electrophysiology Laboratory, Likoff Cardiovascular Institute, Hahnemann University and Hospital, Philadelphia, Pennsylvania*

Wayne Grogan, M.D.
*Fellow in Electrophysiology, Cardiovascular Section, Hospital of the University of Pennsylvania, Philadelphia, Pennsylvania*

Eric L. Hagestad, B.S.
*Doctoral Candidate, Harvard Medical School, Department of Physiology and Biophysics, Boston, Massachusetts*

Alden H. Harken, M.D.
*Professor and Chairman, Department of Surgery, University of Colorado, Denver, Colorado*

Joseph Horgan, M.D.
*Cardiology Fellow, Division of Cardiology, University of Miami School of Medicine, Miami, Florida*

Leonard N. Horowitz, M.D.
*Associate Professor of Medicine; Director, Clinical Cardiac Electrophysiology Laboratory, Likoff Cardiovascular Institute, Hahnemann University and Hospital, Philadelphia, Pennsylvania*

Mark E. Josephson, M.D.
*Robinette Foundation Professor of Medicine (Cardiovascular Disease), University of Pennsylvania School of Medicine; Chief, Cardiovascular Section, Hospital of the University of Pennsylvania, Philadelphia, Pennsylvania*

William B. Kannel, M.D., M.P.H
*Professor of Medicine; Chief, Section of Preventive Medicine and Epidemiology, Division of Medicine, Boston University Medical Center, Boston, Massachusetts*

Martin S. Kanovsky, M.D.
*Clinical Assistant Professor of Medicine, George Washington University School of Medicine; Cardiologist, The Washington Clinic; Attending Physician, George Washington University Medical Center, The Washington Hospital Center, Washington, D.C.*

Kenneth M. Kessler, M.D.
*Associate Professor of Medicine; Director, Non-Invasive Diagnostic Cardiology, University of Miami School of Medicine, Miami, Florida*

Michael G. Kienzle, M.D.
*Fellow in Electrophysiology, Cardiovascular Section, Hospital of the University of Pennsylvania, Philadelphia, Pennsylvania*

Joseph Kmonicek, M.D.
*Instructor, Cardiology Division, Jefferson Medical College, Thomas Jefferson University Hospital, Philadelphia, Pennsylvania*

Lawrence I. Laifer, M.D.
*Resident, Division of Cardiology, Department of Medicine, Albert Einstein College of Medicine, Bronx, New York*

Maurice Lev, M.D.
*Director of Laboratories, Deborah Heart and Lung Center, Browns Mills, New Jersey; Clinical Professor of Pathology, Temple University Medical School, Philadelphia, Pennsylvania; Clinical Professor of Pathology, The Pennsylvania State University, The Milton S. Hershey Medical Center, Hershey, Pennsylvania*

Richard M. Luceri, M.D.
*Assistant Professor of Medicine; Director, Clinical Arrhythmias and Pacemaker Program, University of Miami School of Medicine, Miami, Florida*

Francis E. Marchlinski, M.D.
*Assistant Professor of Medicine, University of Pennsylvania School of Medicine; Director, Arrhythmia Evaluation Center; Co-Director, Clinical Electrophysiology Laboratory, Hospital of the University of Pennsylvania, Philadelphia, Pennsylvania*

Daniel L. McGee, Ph.D.
*Senior Statistician, Agent Orange Project, Centers for Disease Control, Atlanta, Georgia*

Jawahar Mehta, M.D.
*Associate Professor of Medicine, Division of Cardiology; Director, Coronary Care Unit, University of Florida College of Medicine, Gainesville, Florida*

Eric L. Michelson, M.D.
*Chief, Clinical Research, Lankenau Medical Research Center; Associate Professor of Medicine (Cardiology), Jefferson Medical College, Thomas Jefferson University, Philadelphia, Pennsylvania*

John M. Miller, M.D.
*Fellow in Electrophysiology, Cardiovascular Section, Hospital of the University of Pennsylvania, Philadelphia, Pennsylvania*

Joel Morganroth, M.D.
*Professor of Medicine and Pharmacology; Director, Sudden Death Prevention Program, Likoff Cardiovascular Institute, Hahnemann University and Hospital, Philadelphia, Pennsylvania*

Robert J. Myerburg, M.D.
*Professor of Medicine and Physiology; Director, Division of Cardiology, University of Miami School of Medicine, Miami, Florida*

Ioannis P. Panidis, M.D.
*Assistant Professor of Medicine; Associate Director, Cardiac Ultrasound Laboratory, Likoff Cardiovascular Institute, Hahnemann University, Philadelphia, Pennsylvania*

Philip J. Podrid, M.D.
*Research Associate in Cardiology, Harvard School of Public Health; Associate Physician in Medicine, Brigham and Women's Hospital, Boston, Massachusetts*

Dan M. Roden, M.D.
*Assistant Professor of Medicine and Pharmacology, Vanderbilt Unversity School of Medicine, Nashville, Tennessee*

Denis Roy, M.D.
*Staff Cardiologist, Montreal Heart Institute, Montreal, Quebec, Canada*

Lyle A. Siddoway, M.D.
*Postdoctoral Fellow, Divisions of Cardiology and Clinical Pharmacology, Department of Medicine, Vanderbilt University School of Medicine, Nashville, Tennessee*

Michael B. Simson, M.D.
*Samuel Bellet Associate Professor of Medicine, University of Pennsylvania School of Medicine; Director, Medical Intensive Care Unit, Hospital of the University of Pennsylvania, Philadelphia, Pennsylvania*

Scott R. Spielman, M.D.
*Associate Professor of Medicine; Associate Director, Clinical Cardiac Electrophysiology Laboratory, Likoff Cardiovascular Institute, Hahnemann University and Hospital, Philadelphia, Pennsylvania*

Richard Trohman, M.D.
*Electrophysiology Research Fellow, Division of Cardiology, University of Miami School of Medicine, Miami, Florida*

Joseph A. Vassallo, M.D.
*Fellow in Electrophysiology, Cardiovascular Section, Hospital of the University of Pennsylvania, Philadelphia, Pennsylvania*

Richard L. Verrier, Ph.D.
*Assistant Professor of Physiology, Harvard School of Public Health; Assistant Professor of Medicine, Harvard Medical School, Brigham and Women's Hospital; Director, Cardiovascular Laboratories, Harvard School of Public Health, Boston, Massachusetts*

Victoria L. Vetter, M.D.
*Assistant Professor of Pediatrics, University of Pennsylvania School of Medicine; Associate Cardiologist, Division of Cardiology; Director, Pediatric Electrophysiology Laboratory, The Children's Hospital of Philadelphia, Philadelphia, Pennsylvania*

Harvey L. Waxman, M.D.
*Assistant Professor of Medicine, Cardiovascular Section, Hospital of the University of Pennsylvania, Philadelphia, Pennsylvania*

Charles R. Webb, M.D.
*Assistant Professor of Medicine; Senior Attending Physician, The Clinical Cardiac Electrophysiology Laboratory, Likoff Cardiovascular Institute, Hahnemann University and Hospital, Philadelphia, Pennsylvania*

Lewis Wetstein, M.D.
*Assistant Professor of Surgery, Division of Thoracic and Cardiac Surgery, Medical College of Virginia, Richmond, Virginia*

Raymond L. Woosley, M.D., Ph.D.
*Associate Professor of Medicine and Pharmacology, Vanderbilt University School of Medicine, Nashville, Tennessee*

Liaqat Zaman, M.D.
*Assistant Professor of Medicine, University of Miami School of Medicine, Miami, Florida*

# Contents

# The Pathology of Sudden Death*

## Saroja Bharati, M.D., and Maurice Lev, M.D.

This chapter deals with the abnormalities in the conduction system and the surrounding structures that may be related to sudden death. We will describe our experience with the pathology found in the sinoatrial (SA) node, the atrioventricular (AV) node, the AV bundle, the bundle branches, the myocardium, the valves, the endocardium, and the anomalous AV connections (in cases of pre-excitation). Our discussion will include case histories of patients in whom we have studied the conduction system.

## ABNORMALITIES IN THE SINOATRIAL REGION

### Trauma to the SA Node[1]

A 35-year-old woman was believed to have had heart disease since the age of 21. Diagnostic cardiac catheterization studies revealed moderate mitral insuffficiency with marked left ventricular hypertrophy. The pulmonary artery, right ventricular, left ventricular end-diastolic, and pulmonary wedge pressures were elevated. A diagnosis of cardiomyopathy was made. The patient was asymptomatic up to age 35. At that time, she was involved in an automobile accident, and she was unconscious for an unknown period of time. Later, she complained of pain in the right back and the chest. This pain was found to be due to fracture of the right clavicle. Five days later, she collapsed and was found to be in ventricular tachycardia. Subsequent electrocardiograms disclosed paroxysmal atrial tachycardia with varying block and, later, sinus bradycardia with wandering pacemaker from SA node to the AV junction. Twenty-eight days after the accident, she was found dead in bed.

At autopsy, the heart was enlarged, with hypertrophy of both atria and ventricles. At the junction of the left atrium and inferior mitral leaflet close to the posterior commissure, there was a white plaque-like formation measuring 1.5 cm in greatest dimension. This plaque was firm and, on section, showed a tumor-like lesion measuring 0.3 to 0.4 cm in diameter. On section, this plaque was found to consist of benign osteoid tissue. The mitral orifice was enlarged. The coronary arteries revealed moderate atherosclerosis.

Examination of the conduction system revealed a large area of hemorrhage and necrosis in the SA node (Fig. 1), accompanied by macrophages, fibroblasts, and mononuclear cells. Fat tissue partially isolated but did not completely separate the node from the adjacent myocardium. The adjacent epicardium revealed chronic inflammation and hemorrhage. An organiz-

*Aided by Grant HL 30558-02 from the National Institutes of Health, The National Heart, Lung and Blood Institute, Bethesda, Maryland.

1

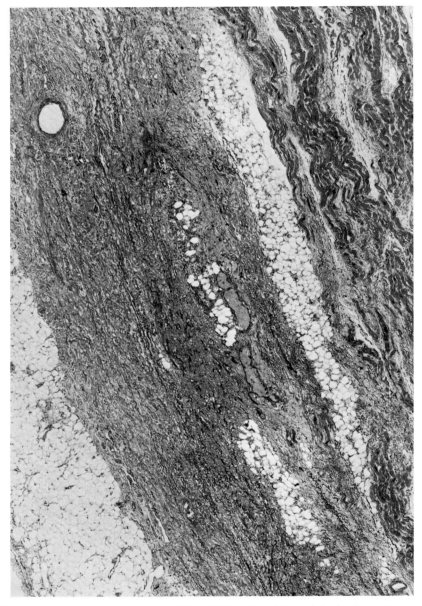

**Figure 1.** Sinoatrial node showing hemorrhage, with partial isolation of the node by fat tissue. Hematoxylin-eosin stain × 45. (From Bharati et al,[1] with permission.)

ing thrombus was present in the adjacent atrial cavity. The approaches to the SA node showed considerable focal vacuolar and eosinophilic degeneration of muscle cells and moderate fatty infiltration, with a fine infiltration of mononuclear and neutrophilic cells. The atria showed moderate degenerative changes and slight to moderate fibrosis, with chronic organizing pericarditis over the right atrium. The same changes were present in the atrial septum (atrial preferential pathways). The remainder of the conduction system revealed insignificant changes. The ventricles contained spotty areas of old fibrosis.

The bradycardia this patient exhibited for several years before the accident probably was related anatomically to the partial separation of the SA node by fatty tissue. The atrial preferential pathways and the approaches to the SA node also revealed some chronic changes. The atrial arrhythmias associated with the collapse of the patient subsequent to the automobile accident were probably related to the hemorrhage in the SA node. This hemorrhage was most likely traumatic in nature. Thus, nonsurgical blunt trauma to the chest wall may result in hemorrhage in the SA node, which may cause various types of atrial arrhythmias and may terminate in sudden death. Likewise, one may hypothesize that if extensive hemorrhage were to occur (as a result of any type of nontraumatic injury to the chest wall) in the region of the AV node, AV bundle, or bundle branches, various types of tachyarrhythmias or bradyarrhythmias or both might result and lead also to sudden death.

## Sick Sinus Syndrome in Younger Age Groups[2]

Although the sick sinus syndrome in young individuals is uncommon and generally well tolerated, it may precipitate a bradyarrhythmic or tachyarrhythmic syndrome that could result in sudden death.

A 16-year-old boy had a harsh systolic murmur at birth. At 11 months, cardiac catheterization revealed a left-to-right shunt at the ventricular level. At 6 years of age, the murmur was not audible, and at 13 years of age, repeat cardiac catheterization was found to be normal. At the age of 5 years, the boy had syncopal attacks and convulsions. Apparently he was asymptomatic thereafter. However, at the age of 14 years, he was evaluated for bradyarrhythmias. He died suddenly at age 16. At 2 years of age, electrocardiograms disclosed sinus tachycardia interrupted by sinus pauses of 1.3 to 1.4 sec. Subsequent electrocardiograms at the ages of 7½ and 8½ years showed normal sinus rhythm. At age 13 years, electrocardiograms showed brief runs of supraventricular tachycardia followed by pauses of 1.5 to 1.7 sec, terminated by junctional escape rhythm, with rates of 40 to 50 beats per min. An electrophysiologic study at the age of 14 years revealed a junctional escape rhythm (cycle length of 1040 msec) that controlled both the atria and ventricles (H–V interval 40 msec). The SA recovery time, determined by atrial pacing, was prolonged. After administration of atropine, the SA recovery time increased. After the study, the patient failed to keep his medical appointments but was reported to have pulse rates of 70 to 90 beats per min during school examinations.

At postmortem examination, there was gross evidence of spontaneously closing ventricular septal defect. The SA nodal artery showed no changes, and there were only minimal changes in the SA node itself. However, the approaches to the SA node showed marked fibrosis (Fig. 2), and diffuse fibrosis was found in the anterior, middle, and inferior preferential pathways. Likewise, the approaches to the atrioventricular node revealed considerable fibrosis. The sinusoids and lymphatics were dilated. The AV node showed moderate fibrosis. The AV bundle was markedly septated. The left bundle branch was disrupted at the region of the bifurcation. This latter region, which revealed considerable fibroelastosis, was the location of the closing ventricular septal defect. The summit of the ventricular septum revealed marked fibrosis, especially in the region of the ventricular septal defect. Likewise, the right bundle branch revealed fibrosis at the region of the closing ventricular septal defect.

In summary, the approaches to the SA node and AV node, and the atrial preferential pathways, were altered by fibrosis in this case. This fibrosis apparently resulted in sick sinus syndrome. The cause of this fibrosis is unknown.

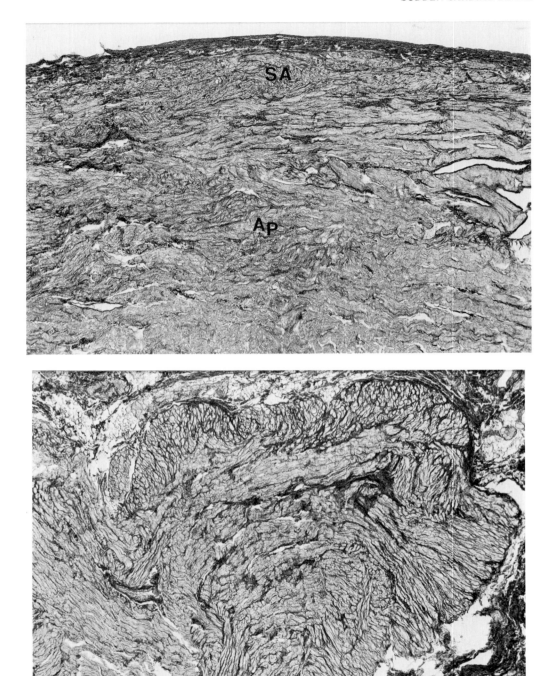

**Figure 2.** *(Top)* Sinoatrial node and approaches; *(bottom)* superior approaches to SA node showing marked fibrosis. Ap = approaches to sinoatrial node; SA = Sinoatrial node. Weigert-van Gieson stain × 45 (both top and bottom). (From Bharati et al,[2] with permission.)

4

### Sick Sinus Syndrome in the Aged[3]

This disorder may manifest itself clinically as the tachycardia-bradycardia syndrome. The latter consists of paroxysmal atrial fibrillation, flutter, or tachycardia followed by SA block or sinus arrest, resulting in Stokes-Adams attacks.

A 74-year-old white man with senile dementia was hospitalized for dizziness and syncope. At admission, the electrocardiogram revealed paroxysmal atrial fibrillation, followed by atrial arrest and depression of the AV junctional pacemaker. In addition to the cardiac rhythm abnormalities, the electrocardiogram revealed evidence of recent ischemia of the anterior, lateral, and posterior walls superimposed on a pattern of left ventricular hypertrophy. Because of the patient's severe senile dementia, a pacemaker was not implanted. The patient died suddenly the following day.

At autopsy, there was a recent thrombus in the left circumflex coronary artery, a huge recent infarct of the proximal two thirds of the posterior ventricular septum, and rupture of the posterior and lateral walls. Some arterioles in the SA node showed marked narrowing, acute degeneration, or necrosis. There was also mononuclear cell infiltration, with focal areas of fibrinoid necrosis of collagen. The approaches to the SA node showed considerable fibrosis and elastosis. Chronic pericarditis was present, involving the adjacent myocardium and the nerve trunks. Examination of the SA nodal artery revealed acute degeneration but no narrowing. There were acute and chronic inflammation, arteriolosclerosis, and necrosis in the approaches to the AV node. Acute degeneration of the AV nodal artery was found. The AV node showed chronic inflammation and proliferation of sheet cells. The AV bundle showed acute degeneration as well. Thus, the sudden death in this patient, although produced by the recent infarct, may have been related to the sick sinus syndrome. This syndrome in the aged is often accompanied by ischemic heart disease.

## ABNORMALITIES IN THE AV NODAL REGION

### Sudden Death Caused by a Benign Tumor (Mesothelioma) of the AV Node[4]

Although mesothelioma of the AV node is benign, it may cause sudden cardiac death related to its location. We have encountered two such cases in our material. We will discuss one particular case in some detail.

A 16-year-old girl, gravida 1, para 1, was hospitalized for cardiac catheterization and evaluation for pacemaker insertion. Six weeks before admission, she gave birth to a normal infant. Immediately postpartum, her heart rate fell to 35 beats per min and her electrocardiogram disclosed 2:1 AV block, with intermittent complete heart block. She was transferred to the coronary care unit and eventually discharged on isoproterenol, with the intention of having her return in 6 weeks for further evaluation of her cardiac condition. Her history revealed that she had two episodes of syncope during her pregnancy. These episodes were apparently similar to the three or four syncopal episodes she had experienced at 9 and 11 years of age in school.

At the time of hospitalization, she had a regular heart rate of 45 beats per min, and the electrocardiogram revealed complete heart block with atrial rates between 70 and 100 beats per min. The ventricular escape rate averaged 45 beats per min. The escape rhythm was junctional with a narrow QRS complex of normal morphologic features. His bundle electrograms revealed complete block proximal to the His bundle. The escape beats were all preceded by His bundle potentials with a normal H–V interval of 40 msec. Diagnostic cardiac catheterization disclosed normal pressures. The patient had an asystolic cardiac arrest during cardiac catheterization, and she could not be resuscitated.

The conduction system of the heart revealed that the distal portion of the atrial septum was replaced by a tumor mass. The AV node was almost completely replaced by the tumor

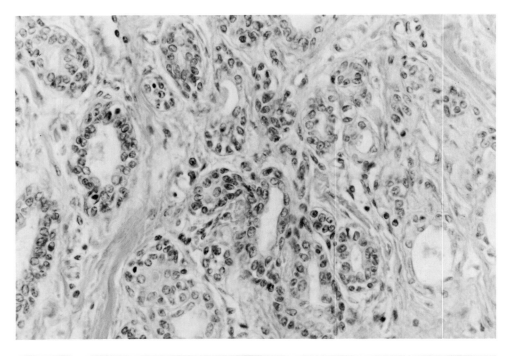

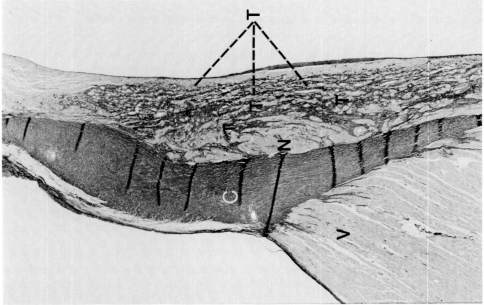

**Figure 3.** (*Left*) Tumor (mesothelioma) involvement of the atrioventricular node. N = AV node; C = central fibrous body; V = ventricular septum; T = tumor. Weigert-van Gieson stain × 9.75. (*Right*) Tumor involvement of the AV node. Hematoxylin-eosin stain × 375 (Right-hand figure from Bharati et al,[4] with permission.)

6

(Fig. 3, left). The penetrating portion of the bundle was partially replaced by tumor. More distally, there was no tumor but there was some degeneration. The tumor consisted of cells arranged in masses or cysts. These cells differed very little in size and shape and generally did not exhibit any mitotic figures (Fig. 3, right).

The origin of this tumor is in dispute today. Some believe that it is of endodermal origin, and others that it is mesothelial in origin. We simply designate it as the AV nodal tumor. It is slow growing and may present initially as first-degree AV block and then proceed to 2:1 block, intermittent complete AV block, and, finally, complete AV block.

## ABNORMALITIES IN THE HIS BUNDLE

### Congenital Abnormalities of the His Bundle and Sudden Death

#### Fragmented or Septated His Bundle[5]

A 13-year-old boy had documented recurrent ventricular tachycardia for several years. Although most of the episodes were brief and well tolerated, several prolonged episodes resulted in weakness and epigastric pain and eventually required cardioversion. The episodes of ventricular tachycardia recurred despite medical treatment.

Physical examination during sinus rhythm was normal, as were chest x-rays, echocardiogram, and electrocardiographic stress test. Right heart cardiac catheterization was normal except for mildy elevated pulmonary artery and right ventricular systolic pressures.

The electrocardiogram during sinus rhythm revealed P–R interval of 0.16 sec, narrow QRS complexes with normal morphology except for Q waves in lead III, and left ventricular hypertrophy by voltage criteria. Ventricular tachycardia was characterized by rates of 150 to 200 beats per min, left bundle branch block morphology, and AV dissociation with capture and fusion beats. Some rhythm strips demonstrated intermittent, unsustained bursts of ventricular tachycardia. Electrophysiologic studies revealed normal P–A and A–H intervals, but the H–V interval was prolonged (65 msec). AV nodal function was normal. The ventricular tachycardias could not be initiated with right ventricular incremental pacing or extrastimulus testing. The left bundle branch pattern of the tachycardia was most consistent with an origin in the right ventricle or via the right bundle branch, but a left ventricular origin could not be ruled out. Because the tachycardia was self-limiting during sinus rhythm and not reproducible in the catheterization laboratory, a re-entrant mechanism for the tachycardia could not be proven. The patient died suddenly.

Histologically, the node formed the bundle abruptly, and it was difficult to differentiate the node from the bundle. The bundle was markedly septated (Fig. 4). What remained on the right side of the bundle became the right bundle branch. The first part of the right bundle branch was divided into three segments that later came together. There was moderate fibrosis of both bundle branches, and the AV node was partially engulfed in the central fibrous body. In addition, there was marked fatty infiltration of the atria and the right ventricle, with recent and old scars noted on the summit of the ventricular septum.

It is not clear in this case what mechanism accounted for the ventricular tachycardia that resulted in sudden death. Inasmuch as His bundle potentials were not demonstrated before the tachycardia beats, re-entry at the level of the His bundle is unlikely. It is also unlikely that the septated right bundle with preferential delivery to the right bundle branch could have occurred becuse the extrastimulus technique did not demonstrate a re-entry mechanism. Conceivably, an enhanced automaticity of the abnormally formed conduction system could have been responsible for re-entry, but this again is only speculative. The fibrotic areas in the ventricular septum or the fatty infiltration or both could have been the site for re-entry in this case.

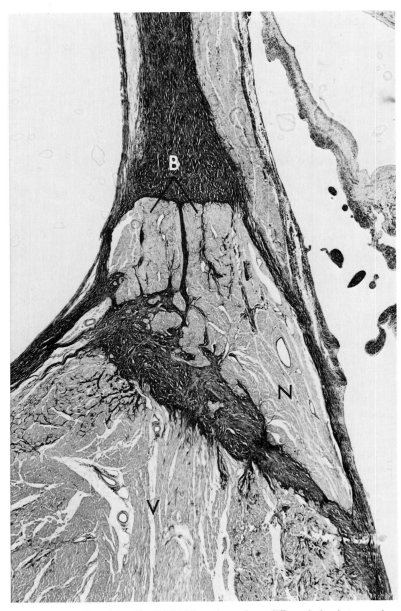

**Figure 4.** Atrioventricular node and bundle of His. There is no sharp differentiation between the node, which is partly engulfed in the central fibrous body, and the markedly septated bundle of His. N = atrioventricular node; B = bundle of His; V = ventricular septum. Weigert-van Gieson stain × 30. (From Bharati et al,[5] with permission.)

Recurrent right ventricular tachycardia with no clinically apparent organic heart disease and essentially negative diagnostic right and left heart catheterization studies (including coronary arteriography) has been well documented in the literature. Although there is no clinically demonstrable, organic heart disease in such individuals, it is evident that sudden death may occur in some of them. Loop formation in the His bundle and fragmented His bundle have been implicated in the literature as causes of sudden death.

## Acquired Abnormalities in the Bundle of His and Sudden Death

### Calcific Impingement of the Bundle of His Resulting in Split His Bundle Potentials[6]

Degenerative changes, such as fibrosis or calcium deposition or both, may occur in the bundle of His. These disorders may give rise clinically to AV block and can result in sudden death.

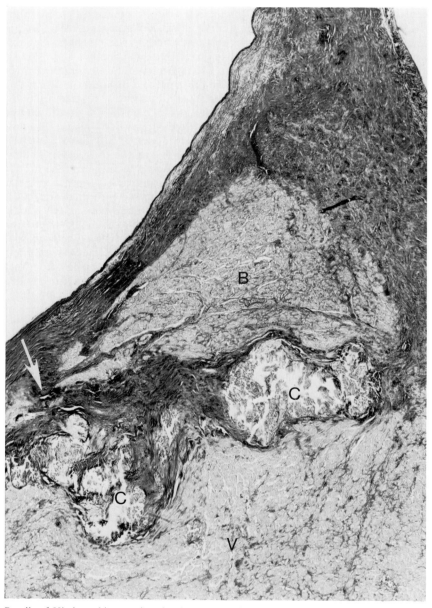

**Figure 5.** Bundle of His branching portion showing compression of lower part by calcium. Note the left bundle branch interrupted by fibroelastic tissue (arrow). B = bundle; C = calcium; V = ventricular septum. Weigert-van Gieson stain × 45. (From Bharati et al,[6] with permission.)

A 67-year-old man was admitted with a 24-hour history of dyspnea and congestive heart failure. He was treated medically, and with temporary transvenous pacing he became asymptomatic within 72 hours after admission. The initial electrocardiogram revealed complete heart block. The escape rhythm was characterized by a right bundle branch block pattern. A few days later, the electrocardiogram revealed sinus rhythm, first-degree AV block, and right bundle branch block. The QRS complex was almost identical to the previous escape rhythm. His bundle recordings revealed split His bundle potentials with intact AV conduction. At a pacing rate of 130 beats per min, a 2:1 block was noted between H and H-prime, the H to H-prime of conducted beats being 100 msec. H-prime–V remained constant during sinus rhythm and at all paced rates. The temporary pacemaker was removed following electrophysiologic studies. The patient was asymptomatic when he was discharged. Three months later, he complained of chest pain and dyspnea, and he died suddenly.

The conduction system revealed calcific impingement on and degenerative changes within the bundle of His (Fig. 5), with healthy bundle proximal and distal to the lesion. In addition, the left bundle branch was separated from the bundle by fibroelastotic tissue that extended throughout its course. There were marked fibrosis and calcification of the summit of the septum. The first part of the right bundle branch showed moderate fibrosis that became marked in the second portion. If one accepts H as being a His bundle electrogram, then H-prime is presumably a His bundle potential recorded distal to His or else a right bundle branch electrogram. If H-prime were a proximal right bundle branch potential, then the site of the right bundle branch must be distal to the recording site, inasmuch as H-prime was not delayed relative to the QRS complex. The prolongation of H to H-prime with single and coupled atrial pacing would then reflect a prolongation of conduction time between the His bundle and the proximal right bundle branch. This abnormality would not effect distal complete right bundle branch block. However, H-prime would move into the QRS complex. The fact that H-prime remained constant as H to H-prime lengthened, suggests that H-prime was recorded with the His bundle. Prominent atrial and ventricular electrograms were recorded from the catheter electrode when H and H-prime were recorded, suggesting that the catheter was in the usual position for recording His bundle and not right bundle branch activity. The H-prime–V interval was within normal range for H–V interval despite the severe pathologic changes in the left bundle branch. Serial sections were consistent with H-prime being recorded from either the distal His bundle or the right bundle branch, inasmuch as the beginning of the right bundle branch was intact, and the functional integrity of the distal portion of the bundle appeared to be intact in its superior half (away from the calcium deposition).

The presence of a calcific lesion impinging upon the His bundle, with healthy bundle tissue proximal and distal to the lesion, may result in either complete AV block or split His bundle potentials with intact AV conduction. Patients with this type of pathology may die suddenly.

## BUNDLE BRANCH SYSTEM DISEASE AND SUDDEN DEATH

### Congenital Abnormalities[7]

Congenital bundle branch system disease may rarely be of familial etiology. We have studied a case of familial congenital bundle branch system disease in which the first child had complete heart block at the age of 2 years and died at age 10 years of ventricular fibrillation. The second sibling at age 15 years had right bundle branch block with left axis deviation and at age 17 years had complete heart block. The third sibling at age 17 years had normal AV conduction but prolonged AV conduction time with incomplete right bundle branch block.

The first patient was referred at the age of 2 years for evaluation of a heart murmur. Physical examination was noncontributory except for a grade II/VI systolic murmur along the left sternal border. The electrocardiogram showed an axis of +80 degrees, complete AV block, left bundle branch block pattern, and a ventricular rate of 55 beats per min. The atrial rate was 110 beats per min. She remained asymptomatic for 8 years, with an unchanged electrocardiogram. At age 10 years while riding a bicycle, she had a Stokes-Adams attack and was taken to the hospital emergency room where she was found to have ventricular fibrillation. Cardioversion was successful and a temporary pacemaker was inserted, but she died suddenly of ventricular fibrillation 48 hours later.

Serial section studies of the conduction system of this patient (first sibling) showed atrophy of the branching portion of the AV bundle with almost complete absence of the left bundle branch (Fig. 6) and absence of the beginning of the right bundle branch. In addition, there

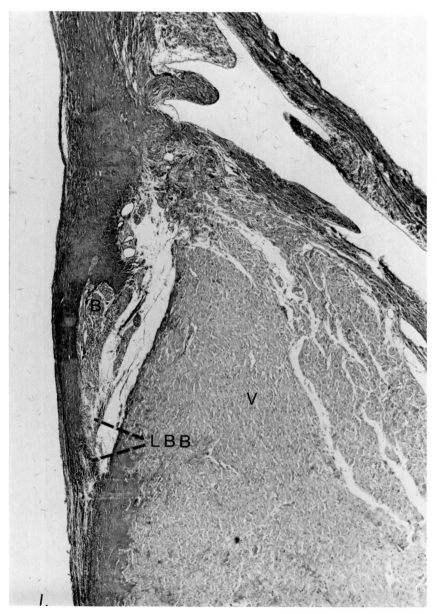

**Figure 6.** AV bundle branching portion showing only remnant of bundle and large spaces and remnant of left bundle branch. B = remnant of AV bundle; LBB = remnant of left bundle branch; V = ventricular myocardium. Weigert-van Gieson stain × 39. (From Husson et al,[7] with permission.)

11

was evidence of acute myocarditis, and the heart was massively hypertrophied with diffuse fibroelastosis. The findings in the bundle branches were most likely of congenital origin inasmuch as the child was found to have heart block at the age of 2 years, and she had no evidence of myocarditis at that time. In addition, there was fibrosis of the summit of the ventricular septum, with arteriolosclerosis localized in this region. It is most likely that the occurrence of acute myocarditis 8 years after the known presence of AV block probably hastened the death of the patient from ventricular fibrillation. The findings suggest that patients with heart block may be susceptible to myocarditis, which may result in sudden death. However, even in the absence of myocarditis, the complete absence of the beginning of the left bundle branch and the right bundle branch could have resulted in sudden death.

From our studies and those reported elsewhere, we might generalize that there are inherited congenital abnormalities of the conduction system and inherited tendencies toward congenital or neonatal degeneration of parts of the conduction system. These developmental abnormalities or tendencies may arise in the conduction system or in the surrounding tissue, secondarily involving the conduction system, or may arise in the blood or nerve supply to the conduction system. These conditions in any combination could trigger a ventricular arrhythmia and may eventuate in sudden death.

## Acquired Degenerative Abnormalities of the Conduction System

### Sclerosis of the Left Side of the Cardiac Skeleton, with Involvement of the Bundle Branches, and Sudden Death[8]

A 72-year-old man with a history of hypertension was hospitalized for syncopal attacks and bradycardia. He was treated with a permanent transvenous pacemaker. The patient was next seen 4 years later with congestive heart failure and bradycardia. He was hospitalized and treated with a temporary transvenous pacemaker. A few days later, a permanent pacemaker was implanted without difficulty. The following day, the patient developed hypotension and ventricular tachyarrhythmias, and died suddenly.

The electrocardiograms taken prior to initial pacemaker insertion revealed complete AV block with an atrial rate averaging 70 beats per min, and ventricular rates of 50 beats per min. There was also wandering of the supraventricular pacemaker with varying atrial cycle lengths and P wave contours. The QRS duration was greater than 0.1 sec and usually of right bundle branch block pattern. Electrocardiograms taken 4 years later revealed complete AV block with atrial rates averaging 70 beats per min, and ventricular rates of 38 beats per min. There was sinus arrhythmia with pauses suggestive of either SA block or arrest. Ventricular complexes were wide and primarily of right bundle branch block pattern. There was some variation in QRS configuration, with occasional premature ventricular beats. No pacemaker spikes were seen. Electrophysiologic studies revealed complete AV block distal to the His bundle, wide QRS complex, and a P–H interval of 135 msec (P–A of 30 msec and A–H of 105 msec).

At postmortem examination, there was no evidence of atherosclerotic narrowing of the coronary arteries. Examination of the conduction system revealed relatively insignificant AV nodal lesions but major destructive lesions of both bundle branches (Fig. 7). In addition, there were arteriolosclerosis, mononuclear cell infiltration, and fibroelastosis of the SA nodal approaches. There was also fibrosis of the summit of the ventricular septum, which was quite marked anteriorly and to the right. Thus, this was a case of sclerosis of the summit of the ventricular septum, accentuated by the hypertensive heart disease, resulting in degenerative changes at the beginning of the bundle branches. The changes in the SA nodal approaches alone, or in combination with the changes in the bundle branches, could have caused the sudden death in this case.

12

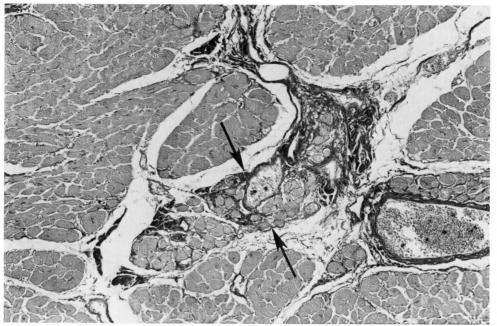

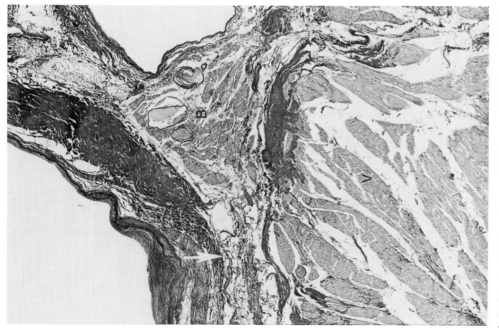

**Figure 7.** *(Left)* Fibroelastosis replacement of the connection between the left bundle branch (arrow) and the branching portion of the AV bundle. V = ventricular musculature; B = branching portion of the AV bundle. Weigert-van Gieson stain × 39. *(Right)* Fibroelastosis of the second portion of the right bundle branch (arrow). Weigert-van Gieson stain × 130. (From Rosen et al,[8] with permission.)

13

## Masquerading Bundle Branch Block[9]

A 75-year-old man with known hypertensive disease was treated for congestive heart failure. An electrocardiogram revealed atrial fibrillation, with ventricular premature beats. The standard limb and unipolar leads showed left bundle branch block pattern, whereas the precordial leads showed right bundle branch block pattern. The patient died suddenly.

Examination of the coronary arteries revealed moderate sclerosis with only slight narrowing. The heart was considerably hypertrophied and enlarged. Microscopic examination revealed generalized arteriolar narrowing. Throughout the myocardium of the free walls of the left ventricle there was slight to moderate subepicardial and perivascular fibrosis, with dispersion of small microscopic scars and occasional organizing infarcts. These changes were more marked in the posterior wall. The SA node showed degeneration, and the approaches revealed moderate fibrosis. Moderate fibrosis was evident also in the approaches to the AV node. However, the AV node was normal. The penetrating bundle revealed minimal fibrosis. The branching part of the bundle of His showed marked elastosis at the region of the bifurcation and compression by a calcified mass on the summit of the ventricular septum. There was marked fibrosis at the origin in the right bundle branch, and the left bundle branch revealed slight fibrosis throughout. Thus, we found incomplete widespread damage to both bundle branches, with marked damage to the septal, myocardial, and free walls of the left ventricle. The masquerading bundle branch block probably was related to the hypertensive heart disease and sclerosis of the left side of the cardiac skeleton. Such lesions may be responsible for sudden death in some elderly patients.

## DISEASE IN THE MYOCARDIUM AND ITS RELATIONSHIP TO SUDDEN DEATH

These disorders may be divided into (1) aging phenomena that may occur on the *right* side of the summit of the ventricular septum in young people; (2) dysplasia of the right ventricular myocardium, which may be considered a type of partial Uhl's or Uhl's anomaly; (3) idiopathic hypertrophic subaortic stenosis (IHSS); (4) infiltrative diseases of the myocardium; and (5) myocarditis.

### Sudden Death in Three Teenagers[10]

We studied the conduction system of three teenagers who apparently were in good health but died suddenly. The first patient, a 15-year-old boy, was known to have right ventricular premature beats. He collapsed suddenly while playing soccer. Postmortem examination revealed marked premature aging of the ventricular summit, sclerosis of the cardiac skeleton extending to the *right side of the summit* (Fig. 8, top left), and fibrosis of the right and left bundle branches. The second teenager, a 17-year-old high school student and a trained athlete, died during football scrimmage. Autopsy revealed moderate mitral valve prolapse and marked premature aging of the summit, especially on the right ventricular side (Fig. 8, top right), and secondary involvement of the trifascicular conduction system, with mononuclear cell infiltration. The third patient, a 19-year-old honor college student, died suddenly at home. Autopsy revealed mitral valve prolapse, thrombosis of the SA nodal artery, and premature aging and sclerosis of the summit of the ventricular septum, especially involving the right ventricular side with involvement of the bundle (Fig. 8, bottom) and trifascicular conduction system.

In summary, unexpected deaths in three teenagers occurred with demonstrable pathologic findings in the heart. Two of the three patients had mitral valve prolapse, one of whom also had thrombosis or embolism of the SA nodal artery. All three had sclerosis not only of the left side but also of the *right side of the ventricular septum,* with varying involvement of the

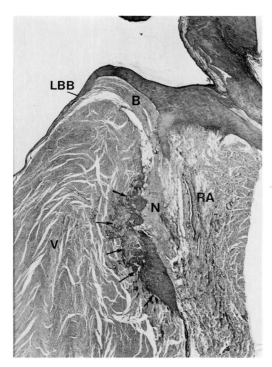

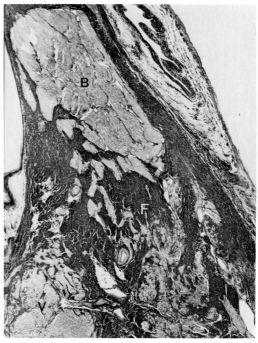

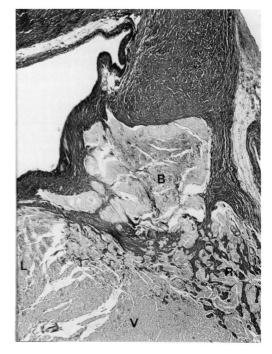

**Figure 8.** *(Top left)* Case 1—Summit of the ventricular septum showing fibrosis on the right ventricular side (arrows). B = bundle of His; LBB = left bundle branch; N = AV node; RA = right atrium; V = ventricular septum. Weigert-van Gieson stain × 10. *(Top right)* Case 2—Summit of the ventricular septum showing fibrosis, particularly on the right ventricular side. B = penetrating part of the bundle of His; V = ventricular septum; F = fibrosis. Weigert-van Gieson stain × 30. *(Bottom)* Case 3—Septated penetrating part of the bundle of His with fine fibrosis. L = left ventricular side; R = right ventricular side; V = ventricular septum; B = bundle of His. Weigert-van Gieson stain × 45. (From Bharati et al,[10] with permission.)

conduction system. The anatomic substrate demonstrated in these three patients could account for bradyarrhythmia or tachyarrhythmia or both, resulting in sudden death.

## Hypoplasia of the Right Ventricular Myocardium and Sudden Death (Uhl's or Partial Uhl's Anomaly)[11]

A 20-year-old woman died suddenly after having recurrent ventricular tachycardia for 5 years. An electrocardiogram showed two distinct varieties of ventricular tachycardia, both characterized by a left bundle branch block pattern. Pathologic examination of the heart revealed the anterior wall of the right ventricle to be largely replaced by fat, except for the trabeculae. The trabeculae showed fibrosis (Fig. 9, top) and focal necrosis, with an infiltration of mononuclear cells. The posterior wall of the right ventricle revealed considerable fibrosis, mostly in the epicardial region of the myocardium, with severe fatty infiltration between epicardium and endocardium. At the apex of the right ventricle, most of the myocardium was replaced by fat, except the trabecular area. The left ventricular myocardium showed focal areas of necrosis and fibrosis, and an infiltration of mononuclear cells and neutrophils. The SA node revealed slight fatty infiltration, with mononuclear cells in some nerve ganglia. The AV bundle was septated (Fig. 9, bottom), and the branching bundle was situated on the left ventricular side. There was slight to moderate fibrosis in the proximal portion of the branching bundle. The entire right bundle branch was intramyocardial, and moderate to severe fibrosis of the periphery of the right bundle and the left bundle branches was present. The summit of the ventricular septum showed distinct large and small areas of necrosis and organization and infiltration of mononuclear cells. The right side of the ventricular septum revealed necrosis of the muscle and considerable infiltration of mononuclear cells, severe fatty infiltration, and severe fibrosis.

We believe that the pathologic changes found in this patient were not entirely due to myocarditis. It is unlikely that a myocarditis could produce a hypoplasia of the myocardium of the right ventricle. We believe that in Uhl's or partial Uhl's anomaly, in addition to marked fatty infiltration, one may find inflammatory changes, especially in adults. In this particular patient, we must also take into account that she had frequently undergone cardioversion and she had an attempted insertion of a pacemaker and received various drugs to control her arrhythmia. The ventricular tachycardia probably originated at the site where there were mixtures of altered and intact ventricular myocardial cells. The altered cells could have provided the substrate for re-entry or increased automaticity, either of which could have been responsible for ventricular tachycardia. Another possible origin of ventricular tachycardia could have been the region of the septated bundle found in this patient. Thus, sudden death may occur in cases of Uhl's or partial Uhl's anomaly, in which marked fatty infiltration and replacement of myocardium may be associated with abnormalities of the conduction system and probably superimposed myocarditis. It is not known why this anomaly occurs most frequently in young women.

## Idiopathic Hypertrophic Subaortic Stenosis and Sudden Death[12]

It is well known that idiopathic hypertrophic subaortic stenosis (IHSS) is frequently associated with various types of arrhythmias and sudden death. A 25-year-old white woman had IHSS proved by cardiac catheterization. An electrocardiogram revealed left bundle branch block. Electrophysiologic studies revealed normal P–A and P–H intervals, but the H–V interval was prolonged (70 msec). The width of the His spike was 20 msec. A reproducible split His potential was demonstrated with the atrial extrastimulus technique. Because the patient was symptomatic, a permanent pacemaker was inserted. One week later, the patient died suddenly.

16

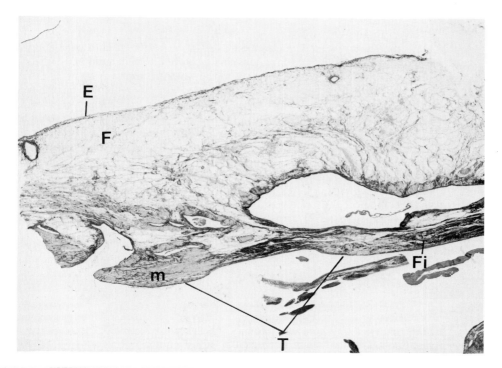

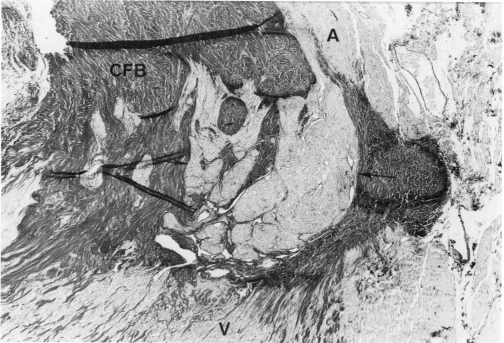

**Figure 9.** *(Top)* Right ventricular myocardium, anterior wall, showing replacement of muscle by fat. Trabeculation shows fibrosis. E = epicardium; F = fat tissue; T = trabeculation; m = muscle; Fi = fibrosis. Weigert-van Gieson stain × 16. *(Bottom)* Septated penetrating portion of bundle of His, horizontal section. Arrows point to the septated bundle. A = atrial septum; CFB = central fibrous body; V = ventricular septum. Weigert-van Gieson stain × 45. (From Bharati et al,[11] with permission.)

Examination of the heart revealed characteristic features of IHSS. There were a markedly thickened and sigmoid ventricular septum and a small, heavily trabeculated lumen. Histologically, myocardial disarray was present not only in the myocardium but in the beginning of the bundle and the bundle branches as well. It was noteworthy that the His bundle was situated on the right side of the ventricular septum. Although it was intact at its origin, it showed marked fibrotic changes more distally. The bundle extended over the markedly hypertrophied ventricular septum to reach the left ventricular side, where it gave off the left bundle branch. The beginning of the left bundle branch was markedly disrupted as it traversed the septum. The right bundle branch was moderately fibrosed.

We hypothesized that the congenitally abnormal architecture of the left side of the septum produced a secondarily abnormal central fibrous body, flattening of the AV node and the bundle, and displacement of the bundle to the right side. The abnormal septum resulted in arteriolosclerosis, which is found in many cases of IHSS. Thus, ischemia may have accentuated fibrosis of the bundle and bundle branches. The left bundle branch was probably traumatized as it went over the hump of the septum into the markedly trabeculated left side of the septum. Thus, we believe that in IHSS, not only is the ventricular septum abnormal but the central fibrous body either primarily or secondarily also shares in this abnormality. The disorganization of the myocardium also involves the specialized myocardium. Sudden death, which is frequently encountered in IHSS, may be due to either tachyarrhythmias or bradyarrhythmias, related to the aforementioned abnormalities. Despite the fact that the patient had a permanent pacemaker, she died suddenly. In this particular case, the sudden death could have been due also to sudden left ventricular outflow obstruction.

## Infiltrative Cardiomyopathy with Conduction Disease and Sudden Death[13]

Infiltrative cardiomyopathy may be complicated by conduction defects, ventricular arrhythmias and sudden death. A 34-year-old man of Italian ancestry was hospitalized because of vertigo and syncopal episodes. The neurologic evaluation was normal. He was noted to have bradycardia, and the electrocardiogram revealed AV block. Initially, a temporary pacemaker was inserted and, subsequently, a permanent transvenous demand pacemaker was implanted. The patient complained of fast heart beating. Electrocardiographic monitoring revealed short episodes of wide QRS tachycardia (rate of 180 beats per min). A subsequent electrocardiogram revealed right bundle branch block, first-degree and intermittent third-degree AV block, and recurrent unifocal and paroxysmal ventricular tachycardia. Electrophysiologic studies disclosed normal sinus rhythm with prolonged A–H (175 msec) and H–V (60 msec) intervals and extrastimulus induction of rapid ventricular firing. The patient was discharged on procainamide, which was later changed to propranolol because of recurrent episodes of ventricular tachycardia observed during exercise. A year and a half later, while riding a bicycle, he collapsed and died suddenly.

Postmortem examination revealed a sarcoid aneurysm of the posterior left ventricle and granulomatous infiltration of the AV node, His bundle and branching bundle (Fig. 10), and bundle branches. Sarcoidosis involves the heart in approximately 13 to 25 percent of cases. Usually, this disorder is associated with lymph node and lung involvement. The involvement of the heart may result in heart block, ventricular arrhythmias, and sudden death. The posterior wall of the left ventricle has a predilection for the aneurysmal formation. Thus, infiltrative diseases such as sarcoidosis, amyloidosis, or even marked fatty infiltration may result in ventricular arrhythmias and sudden death.

## Myocarditis and Sudden Death[14]

It is well known that myocarditis of any etiology, with or without involvement of the conduction system, may result in sudden death in its acute phase. Uncommonly, one may find a

18

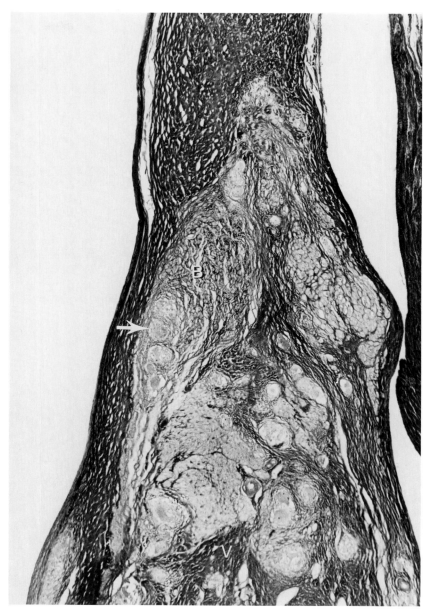

**Figure 10.** Photomicrograph of the branching bundle showing sarcoid involvement (arrow). V = ventricular septum; B = branching bundle. Weigert-van Gieson Stain × 45.

smoldering type of myocarditis. In some cases, myocarditis may involve only neural elements of the heart, producing ganglionitis or neuritis, which may result in sudden death.

A 46-year-old woman was hospitalized because of syncope. The general and neurologic examinations were normal. The electrocardiogram revealed sinus rhythm, second-degree AV block with 3:1 conduction, and left posterior hemiblock. She had repeated syncopal episodes in the next couple of years during which time the electrocardiogram revealed intermittent complete heart block. Despite cardiac pacemaker implantation, the patient died suddenly.

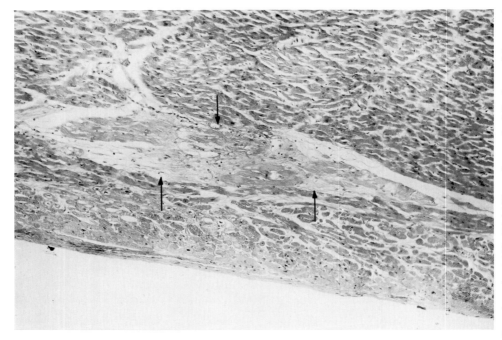

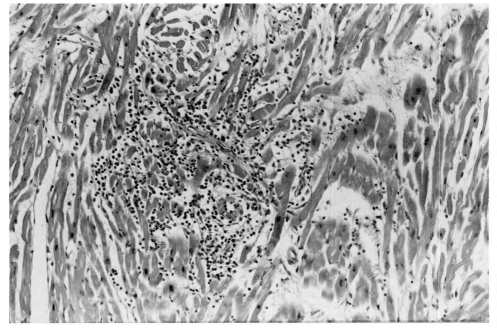

**Figure 11.** *(Left)* Photomicrograph of myocardium showing myocarditis. Hematoxylin-eosin stain × 190. *(Right)* Photomicrograph of distal part of the second portion of the right bundle branch (arrows) showing cellular necrosis and an infiltration of mononuclear cells. Arrows point to right bundle branch. Hematoxylin-eosin stain × 105. (From Harris et al,[14] with permission.)

The pathologic examination revealed organizing myocarditis (Fig. 11, left), with fibrosis of the summit of the ventricular septum associated with severe, old destruction of the origin of the left bundle branch and more recent, partial destruction of the right bundle branch. There was superimposition of acute degeneration and inflammatory changes, mostly of the branching portion of the AV bundle at the bifurcation and the bundle branches (Fig. 11, right).

Involvement of the conduction system resulting in AV block has frequently been reported in acute myocarditis. This condition is considered evanescent if the patient recovers. Chronic AV block produced by a previous myocarditis is rare. In this particular case, we were dealing with a smoldering type of myocarditis of 2 years' duration with no known acute phase. In addition to the myocarditis, the patient had fibrosis of the summit of the ventricular septum.

## MITRAL VALVE PROLAPSE[15]

It is well recognized that mitral valve prolapse may result in sudden death. Although the mechanism of sudden death in these cases is presently unknown, we believe that at least in some cases, this event may be related to abnormalities in the conduction system.

A 45-year-old male physician had a long history of palpitations. The electrocardiogram revealed sinus rhythm, normal P–R and Q–T intervals, Q waves in lead 3, and normal QRS morphology. A 24-hour Holter monitor disclosed frequent premature ventricular beats and several episodes of rapid, unsustained (3 to 5 beats) ventricular tachycardia. He refused further medical checkups and died suddenly a year later.

Postmortem examination of the mitral valve revealed the characteristic features of a floppy mitral valve, but, in addition, there was marked calcification at the anulus (Fig. 12, left). The anulus was elongated, and the valve was anchored more toward the left atrial side. The conduction system revealed marked fatty infiltration in the approaches to the SA and AV nodes and the atrial preferential pathways. The AV node was compressed by the enlarged left atrium, the mitral orifice, and by calcium. The central fibrous body was abnormally formed, and the branching bundle was situated on the right side of the summit of the ventricular septum (Fig. 12, right). The right side of the bundle continued as the right bundle branch. Some of the fibers of the left bundle branch terminated just beneath the summit of the ventricular septum. In addition, the summit of the ventricular septum, especially the right side, revealed premature aging phenomenon (fibrosis) with arteriolosclerosis (see Fig. 12, right). The right-sided bundle alone, with or without fibrosis found on the summit of the ventricular septum, could have resulted in a re-entry mechanism that might have produced sudden death in this young physician.

## PRE-EXCITATION AND SUDDEN DEATH[16]

Pre-excitation syndromes may result in sudden death. We studied two cases associated with idiopathic myocardial hypertrophy and diffuse fibroelastosis of the left ventricle. The first case was a 13-year-old girl who died of cardiac arrest. The electrocardiogram revealed Type B pre-excitation and a leftward and inferior 20-msec vector suggesting a right free wall anomalous pathway. The patient had a mitral anuloplasty at age 33 months because of marked left ventricular failure. Her postoperative course was uncomplicated. Subsequently, she complained of short-lived episodes of palpitations and, at the age of 13 years, she had an unexpected cardiac arrest while in church and died suddenly. In this case, there were two small anomalous pathways in the right free wall (Fig. 13, top).

The second patient was a 26-year-old man who had a history of cardiovascular disease dating back to childhood when a heart murmur was noted. He was hospitalized at age 19 years with a syncopal episode and a history of paroxysmal tachycardia. Wolff-Parkinson-White syndrome was discovered at that time. He got along well until the age of 24 years when he had recurrent paroxysmal tachycardia and chest pain. Cardiac catheterization

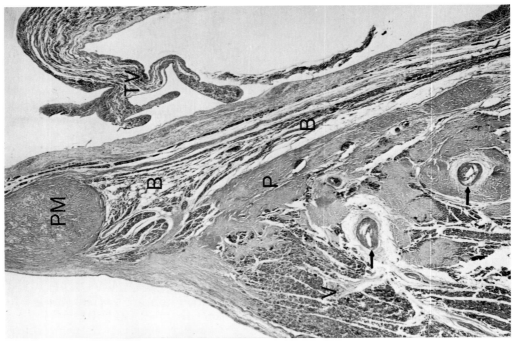

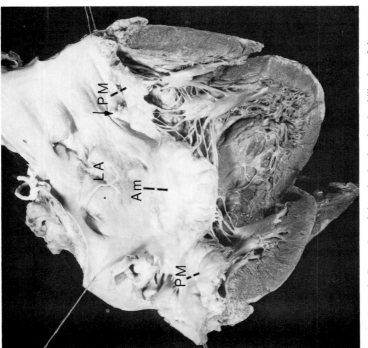

**Figure 12.** *(Left)* Gross view of the mitral valve showing billowing of the posterior and anterior leaflets, prolongation of posterior leaflet, and calcification of the anulus of the posterior leaflet. The calcification elevates the posterior leaflet, and the calcification extends into the left atrium (arrow). LA = left atrium; PM = posterior mitral leaflet; Am = anterior mitral leaflet. *(Right)* Beginning of the penetrating portion of the bundle of His extending downward on the right side of the summit of the ventricular septum. A prong of connective tissue extends from the parsmembranacea downward to the right side of the summit. The large arterioles (arrows) show marked arteriolosclerosis. PM = parsmembranacea; P = prong to right of summit of ventricular septum; B = bundle of His; V = summit of ventricular septum; TV = tricuspid valve. Hematoxlyin-eosin stain × 30. (From Bharati et al,[15] with permission.)

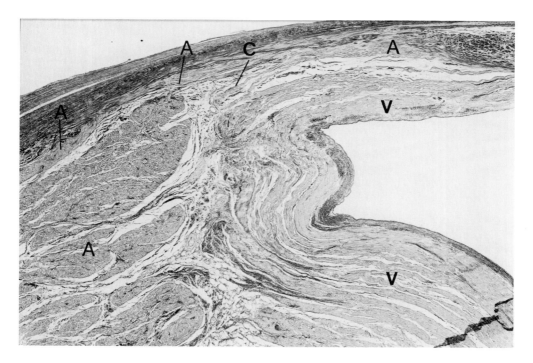

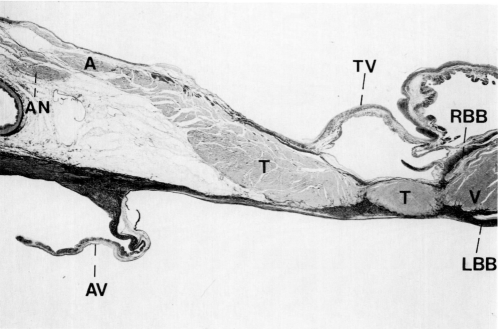

**Figure 13.** *(Top)* Case 1—Bypass tract in the right free wall. A = atrial musculature; C = connection; V = ventricular musculature. Weigert-van Gieson stain × 40. *(Bottom)* Case 2—Bypass tract in anterior portion of atrial septum and in bulbar septum. A = atrial musculature; AN = anterior nodal structure; AV = aortic valve; I = infundibular musculature; LBB = left bundle branch; RBB = right bundle branch; T = bypass tract; TV = tricuspid valve; V = ventricular musculature at summit of ventricular septum. Weigert-van Gieson stain × 17.25. (From Bharati et al,[16] with permission.)

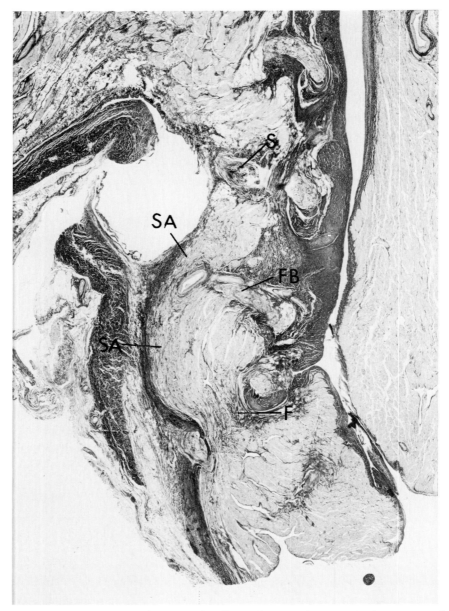

**Figure 14.** Case 1—Sinoatrial node and its approaches. Sutures interrupt the approaches in one area, and there is fibrosis at the opposite approaches. S = suture interrupting the approaches; F = fibrosis of the approaches; SA = sinoatrial node; FB = foreign body reaction in the node. Weigert-van Gieson stain × 43. (From Bharati el al,[18] with permission.)

revealed congestive cardiomyopathy and mitral regurgitation. He subsequently had recurrent congestive heart failure and paroxysmal tachycardia, and he died suddenly at home. In this particular case, there were no anomalous pathways found in the right anterior free wall. However, the right atrium was in continuity with the infundibular muscular septum anterior to the membranous septum. This anomalous pathway had continuity with an anterior AV nodal type of structure in the right atrium (Fig. 13, bottom).

Thus it is clear that the various types of anomalous connections between the atria and the ventricles and/or the conduction system may provoke supraventricular or ventricular arrhythmias and result in sudden death in cases of Wolff-Parkinson-White syndrome.

## SUDDEN DEATH IN POSTOPERATIVE CONGENITAL HEART DISEASE

### Postoperative Tetralogy of Fallot[17]

Although the cause of sudden death many years after surgery in cases of totally corrected tetralogy of Fallot is presently unknown, we believe the following factors may result in sudden death: (1) The infundibular pulmonary resection and outflow tract reconstruction with the Dacron prosthesis in some cases may result in a right ventricular aneurysm in the anterior wall. (2) There is usually fibroelastosis of this region, which may result in ventricular tachyarrhythmias and sudden death. (3) Many of these patients have pulmonary regurgitation. (4) The involvement of the conduction system, especially the right bundle branch, during closure of ventricular septal defect may result in right bundle branch block pattern in some cases. (5) The fibrosis or fibroelastosis or both that occur in the right ventricle postoperatively may involve the undamaged portions of the right bundle branch and may facilitate the production of complete right bundle branch block pattern over the course of time. (6) The involvement of the left bundle branch in some cases owing to the effects of the fibroelastosis on the left ventricular aspect may result in complete AV block, which may result in sudden death.

### Mustard Procedure for Transposition[18]

It is well established that various types of atrial arrhythmias occur postoperatively in the Mustard procedure, which may lead to sudden death. We studied two cases of sudden death occurring 2 years after the Mustard procedure. The first child manifested sinus rhythm alternating with junctional rhythm during the first year of life. The second child, 2 months before death, had first-degree AV block that progressed to second-degree AV block with 2:1 conduction alternating with junctional rhythm and AV dissociation. Examination of the conduction system in both cases revealed the approaches to the SA node (Fig. 14) and AV node to be markedly fibrosed. In addition, in the first case, the SA node was interrupted by sutures, and in the second, the SA node was considerably fibrosed. Also in the second case, the superior approaches to the AV node were markedly involved by fibrous tissue. The arrhythmias produced and the probable cause of sudden death in both cases could be related to surgical injury to the approaches to the SA and AV nodes. There are other cases of congenital heart disease in which sudden death occurred several years after surgical correction.

### SUMMARY AND CLASSIFICATION OF SUDDEN DEATH
### FROM OUR MATERIAL

Based on our material, we classify sudden death according to the lesions we find in the conduction system and various parts of the heart as follows:

1. Lesions in the SA node
   A. Trauma to the SA node
   B. Sick sinus syndrome
      1. In adolescence, etiology—congenital?
      2. In old age, tachycardia-bradycardia syndrome—acquired
2. Lesions in the AV node and its approaches—benign tumor of the AV node—mesothelioma

3. Lesions in the AV bundle
   A. Congenital—fragmented or septated bundle
   B. Acquired—calcific impingement with split His
4. Lesions in the bundle branches
   A. Congenital—familial
   B. Acquired
      1. Sclerosis of the left side of the cardiac skeleton
         a. Bilateral bundle branch block
         b. Masquerading bundle branch block
5. Lesions in the myocardium
   A. Sclerosis of the right side of the cardiac skeleton with involvement of the bundle branches
   B. Uhl's and partial Uhl's anomaly
   C. IHSS
   D. Infiltrative cardiomyopathy
   E. Myocarditis
6. Mitral valve prolapse
7. Accessory pathways—pre-excitation
8. Various lesions related to postoperative congenital heart disease
   A. Tetralogy of Fallot
   B. Mustard procedure for complete transposition

From the literature,[10,19-21] it is well known that ischemic heart disease is the most common cause of sudden death in the middle-aged and the older age groups. It is also known that congenital anomalies of the coronary arteries,[22-24] cardiac tumors,[25] Q–T prolongation,[25] acute aneurysm of the aortic cusp with thrombus,[26] and various types of muscular dystrophies[27] may result in sudden death.

## REFERENCES

1. BHARATI, S, CHERVONY, A, GRUHN, J, ET AL: *Atrial arrhythmias related to trauma to sinoatrial node.* Chest 61:331, 1972.

2. BHARATI, S, NORDENBERG, A, BAUERNFEIND, R, ET AL: *The anatomic substrate for the sick sinus syndrome in adolescence.* Am J Cardiol 46:163, 1980.

3. KAPLAN, BM, LANGENDORF, R, LEV, M, ET AL: *Tachycardia-bradycardia syndrome (so-called "sick sinus syndrome").* Am J Cardiol 31:497, 1973.

4. BHARATI, S, BICOFF, JP, FRIDMAN, JL, ET AL: *Sudden death caused by benign tumor of the atrioventricular node.* Arch Intern Med 136:224, 1976.

5. BHARATI, S, BAUERNFEIND, R, SCHEINMAN, M, ET AL: *Congenital abnormalities of the conduction system in two patients with tachyarrhythmias.* Circulation 59:593, 1979.

6. BHARATI, S, LEV, M, DELON, W, ET AL: *Pathophysiologic correlations in two cases of split His bundle potentials.* Circulation 49:615, 1974.

7. HUSSON, GS, BLACKMAN, MS, ROGERS, MC, ET AL: *Familial congenital bundle branch system disease.* Am J Cardiol 32:365, 1973.

8. ROSEN, KM, RAHIMTOOLA, SH, GUNNAR, RM, ET AL: *Site of heart block as defined by His bundle recordings.* Circulation 45:965, 1972.

9. UNGER, PN, LESSER, ME, KUGEL, VH, ET AL: *The concept of "masquerading" bundle-branch block: An electrocardiographic-pathologic correlation.* Circulation 17:397, 1958.

10. BHARATI, S, BAUERNFEIND, R, MILLER, LB, ET AL: *Sudden death in three teenagers: Conduction system studies.* J Am Coll Cardiol 1:879, 1983.

11. BHARATI, S, FELD, AW, BAUERNFEIND, R, ET AL: *Hypoplasia of the right ventricular myocardium with ventricular tachycardia.* Arch Pathol Lab Med 107:249, 1983.

12. BHARATI, S, MCANULTY, JH, LEV, M, ET AL: *Idiopathic hypertrophic subaortic stenosis with split His bundle potentials.* Circulation 62:1373, 1980.

13. BHARATI, S, LEV, M, DENES, P, ET AL: *Infiltrative cardiomyopathy with conduction disease and ventricular arrhythmia: Electrophysiologic and pathologic correlations.* Am J Cardiol 45:163, 1980.

14. HARRIS, R, SIEW, S, AND LEV, M: *Smoldering myocarditis with intermittent complete A-V block and Stokes-Adams syndrome.* Am J Cardiol 24:880, 1969.

15. BHARATI, S, GRANSTON, AS, LIEBSON, PR, ET AL: *The conduction system in mitral valve prolapse syndrome with sudden death.* Am Heart J 101:667, 1981.

16. BHARATI, S, STRASBERG, B, BILITCH, M, ET AL: *Anatomic substrate for pre-excitation in idiopathic myocardial hypertrophy with fibroelastosis of the left ventricle.* Am J Cardiol 48:47, 1981.

17. BHARATI, S AND LEV, M: *The myocardium, conduction system, and general sequelae after surgery for congenital heart disease.* In ENGLE, MA AND PERLOFF, JK (EDS): *Congenital Heart Disease After Surgery.* Yorke Medical Books, New York, 1983, pp 247–260.

18. BHARATI, S, MOLTHAN, ME, VEASY, G, ET AL: *Conduction system in two cases of sudden death two years after the Mustard procedure.* J Thorac Cardiovasc Surg 77:101, 1979.

19. HINKLE, LE, JR AND THALER, HT: *Clinical classification of cardiac deaths.* Circulation 65:457, 1982.

20. FRIEDMAN, GD, KLATSKY, AL, AND SIEGELAUB, AB: *Predictors of sudden cardiac death.* Circulation 51:164, 1974.

21. WEAVER, DW, LORCH, GS, ALVAREZ, HA, ET AL: *Angiographic findings and prognostic indicators in patients resuscitated from sudden cardiac death.* Circulation 54:895, 1976.

22. MARON, BJ, ROBERTS, WC, MCALLISTER, HA, ET AL: *Sudden death in young athelets.* Circulation 62:218, 1980.

23. JOKL, E AND MCCLELLAN, JT: *Exercise and cardiac death.* JAMA 213:1489, 1970.

24. LYNCH, P: *Soldiers, sport and sudden death.* Lancet 1:1235, 1980.

25. JAMES, TN: *Chance and sudden death.* J Am Coll Cardiol 1:164, 1983.

26. MANT, AK: *Sudden death due to unusual cardiac pathology.* Forensic Sci 8:7, 1976.

27. JAMES, TN AND MARSHALL, TK: *De Subitaneis Mortibus 18: Persistent fetal dispersion of the atrioventricular node and His bundle within the central fibrous body.* Circulation 53:1026, 1976.

# Electrophysiology of Experimental Models of Sudden Death

*Eric L. Michelson, M.D.*

Several animal models have been developed for the purpose of studying the electrophysiology of arrhythmias that contribute to sudden cardiac death in humans. Sudden cardiac death is a complex problem. The majority of afflicted patients have coronary artery disease, but only a minority have evidence of acute infarction as the antecedent, precipitating event. Malignant ventricular arrhythmias, specifically ventricular tachycardia and fibrillation, are the immediate cause of death in most cases.

The complexity of the problem of sudden cardiac death poses a challenge in designing appropriate animal models. Ideally, an experimental animal model represents a less complex system while still exhibiting specific critical characteristics of the human situation. Then, by evaluating selected characteristics under controlled experimental conditions, it is possible to gain insight into the functioning of the human system. The specific characteristics of an animal model are therefore determined by the experimental questions that are to be answered or the hypotheses to be tested. A valid model must be a reasonable analog of the human system; yet it must be sufficiently simple so that most variables can be controlled. The complexity of the problem of sudden cardiac death implies that no one animal model will provide all answers.

The bulk of this chapter will be restricted to a consideration of several recent *in vivo* canine electrophysiologic experiments that have clarified some of the mechanisms of arrhythmias associated with sudden cardiac death in man. There are three major periods of ventricular arrhythmias that occur in the dog following occlusion of a major coronary artery. In this discussion, these periods will be referred to as acute, subacute, and chronic. They are distinguished both by the time of onset of the arrhythmias and by specific characteristics of the arrhythmias.

## ACUTE ARRHYTHMIAS

The vast majority of studies have been done in animals made acutely ischemic by the occlusion of a major coronary artery, although recently there has been considerable interest in the lethal consequences of acute coronary artery reperfusion following transient ischemia. The electrophysiologic derangements that follow either acute myocardial ischemia or the restoration of blood flow to an acutely ischemic area apparently each involve the superimposition of multiple arrhythmia mechanisms, including ectopic impulse formation and re-entry phenomena. Within minutes after acute occlusion of a proximal artery, malignant ventricular arrhythmias occur. The acute period of vulnerability to arrhythmias persists for approximately 30 minutes and often leads to ventricular fibrillation (VF).[1] A number of factors influence the susceptibility to VF, including the mass of myocardium at risk, the presence of previous ischemic damage, heart rate, neurohumoral factors, and various autonomic mediators. A larger mass, faster heart rate, high catecholamine levels, and "stress" may all predispose to VF. There is evidence that the mechanism of the arrhythmias in this acute period is due to slow conduction and re-entry within the ischemic epicardium.[2-8] Immediately following coronary occlusion, there is a brief period of accelerated conduction within the ischemic zone.[8] This is followed by a dramatic slowing of conduction. Very slowly conducting activity may persist in the ischemic area sufficiently long to exit and re-excite the heart after the refractory period in the normal zone has subsided. During these arrhythmias, the Purkinje system at the border of the ischemic zone is activated first, suggesting that the exit point for re-excitation of the heart may be by way of subendocardial Purkinje system.[9] An additional mechanism for the acute arrhythmias has been suggested by studies in both the dog and pig.[10] Ectopic impulses may be evoked at the border zone by electrotonically induced depolarization owing to the current of injury that flows between the normal and ischemic myocardium.

In addition, recent evidence indicates that even in the initial 30-minute period of acute ischemia, arrhythmias occur in two phases: "immediate" and "delayed." The immediate phase occurs within 2 to 12 minutes, and the delayed phase occurs from 14 to 30 minutes after ligation of the left anterior descending coronary artery.[6] The delayed ventricular arrhythmias have as high an incidence of VF as the immediate ventricular arrhythmias but are not accompanied by epicardial conduction delay.[6] Presumably, either more localized subendocardial re-entry or focal excitation (automaticity) is the mechanism for these "delayed"-phase arrhythmias during acute ischemia.

### Acute Coronary Reperfusion

Release of an acute coronary artery occlusion is also associated with malignant ventricular arrhythmias. The incidence of VF is highest if release occurs after 20 to 30 minutes of occlusion when ischemic alterations are apparently maximal and infarction still minimal.[11] Again, susceptibility to VF is heightened if the mass of ischemic myocardium is large and reperfusion is abrupt, and is also influenced by heart rate, and neurohumoral and autonomic alterations. The mechanisms for these arrhythmias are also complex; both re-entry and altered automaticity have been implicated.[12,13] Re-entrant mechanisms are at least contributory to the malignant arrhythmias occurring instantaneously within the first minute following abrupt reperfusion; whereas more benign automatic mechanisms predominate minutes later when nonsustained ventricular tachycardia (VT) occurs, but VF is less common. No direct information is yet available in man with respect to either acute coronary occlusion or reperfusion phenomena to verify the applicability of these findings to the human situation. However, the occurrence of short paroxysms of VT is a common concomitant of successful reperfusion during streptokinase infusion in patients with evolving myocardial infarction.

Both the acute occlusion and reperfusion models of myocardial ischemia offer direct, but severe, tests for any potential antiarrhythmic drug. Notably, a recent critical view of the literature[14] suggests that none of the presently available antiarrhythmic agents has shown optimal efficacy in preventing the lethal ventricular arrhythmias that occur following either the experimental occlusion or reperfusion of a major coronary artery. As further detailed in this recent review, the interpretation of antiarrhythmic drug studies using acute coronary occlusion models is potentially hazardous unless one takes into careful consideration the techniques of occlusion, anesthetic, heart rate, site of occlusion, mass of myocardium at risk, species, and the considerable biologic variability among individual animals based on anatomic heterogeneity, among other factors.

## SUBACUTE ARRHYTHMIAS

Approximately 6 to 24 hours after experimental coronary artery occlusion, a subacute period of spontaneous arrhythmias appears.[15] These arrhythmias include frequent ventricular premature beats (VPBs) and incessant runs of ventricular tachycardia at rates mildly to moderately faster than the sinus rate, and they persist for up to 72 hours. Ventricular fibrillation occurs only rarely during this phase. The mechanism for those arrhythmias is different from the ventricular arrhythmias of the acute period. Purkinje fibers removed from the infarcted region 24 hours after coronary occlusion exhibit enhanced automaticity.[16,17] Studies using multiple recording and stimulation techniques in anesthetized dogs following left anterior descending coronary artery occlusion[4,18] or septal coronary artery occlusion[19] have localized the origin of the arrhythmias to surviving subendocardial Purkinje fibers overlying the infarcted myocardium. The arrhythmias may be overdriven by electrical pacing and can be unmasked by slowing of the heart rate. Although potentially malignant re-entrant ventricular arrhythmias may be induced during this period, the dominant rhythm disturbance appears to be due to enhanced automaticity in the Purkinje system.[20] In humans, accelerated idioventricular rhythms that occur during this period following myocardial infarction appear to have a similar mechanism.[21] Finally, there is also recent evidence suggesting an alternative arrhythmia mechanism, so-called "slow channel"–mediated rhythms related to "after-depolarizations."[20] The relevance of these findings to the human situation is even less well defined at present.

Models of subacute myocardial infarction have also been used widely for evaluating the potential antiarrhythmic efficacy of investigational drugs. Traditionally, most drugs studied for their potential antiarrhythmic activity have been chosen for their local anesthetic, or membrane depressant, properties, to which "fast channel"–mediated, "automatic" arrhythmias are often most sensitive. Thus, virtually every potential, conventional antiarrhythmic agent when administered in an appropriate dosage has been successful in suppressing these arrhythmias. However, it is not at all clear that the effects of a potential antiarrhythmic drug on these arrhythmias will have any bearing on the ultimate utility of such an agent in preventing VF and sudden coronary death.[14]

## "LATE" AND "CHRONIC" VENTRICULAR TACHYARRHYTHMIAS

Historically, the arrhythmias occurring late or chronically after an experimental coronary occlusion were not well studied. It had been thought that by the fourth day following even an extensive myocardial infarction in dogs, arrhythmias were no longer present. In this respect, dogs were considered much different than man, and thus were believed to be most unsuitable as a model for studying chronic ventricular arrhythmias. It was hypothesized that either the absence of other diseased coronary vessels, or alternatively the rich supply of anastomosing and preformed collateral vessels, limited the chronic consequences of an acute infarction in the dog model. However, the application of methods of programmed stimulation and cardiac pacing to the study of chronically infarcted animals has led to recent noteworthy advances.

In an extensive series of studies, El-Sherif and colleagues[22,23] demonstrated delayed, slowly conducting, fractionated electrical activity within areas of damaged canine myocardium at 3 to 5 days following an acute occlusion of the left anterior descending coronary artery. During rapid pacing, or following the introduction of appropriately timed premature beats, this fractionated activity was delayed further, spanning diastole. When fractionated activity was "continuous" throughout the cardiac cycle, as revealed by composite epicardial electrograms, runs of ventricular tachyarrhythmias were observed, suggesting a re-entrant mechanism. Similar observations had been made previously by Durrer and associates,[24] Waldo and Kaiser,[2] and Boineau and Cox[3] in the setting of acute canine myocardial infarction, and subsequently in patients with sustained ventricular tachyarrhythmias studied in the clinical electrophysiologic laboratory by Josephson and coworkers.[25,26]

## Chronic Coronary Artery Occlusion/Reperfusion Models

Subsequently, a number of investigators working independently have developed models in which dogs are more chronically susceptible to the initiation of sustained ventricular tachyarrhythmias. Initially, Karagueuzian and colleagues[27] reported that occluding the proximal left anterior descending coronary artery and then releasing the occlusion after 2 hours[28-30] rendered dogs much more highly susceptible to the initiation of sustained ventricular tachyarrhythmias than animals subjected to routine coronary artery occlusion procedures. Using methods adapted from the clinical electrophysiologic laboratory, that is, ventricular pacing with the introduction of a single ventricular extrastimulus in awake animals, sustained ventricular tachyarrhythmias could be initiated on days 3 to 5 following the acute infarction, but not thereafter. More recent studies[31] have focused on further elucidation of arrhythmia mechanisms, particularly with respect to localizing potential sites of re-entrant phenomena. Re-entry appears to be the predominant mechanism, often localized to a surviving rim of epicardial tissue.

In our own laboratory, at the Lankenau Medical Research Center and in close collaboration with the School of Veterinary Medicine at the University of Pennsylvania, we have also had considerable experience using a canine occlusion/reperfusion model of chronic myocardial infarction.[32-37] Routinely, the left anterior descending coronary artery is occluded either just proximal or distal to the first large diagonal branch using a two-stage Harris procedure, followed 2 hours later by release of the occlusion. In animals with extensive preformed collateral or anastomosing vessels, we also ligate permanently at least two or three of the more prominent anastomosing epicardial vessels at the cardiac apex. This procedure often results in dogs with heterogeneous, mottled infarctions with close interspersing of normal and abnormal tissue transmurally, confirmed both histopathologically and electrophysiologically.[32] For example, on a millimeter-to-millimeter basis, there is often marked interspersing of apparently normal, viable, surviving myocardium and tissues having widely disparate properties of excitability, refractoriness, and conduction.

Serious arrhythmias rarely occur spontaneously in these animals following the third day after infarction. However, these dogs are highly susceptible to sustained ventricular tachyarrhythmias using programmed stimulation. The best evidence available from extensive electrophysiologic studies suggests that the arrhythmias inducible by programmed pacing in this model are re-entrant and use abnormal but surviving myocardial tissue as part of a localized re-entrant circuit.[32,35] To date, for the purpose of doing extensive basic electrophysiologic studies in these animals, including detailed evaluations of regional properties of excitability, refractoriness, and conduction, we have done the majority of our studies in open-chest, barbiturate-anesthetized animals. For the purpose of understanding basic electrophysiology, these methods have been very satisfactory in many respects. However, they present many inherent limitations in extrapolating to the clinical domain of preventing sudden cardiac death.

It is important to note that the major advantage of this model appears to be that using routine methods of programmed pacing, the majority of animals prepared in this manner are reproducibly susceptible to the initiation of sustained ventricular tachyarrhythmias. The arrhythmias can often be initiated during ventricular pacing with the introduction of either one or multiple extrastimuli, and episodes of sustained tachycardia can often be terminated with either programmed pacing or overdrive burst pacing. The tachyarrhythmias so initiated tend to be more rapid than those encountered clinically in man, but are otherwise similar in many of their characteristics.[25,26,38,39] Presumably, this shorter cycle length reflects a combination of factors including the shorter refractory periods of canine ventricular myocardium, smaller hearts, and the influence of catecholamines in these open-chest, barbiturate-anesthetized animals. It should be pointed out, however, that in these same animals studied closed chest with chronically implanted electrodes, similar tachyarrhythmias can be initiated. As indicated above, the major reason for studying these animals open chest is to facilitate detailed electrophysiologic data collection. Notably, although microelectrode studies done on tissue preparations from these animals suggest continued infarct evolution and healing over the first 2 to 4 weeks and longer following the occlusion/reperfusion procedure,[40,41] animals remain highly susceptible to tachyarrhythmia initiation for at least the first 4 weeks following infarction and, anecdotally, in the few animals we have studied, for as long as 2 years in some cases. Undoubtedly, the addition of a reperfusion stage to the usual canine coronary occlusion procedure is sufficient to distort the usual healing process[27-32] such that a chronic anatomic and electrophysiologic milieu develops that is a suitable substrate for re-entry. However, limited ambulatory monitoring has suggested that these dogs are essentially free of serious spontaneous ventricular arrhythmias during normal activities.

Thus, these chronically infarcted animals require an additional insult or stimulus to unmask their susceptibility to sustained VT or VF or both. But not to underestimate their potential susceptibility to arrhythmias under appropriate conditions, even a single appropriately timed premature beat is often sufficient to initiate reproducibly either sustained VT or VF.

Investigators in several laboratories including our own have found promising the potential utility of these chronic canine myocardial infarction–ventricular tachyarrhythmia models in evaluating the electropharmacology of conventional and new investigational antiarrhythmic drugs. First, it is possible to gain insight into the potential efficacy of these agents in preventing pacing-initiated sustained ventricular tachyarrhythmias. Second, it is possible to determine potential electropharmacologic mechanisms of action. The results of these many studies are beyond the scope of this chapter. Notably, the effects of several drugs in these models appear to correlate well with their effects in patients with ischemic heart disease and inducible ventricular tachyarrhythmias. Thus, the potential utility of these models for furthering our understanding of serious arrhythmias and their therapy is considerable.

There are several potential limitations that one must consider in interpreting experimental electrophysiologic studies. For example, in evaluating the electropharmacology of drugs in canine models, one must be aware of potential differences between intravenous and oral dosing (which is also true in man), differences in metabolites between dog and man (e.g., a lack of N-acetyl procainamide metabolites in the dog), and potential inconsistencies secondary to differences in technique from one laboratory to the next. On the other hand, the opportunity to selectively study both the parent compound and individual metabolites can help to elucidate the mechanisms whereby an antiarrhythmic drug may have either salutary or deleterious effects.

To put these models in perspective, animals are susceptible reproducibly to inducible sustained ventricular tachyarrhythmias. The arrhythmias are similar in many respects to those induced in the clinical electrophysiologic laboratory in patients with chronic ischemic heart disease who are susceptible to either recurrent sustained VT or VF.[25,26,33,36,38] The utility of electropharmacologic drug testing in these animals has the most immediate relevance to this subset of patients. These methods are not necessarily applicable to the problem of sudden cardiac death in patients with either cardiomyopathies or isolated "electrical heart disease." Clinically, there is considerable evidence accumulating that the prescription of antiarrhythmic therapy based on the results of programmed electrophysiologic testing may have great utility in predicting either the efficacy or lack of efficacy of a proposed antiarrhythmic regimen.[39,42-44] Accordingly, a drug proven useful in these dogs is potentially of great interest in treating patients susceptible to sustained ventricular tachycardia or fibrillation in the setting of chronic ischemic heart disease, and particularly when the mechanism involves reentrant phenomena. On the other hand, these are not models of spontaneous sudden death, and many interventions or potential therapeutic regimens that may have value in preventing either the inciting ischemic episode or the resultant lethal acute arrhythmia may still be of value in man even if they do not prevent the initiation of sustained ventricular tachyarrhythmias using programmed pacing in these dogs. Moreover, there is also evidence accumulating in man that antiarrhythmic drugs such as amiodarone may be protective with respect to recurrent arrhythmias, and yet still leave the patient susceptible to arrhythmia initiation in the laboratory. Presumably, therefore, there will also be antiarrhythmic drugs that fail in these models but will have ultimate utility in the treatment of patients. In addition, although these models may provide information with respect to the antitachycardia and antifibrillation properties of a new drug, they do not provide direct information with respect to activity versus isolated, frequent, or complex but unsustained ventricular arrhythmias.

Based on our present experience, it is further suggested that new potential antiarrhythmic drugs be evaluated both after intravenous administration and after chronic oral therapy in these animals. Open-chest, anesthetized preparations are most suitable for detailed electropharmacologic testing, whereas closed-chest preparations more closely simulate the human situation. In addition, a number of other confounding variables must also be taken into consideration, including effects mediated by either the central or autonomic nervous system. Interestingly, even dogs prepared in an apparently identical manner and with similar occlusion/reperfusion lesions demonstrate considerable biologic variability with respect to whether VT or VF or no arrhythmia is initiated in any individual animal. In addition, there may be variability from dog to dog with respect to the response of the same drug. In man, the anatomic and pathophysiologic substrates are even more heterogeneous, and the response to even the most effective antiarrhythmic agents still remains inconsistent from patient to patient, and therapy is therefore empiric. Reassuringly, the dosages of antiarrhythmic drugs found effective in suppressing ventricular tachyarrhythmia initiation in these dogs appear similar to those required in man.[42,45,46] However, as noted above, animal studies often do not take into account the potential effects of antiarrhythmic drug metabolites found in man, or other complicating factors such as hypokalemia, concomitant digoxin use, or marked left ventricular dysfunction.

An additional experimental and clinical observation of potential relevance is that some drugs may facilitate VT initiation,[47] decrease rather than increase the cycle length of arrhythmias initiated, or, even worse, make VF more likely. Furthermore, they may even make defibrillation more difficult. This may be particularly true when certain drugs are given intravenously, much more so than with chronic oral therapy. Thus, these chronic ventricular tachyarrhythmia–myocardial infarction models may be of further utility in predicting these potentially deleterious effects of a new antiarrhythmic agent.

It is also worth noting the results of two additional, recent provocative studies further highlighting the potential relevance of chronic canine myocardial infarction models to the study of sudden death prevention. First, Gang and coworkers[48] have modified the occlusion/reperfusion procedure to study the relationship between inducible VT and ventricular "vulnerability." Specifically, they created myocardial infarctions in closed-chest dogs by inflating a balloon catheter in the left anterior descending coronary artery for 2 hours. Using a transvenous electrode catheter, the animals were then studied by programmed electrical stimulation 4 days later. The researchers evaluated the so-called "repetitive ventricular response" threshold, the ventricular fibrillation threshold, and the susceptibility to sustained ventricular tachyarrhythmias using single and double extrastimuli as well as burst ventricular pacing. They found that the VF threshold was markedly reduced 4 days after infarction in dogs capable of sustained tachycardia, whereas in dogs not susceptible to sustained tachycardia, there was no significant change in the mean VF threshold. Similarly, the ventricular repetitive response threshold was also reduced in dogs susceptible to VT; in dogs not susceptible to VT, neither threshold was significantly altered. However, changes in the repetitive response and VF thresholds were not always parallel. Overall, Gang and coworkers[48] believed that the VF threshold was a more reliable indicator of susceptibility to tachyarrhythmias. This is of considerable interest because the VF threshold has been used conventionally as a screen for new potential antiarrhythmic agents capable of preventing sudden arrhythmic death, and suggests further that chronic models of inducible sustained ventricular tachyarrhythmias may also have a role in this respect. In addition, the application of closed-chest coronary occlusion techniques by these and other investigators[49] should further extend the usefulness of various chronic animal models.

A second recent study also warrants comment. Jackman and Zipes[50] have recently reported the feasibility and safety of terminating sustained ventricular tachyarrhythmias using low-energy, synchronized shocks delivered through transvenous, intracardiac catheter electrodes. For this purpose they used dogs studied 3 to 8 days after surviving a 2-hour occlusion-release of the left anterior descending coronary artery with adjunctive ligation of anastomosing vessels at the left ventricular apex. Using this model, they were able to show convincingly the feasibility of transvenous low-energy tachycardia termination and its potential applicability to man. These methods are now undergoing further evaluation in both animals and man.

**Other Chronic Ventricular Tachyarrhythmia Models**

Several other chronic myocardial infarction models have been developed for studying the problem of sudden cardiac death. For example, they include models evaluating the potential arrhythmogenic effects of peri-infarction steroids in dogs, of high-fat diets in pigs subjected to chest irradiation, and of multiple coronary occlusions in the cat. These several models have recently been the subject of another review.[51]

**Chronic Canine Myocardial Infarction Models With Superimposed Acute Ischemia**

A number of laboratories have recently developed even more promising models for studying the electrophysiologic mechanisms and the electropharmacologic prophylaxis of sudden cardiac death in the setting of ischemic heart disease. Patterson and coworkers[52,53] have extended their earlier studies by adding an acute ischemic lesion to dogs with chronic occlusion/reperfusion myocardial infarctions. They have studied chronically instrumented conscious dogs, in which a 30-gauge silver wire is left in the lumen of the left circumflex coronary artery at the time of the infarction procedure. Dogs are studied 4 to 30 days after occlusion/reperfusion of the left anterior descending coronary artery. The intimal surface of the left circumflex artery is then injured by applying a 150-microampere current. A typical sequence ensues, with ST segment changes occurring at a mean of 127 minutes following current application, ventricular tachyarrhythmias shortly thereafter, and VF in nearly every animal by a mean of 133 minutes. Ventricular fibrillation is preceded by the development of delayed electrical activity within the distribution of the circumflex artery, and the development of antecedent ventricular arrhythmias is accompanied by continuous local electrical activity within the subepicardial region of the circumflex disturbution. Notably, such an ischemic lesion of the circumflex coronary artery produced in animals without an antecedent occlusion/reperfusion infarction is not accompanied by malignant ventricular arrhythmias or sudden death. Interestingly, although the beta blocker nadolol was ineffective in preventing pacing-induced initiation of sustained re-entrant ventricular tachyarrhythmias in their dogs with chronic infarctions, nadolol (8 mg/kg, intravenously) was effective in preventing VF after superimposed circumflex artery stimulation in 5 of 12 treated animals, whereas each of 13 untreated dogs developed fatal dysrhythmias following anodal current-induced thrombosis of the circumflex coronary artery.[53] Apparently, the protective effects of nadolol were mediated by its beta-blocking properties in preventing VF, rather than a specific electrophysiologic property. For example, nadolol treatment had no demonstrable effect on excitability, refractoriness, or conduction in either normal or ischemically injured ventricular myocardium in this model. In addition, the ultimate infarct size was also not apparently reduced in animals pretreated with nadolol.

In another series of provocative experiments of considerable potential importance, Harrison and coworkers[54] have studied dogs subjected to ligation of the proximal left anterior descending coronary artery and 75 to 90 percent stenosis of the left circumflex artery just proximal to the posterior descending branch. In their preliminary study, 6 of 10 dogs undergoing this procedure showed angiographic evidence of apical dyskinesis and elevated left ventricular end-diastolic pressure 6 to 8 weeks after the acute myocardial infarction. Two of these six dogs showed spontaneous ventricular ectopic beats or VT or both. Presumably, the substrate of multivessel coronary artery disease is rather analogous to that encountered in most patients resuscitated from sudden cardiac death. Moreover, it is also clear that those patients with recent myocardial infarction who have residual left ventricular dysfunction are also at highest risk for sudden death in the subsequent convalescent period. It is likely, therefore, that this model will also have utility in future electropharmacologic studies.

### Chronic Canine Models/Neural Mechanisms

It is beyond the scope of this chapter to review the vast research relating neural and autonomic influences to the occurrence of sudden cardiac death. These have been studied elaborately in whole animals, in selected tissues, and even on a cellular level.[55-58] Undoubtedly, in man, both the central and autonomic nervous systems are potent mediators of potentially salutary and deleterious arrhythmogenic effects on the heart. Schwartz and Stone have performed a series of experiments to elucidate the mechanisms whereby these effects are mediated and the consequences of various interventions. They have developed multiple models for these purposes.[56,57] Typically, the interaction of a number of clinically relevant factors is evaluated in conscious animals. These include the effects of coronary occlusion, exercise, cessation of exercise, and sympathetic stimulation. Schwartz and Stone[56] have also evaluated the potential of left stellectomy in reducing the incidence of VF associated with acute myocardial ischemia in a variant of this model and have shown a protective effect. This protective effect of left stellectomy supports findings in other models of sudden death studied by these and other investigators. Moreover, there is now considerable interest in further evaluating many potential interventions that affect the autonomic nervous system, particularly in light of the recent beta-blocker heart attack trials, which have shown convincingly the potential protective role of beta blockers in preventing sudden death after recent myocardial infarction.

## OVERVIEW

A number of animal models have recently been developed that have relevance to the problem of sudden cardiac death in humans. These models have importance with respect to understanding both basic electrophysiologic mechanisms and potentially effective therapeutic interventions. However, none of these models is ideal in all respects for studying the problem of sudden death prevention in man.[34,59] Several models, already available, are particularly well suited for specific purposes, usually reflecting the research interests of an individual group of investigators. The methods involved in developing most of these models are sufficiently simple and straightforward to be accessible to most investigators. Models are available using both open-chest, anesthetized animals—more suitable for detailed evaluations of electropharmacologic mechanisms—and conscious, closed-chest animals—more closely resembling the human situation. Several alternative methods, including coronary occlusion/reperfusion, ligation of multiple distal arteries, or coronary occlusion in conjunction with the administration of various drugs (e.g., methylprednisolone), have each been used successfully to produce animals with chronic myocardial infarctions susceptible to sustained ventricular tachyarrhythmias. Arrhythmias can be initiated in these dogs using methods of programmed pacing similar to those used in patients in the clinical electrophysiologic laboratory. In addition, more elaborate models are now available that involve the superimposition of an acute ischemic lesion, with or without the additional stress of physical exertion, on a previous chronic myocardial infarction in conscious animals. The majority of studies to date have been done using canine models of ischemia and infarction, but cats, pigs, guinea pigs, and other animals also appear suitable for study. The electrophysiology of sudden cardiac death in nonischemic models has not been studied as extensively.

The recent availability of multiple, chronic myocardial infarction–ventricular tachyarrhythmia models now provides: (1) an opportunity to determine more precisely arrhythmia mechanisms that may be operative in patients with coronary artery disease susceptible to sudden cardiac death; (2) a means for identifying either invasive or noninvasive (e.g., via signal averaging[60]) electrophysiologic markers that may be helpful in identifying patients at highest risk for sudden death; (3) a more direct way to evaluate the antitachycardia and antifibrillatory potential of new antiarrhythmic drugs; (4) a means for evaluating both the acute and chronic effects of other antiarrhythmic therapies, including cryoablative and surgical techniques; (5) a way to evaluate the potential electrophysiologic consequences of modalities designed to salvage ischemic myocardium; and (6) a means to re-evaluate critically our present clinical methods of programmed pacing.[34,61,62] There are multiple potential limitations in applying any one animal model to the human situation, and thus, each model should be used for a specific purpose. This is particularly relevant in doing electropharmacologic studies, in which great caution must be exercised, particularly with respect to drug dosages, metabolites, and drug interactions.

Moreover, although the value of these models should not be underestimated, their differences from the human situation must be considered. Most of the models studied are nonprimate, and their arrhythmias result from myocardial ischemia and infarctions imposed extrinsically on an otherwise normal coronary anatomy and a previously normal ventricular myocardium; the etiology of the myocardial infarction in most models therefore is nonatherogenic. In open-chest and/or anesthetized animals, further cautions may pertain. Notwithstanding these limitations, the recent innovative development of several elegant models is most encouraging, and undoubtedly will provide answers that may help reduce the tragically high incidence of sudden cardiac death in humans.

## ACKNOWLEDGMENTS

I gratefully acknowledge the contributions and support of my several collaborating investigators, including Daniel David, M.D.; Leonard S. Dreifus, M.D.; Hideo Mitamura, M.D.; E. Neil Moore, D.V.M., Ph.D.; Masahito Naito, M.D.; Ole-Jorgen Ohm, M.D.; and Joseph F. Spear, Ph.D. I also gratefully acknowledge the expert help of Rose Marie Wells with manuscript preparation.

## REFERENCES

1. HARRIS, A AND ROJAS, AG: *Initiation of ventricular fibrillation due to coronary occlusion.* Experimental Medicine and Surgery 1:105, 1943.

2. WALDO, AL AND KAISER, GA: *A study of ventricular arrhythmias associated with acute myocardial infarction in the canine heart.*Circulation 47:1222, 1973.

3. BOINEAU, JP AND COX, JL: *Slow ventricular activation in acute myocardial infarction: A source of reentrant premature ventricular contractions.* Circulation 48:702, 1973.

4. SCHERLAG, BJ, EL-SHERIF, N, HOPE, R, ET AL: *Characterization and localization of ventricular arrhythmias resulting from myocardial ischemia and infarction.* Circ Res 34:372, 1974.

5. WIT, AL AND BIGGER, JT, JR: *Possible electrophysiological mechanisms for lethal arrhythmias accompanying myocardial ischemia and infarction.* Circulation 51,52(Supp III):96, 1975.

6. KAPLINSKY, E, OGAWA S, BALKE, CW, ET AL: *Two periods of early ventricular arrhythmia in the canine acute myocardial infarction model.* Circulation 60:397, 1979.

7. LEVITES, R, BANKA, VS, AND HELFANT, RH: *Electrophysiologic effects of coronary occlusion and reperfusion: Observations on dispersion of refractoriness and ventricular automaticity.* Circulation 52:760, 1975.

8. ELHARRAR, V, FOSTER, PR, JIRAK, TL, ET AL: *Alterations in canine myocardial excitability during ischemia.* Circ Res 40:98, 1977.

9. KAPLINSKY, E, OGAWA, S, BALKE, W, ET AL: *Role of endocardial activation in malignant ventricular arrhythmias associated with acute ischemia.* J Electrocardiol 12:299, 1979.

10. JANSE, MJ, VANCAPELLE, JL, MORSINK, H, ET AL: *Flow of "injury" current and patterns of excitation during early ventricular arrhythmias in acute regional myocardial ischemia in isolated porcine and canine hearts: Evidence for two different arrhythmogenic mechanisms.* Circ Res 47:151, 1980.

11. BALKE, CW, KAPLINSKY, E, MICHELSON, EL, ET AL: *Reperfusion ventricular tachyarrhythmias: Correlation with antecedent coronary artery occlusion tachyarrhythmias and duration of myocardial ischemia.* Am Heart J 101:449, 1981.

12. PENKOSKE, PA, SOBEL, BE, AND CORR, PB: *Disparate electrophysiological alterations accompanying dysrhythmia due to coronary occlusion and reperfusion in the cat.* Circulation 58:1023, 1978.

13. KAPLINSKY, E, OGAWA, S, MICHELSON, EL, ET AL: *Instantaneous and delayed ventricular arrhythmias after reperfusion of acutely ischemic myocardium: Evidence for multiple mechanisms.* Circulation 63:333, 1981.

14. DREIFUS, LS, NAITO, M, AND MICHELSON, EL: *What animal models should be used to define antiarrhythmic efficacy? Acute dog models.* In MORGANROTH, J, MOORE, EN, DREIFUS, LS, ET AL (EDS): *How to Evaluate a New Antiarrhythmic Drug.* Martinus Nijhoff, The Hague, 1981, p 17.

15. HARRIS, AS: *Delayed development of ventricular ectopic rhythms following experimental coronary occlusion.* Circulation 1:1318, 1950.

16. FRIEDMAN, PL, STEWARD, JR, FENOGLIO, JJ, ET AL: *Survival of subendocardial Purkinje fibers after extensive myocardial infarction in dogs.* Circ Res 33:597, 1973.

17. LAZZARA, R, EL-SHERIF, N, AND SCHERLAG, BJ: *Electrophysiological properties of canine Purkinje cells in one-day-old myocardial infarction.* Circ Res 33:722, 1973.

18. HOROWITZ, LN, SPEAR, JF, AND MOORE, EN: *Subendocardial origin of ventricular arrhythmias in 24-hour-old experimental myocardial infarction.* Circulation 53:56, 1975.

19. SPEAR, JF, MICHELSON, EL, SPIELMAN, SR, ET AL: *The origin of ventricular arrhythmias 24 hours following experimental anterior septal coronary artery occlusion.* Circulation 55:844, 1977.

20. EL-SHERIF, N, MEHRA, R, GOUGH, WB, ET AL: *Ventricular activation patterns of spontaneous and induced ventricular rhythms in canine one-day-old myocardial infarction.* Circ Res 51:152, 1982.

21. WELLENS, HJJ, LIE, KI, AND DURRER, D: *Further observations on ventricular tachycardia.* Circulation 49:647, 1974.

22. EL-SHERIF, N, SCHERLAG, BJ, LAZZARA, R, ET AL: *Reentrant arrhythmias in the late myocardial infarction period: I. Conduction characteristics in the infarct zone.* Circulation 55:686, 1977.

23. EL-SHERIF, N, HOPE, RR, SCHERLAG, BJ, ET AL: *Reentrant arrhythmias in the late myocardial infarction period: II. Patterns of initiation and termination of reentry.* Circulation 55:702, 1977.

24. DURRER, D, VANDAM, RT, FREUD, GE, ET AL: *Reentry and ventricular arrhythmias in local ischemia and infarction of the intact dog heart.* Proc K Ned Akad Wet (Biol Med) 74:321, 1971.

25. JOSEPHSON, ME, HOROWITZ, LN, FARSHIDI, A, ET AL: *Recurrent sustained ventricular tachycardia: 1. Mechanisms.* Circulation 57:431, 1978.

26. JOSEPHSON, ME, HOROWITZ, LN, FARSHIDI, A, ET AL: *Sustained ventricular tachycardia: Evidence for protected localized reentry.* Am J Cardiol 42:416, 1978.

27. KARAGUEUZIAN, HS, FENOGLIO, JJ, WEISS, MB, ET AL: *Protracted ventricular tachycardia induced by premature stimulation of the canine heart after coronary artery occlusion and reperfusion.* Circ Res 44:833, 1979.

28. SOBEL, J AND ROSS, J, JR: *Coronary artery reperfusion: II. Reduction of myocardial infarct size at 1 week after the coronary occlusion.* J Clin Invest 51:2717, 1972.

29. MAROKO, PR, LIBBY, P, GINKS, WR, ET AL: *Coronary artery reperfusion: I. Early effects on local myocardial function and the extent of myocardial necrosis.* J Clin Invest 51:2710, 1972.

30. REIMER, KS, LOWE, VE, RASMUSSEN, MM, ET AL: *The wavefront phenomenon of ischemic cell death: I. Myocardial infarct size vs. duration of coronary occlusion in dogs.* Circulation 56:786, 1977.

31. WIT, AL, ALLESSIE, MA, BONKE, FIM, ET AL: *Electrophysiologic mapping to determine the mechanism of experimental ventricular tachycardia initiated by premature impulses.* Am J Cardiol 49:166, 1982.

32. MICHELSON, EL, SPEAR, JF, AND MOORE, EN: *Electrophysiologic and anatomic correlates of sustained ventricular tachyarrhythmias in a model of chronic myocardial infarction.* Am J Cardiol 45:583, 1980.

33. MICHELSON, EL, SPEAR, JF, AND MOORE, EN: *Effects of procainamide on strength-interval relations in normal and chronically infarcted canine myocardium.* Am J Cardiol 47:1223, 1981.

34. MICHELSON, EL, SPEAR, JF, AND MOORE, EN: *Initiation of sustained ventricular tachyarrhythmias in a canine model of chronic myocardial infarction: Importance of the site of stimulation.* Circulation 63:776, 1981.

35. MICHELSON, EL, SPEAR, JF, AND MOORE, EN: *Further electrophysiologic and anatomic correlates in a canine model of chronic myocardial infarction susceptible to the initiation of sustained ventricular tachyarrhythmias.* Anat Rec 201:55, 1981.

36. MICHELSON, EL: *Recent advances in antiarrhythmic drug research: Studies in chronic canine myocardial infarction–ventricular tachyarrhythmia models.* PACE 5:90, 1982.

37. WETSTEIN, L, MICHELSON, EL, SIMSON, MB, ET AL: *Increased normoxic-to-ischemic tissue borderzone as the cause for reentrant ventricular tachycardias.* J Surg Res 32:526, 1982.

38. WELLENS, HJJ, DUREN, DR, AND LIE, KI: *Observations on mechanisms of ventricular tachycardia in man.* Circulation 54:237, 1976.

39. WELLENS, HJJ: *Value and limitations of programmed electrical stimulation of the heart in the study and treatment of tachycardias.* Circulation 57:845, 1978.

40. SPEAR, JF, MICHELSON, EL, AND MOORE, EN: *Cellular electrophysiologic characteristics of chronically infarcted myocardium in dogs susceptible to sustained ventricular tachyarrhythmias.* J Am Coll Cardiol 1:1099, 1983.

41. SPEAR, JF, MICHELSON, EL, AND MOORE, EN: *Reduced space constant in slowly conducting regions of chronically infarcted canine myocardium.* Circ Res 53:176, 1983.

42. HOROWITZ, LN, JOSEPHSON, ME, FARSHIDI, A, ET AL: *Recurrent sustained ventricular tachycardia: 3. Role of electrophysiologic study in selection of antiarrhythmic regimens.* Circulation 58:986, 1978.

43. MASON, JW AND WINKLE, RA: *Accuracy of the ventricular tachycardia–induction study for predicting long-term efficacy and inefficacy of antiarrhythmic drugs.* N Engl J Med 303:1073, 1980.

44. RUSKIN, JN, DiMARCO, JP, AND GARAN, H: *Out-of-hospital cardiac arrest: Electrophysiologic observations and selection of long-term antiarrhythmic therapy.* N Engl J Med 303:607, 1980.

45. WELLENS, HJJ, BAR, FWHM, AND LIE, KI: *Effect of procainamide, propranolol and verapamil on mechanism of tachycardia in patients with chronic recurrent ventricular tachycardia.* Am J Cardiol 40:579, 1977.

46. GREENSPAN, AM, HOROWITZ, LN, AND SPIELMAN, SR: *Large dose procainamide therapy for ventricular tachycardia.* Am J Cardiol 46:453, 1980.

47. PATTERSON, E, GIBSON, JK, AND LUCCHESI, BR: *Postmyocardial infarction re-entrant ventricular arrhythmias in conscious dogs: Suppression by bretylium tosylate.* J Pharmacol Exp Ther 216:453, 1981.

48. GANG, ES, BIGGER, JT, JR, AND LIVELLI, FI, JR: *A model of chronic ischemic arrhythmias: The relationship between electrically inducible ventricular tachycardia and ventricular fibrillation threshold.* Am J Cardiol 50:469, 1982.

49. GEWIRTZ, H AND MOST, AS: *Production of a critical coronary arterial stenosis in closed chest laboratory animals.* Am J Cardiol 47:589, 1981.

50. JACKMAN, WM AND ZIPES, DP: *Low-energy synchronous cardioversion of ventricular tachycardia using a catheter electrode in a canine model of subacute myocardial infarction.* Circulation 66:186, 1982.

51. MICHELSON, EL: *Animal models for the study of antiarrhythmic drugs for the prevention of sudden coronary death: Chronic animal models.* In LUCCHESI, BR, DINGELL, JV, AND SCHWARZ, RB, JR (EDS): *Clinical Pharmacology of Antiarrhythmic Therapy.* Raven Press, New York, 1984, pp 44–70.

52. PATTERSON, E, HOLLAND, K, ELLER, BT, ET AL: *Ventricular fibrillation resulting from ischemia at a site remote from previous myocardial infarction.* Am J Cardiol 50:1414, 1982.

53. PATTERSON, E AND LUCCHESI, BR: *Antifibrillatory actions of nadolol.* J Pharmacol Exp Ther 223:144, 1982.

54. HARRISON, LA, SCHERLAG, BJ, BERBARI, EJ, ET AL: *Left ventricular aneurysm: A canine model.* Circulation 68 (Suppl III): 194, 1983.

55. DeSILVA, RA: *Central nervous system risk factors for sudden cardiac death.* Ann NY Acad Sci 382:143, 1982.

56. SCHWARTZ, PJ AND STONE, HL: *Left stellectomy in the prevention of ventricular fibrillation caused by acute myocardial ischemia in conscious dogs with anterior myocardial infarction.* Circulation 62:1256, 1980.

57. SCHWARTZ, PJ AND STONE, HL: *The role of the autonomic nervous system in sudden coronary death.* Ann NY Acad Sci 382:162, 1982.

58. ZIPES, DP, MARTINS, JB, RUSSY, R, ET AL: *Role of autonomic innervation in the genesis of ventricular arrhythmias.* In ABBOUD, FM, FOZZARD, HA, GILMORE, JP, ET AL (EDS): *Disturbances in Neurogenic Control of the Circulation.* American Physiological Society, Bethesda, MD, 1981, p 225.

59. FOZZARD, HA: *Validity of myocardial infarction models.* Circulation 51&52(Suppl III):131, 1975.

60. SIMSON, MD, EULER, D, MICHELSON, EL, ET AL: *Detection of delayed ventricular activation on the body surface in dogs.* Am J Physiol 241:H363, 1981.

61. MICHELSON, EL, NAITO, M, SPEAR, JF, ET AL: *Comparative effects of cycle length on ventricular refractoriness of normal and chronically infarcted myocardium.* Am J Cardiol 47:391, 1981.

62. MICHELSON, EL, DAVID, D, NAITO, M, ET AL: *Comparative effects of stimulus duration on ventricular refractoriness in normal versus chronically infarcted myocardium: Implications for electrophysiologic studies.* Am J Cardiol 49:958, 1982.

# Role of the Autonomic Nervous System in Sudden Death*

*Richard L. Verrier, Ph.D., and Eric L. Hagestad, B.A.*

Extensive studies in experimental animals and increasing clinical experience with patients resuscitated from sudden death indicate a pervasive involvement of the nervous system in the genesis of fatal cardiac arrhythmias. The objectives of this chapter are to review the current state of knowledge on this subject and to discuss recent developments that are likely to provide novel approaches to the management of malignant arrhythmias.

## AUTONOMIC NERVOUS SYSTEM ACTIVITY AND CARDIAC ARRHYTHMIAS

Webb, Adgey, and Pantridge[1,2] have provided substantial evidence implicating the autonomic neural reflexes in the provocation of cardiac arrhythmias during the early phases of acute myocardial ischemia and infarction. They demonstrated that in 89 patients reached within 30 minutes of onset of symptoms of acute myocardial infarction, only 15 (17 percent) had normal heart rate and arterial blood pressure (Fig. 1). More than one third showed evidence of sympathetic overactivity. Parasympathetic overactivity was present in almost half of the patients. The systolic blood pressure at the initial examination was not greater than 80 mm Hg in nearly one fourth of the patients. Forty-seven percent of patients with bradyarrhythmia had a systolic blood pressure not greater than 80 mm Hg. Eight percent of patients had complete atrioventricular block. The incidence of autonomic disturbance was related to the site of the infarction. Parasympathetic overactivity occurred more frequently in association with posterior wall infarction (see Fig. 1) than with infarctions in other locations.

In experimental animals, Malliani, Lombardi, and coworkers[3,4] have demonstrated that coronary artery occlusion significantly increases the firing frequency of preganglionic cardiac sympathetic fibers. This excitatory response appears to be due to activation of potent cardio-cardiac reflexes (Fig. 2). The reflex response is due in part to excitation of unmyelinated afferent vagal fibers originating in the left ventricle.[3,5,6] This pathway is thought to mediate the depressor effect of acute myocardial ischemia and probably provides the basis for the Bezold-Jarisch reflex.[7,8] The cardiovascular response is the result of combined vagal excitation and reciprocal sympathetic inhibition of sympathetic afferent fibers.

As is the case in humans, the site of myocardial infarction in the feline heart is a major determinant of the hemodynamic and cardiac rhythm changes occurring after coronary

*Supported in part by Grant No. HL-28387 and Grant No. HL-07776 from the National Heart, Lung and Blood Institute, National Institutes of Health, U.S. Public Health Service, Bethesda, Maryland, and The Rappaport International Program in Cardiology.

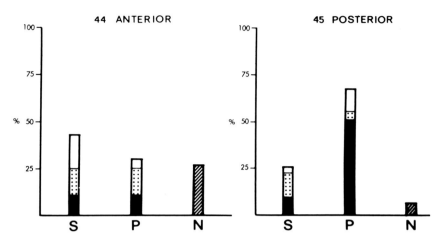

**Figure 1.** Autonomic nervous system disturbances in 89 patients observed within 30 minutes of onset of acute myocardial infarction symptoms. Infarction occurred in the anterior wall in 44 and in the posterior wall in 45 individuals. S = sympathetic overactivity as evidenced by sinus tachycardia and hypertension; P = parasympathetic overactivity as indicated by bradyarrhythmia and hypotension; N = normal heart rate and arterial blood pressure. (From Pantridge,[2] with permission.)

artery occlusion.[9] Left anterior descending (LAD) coronary artery occlusion results in immediate decreases in cardiac output, heart rate, and arterial blood pressure; an increase in total peripheral resistance (TPR); and cardiac rhythm changes including premature ventricular beats, ventricular tachycardia, and occasionally ventricular fibrillation. The decrease in cardiac output and increase in TPR persist in animals surviving a ventricular arrhythmia. By contrast, right coronary occlusion results in a considerably smaller reduction in cardiac output. During recovery from arrhythmia related to right coronary artery occlusion, TPR does not increase, atrioventricular conduction disturbances are common, and sinus bradycardia and hypotension persist. Left circumflex artery ligation results in cardiovascular changes similar to those produced by occlusion of the LAD or the right coronary artery, but less severe.

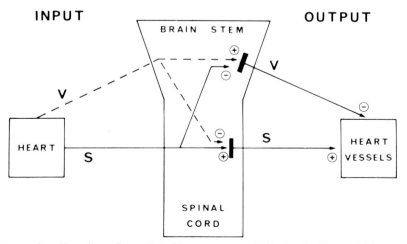

**Figure 2.** Schema of cardiocardiac reflexes elicited by acute myocardial ischemia. (From Malliani and Lombardi,[3] with permission.)

In a recent collaborative study conducted in our laboratory, Lombardi[10] examined the relationship between sympathetic neural activity and susceptibility to ventricular fibrillation (VF) during coronary artery occlusion and release-reperfusion. Preganglionic cardiac sympathetic impulse activity and VF thresholds were separately determined before and during a 10-minute period of LAD coronary artery occlusion and during release-reperfusion in dogs. Within 2 minutes of occlusion, the VF threshold was found to be significantly decreased, corresponding with the period of maximal activation of cardiac sympathetic preganglionic fibers. Both coronary sinus blood flow and oxygen tension decreased significantly. These effects persisted for 5 to 6 minutes, and then returned to control levels despite continued obstruction of the coronary artery. A transient but significant reduction in VF threshold also occurred with release of the occlusion but was not accompanied by increases in sympathetic neural discharge (Fig. 3).

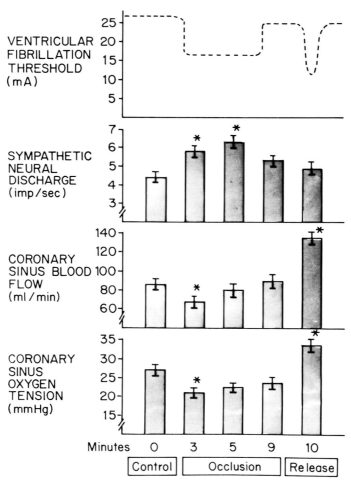

**Figure 3.** Effects of a 10-minute period of left anterior descending coronary artery occlusion and release on neural sympathetic activity, coronary sinus blood flow, and oxygen tension. A schematic representation of the time course of changes in ventricular fibrillation threshold is also displayed. Left anterior descending coronary artery occlusion results in a consistent activation of sympathetic preganglionic fibers, which corresponds with the period of maximal increase in vulnerability to ventricular fibrillation. The concomitant changes in coronary sinus blood flow and reperfusion are also displayed. *p < 0.05 compared with control period. (From Lombardi, Verrier, and Lown,[10] with permission.)

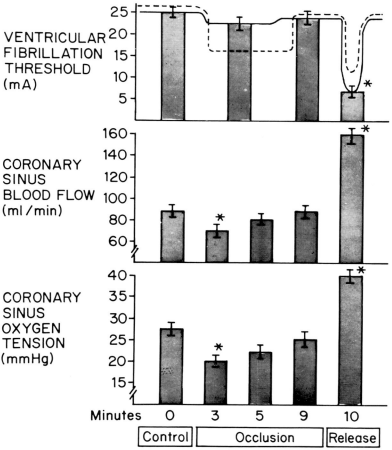

**Figure 4.** Effects of bilateral stellectomy on ventricular fibrillation threshold, coronary sinus blood flow, and oxygen tension induced by a 10-minute period of coronary artery occlusion and release. Stellectomy provides complete protection during coronary artery occlusion without influencing the pattern of change of coronary sinus blood flow and oxygen tension. In contrast, stellectomy enhances the susceptibility to ventricular fibrillation during release-reperfusion. The reactive hyperemic response is also enhanced (see Fig. 1). The dashed and solid lines represent the schematized vulnerability threshold changes in neurally intact and stellectomized dogs respectively. *p < 0.05 compared with control period. (From Lombardi, Verrier, and Lown,[10] with permission.)

Bilateral stellectomy abolished the change in VF threshold observed during coronary artery occlusion but had no effect on coronary sinus oxygen tension or blood flow. These findings indicate that enhanced cardiac sympathetic neural activity contributes to ventricular vulnerability associated with coronary artery obstruction. During the reperfusion phase, stellectomy actually increased rather than decreased vulnerability to ventricular fibrillation (Fig. 4).

The basis for the profibrillatory influence of stellectomy during reperfusion is uncertain. One possibility is that removal of the adrenergic influence on coronary vascular tone following stellectomy augmented the reactive hyperemic response and increased the release of ischemic washout products. There is evidence that a sympathetic alpha-receptor–mediated coronary vasoconstrictor influence operates in both the normal and ischemic heart.[11,12] Schwartz and Stone[13] found that stellectomy increased the hyperemic response following coronary artery occlusion, as shown by an enhancement in repayment of flow debt, a factor that has been recently implicated in reperfusion-induced vulnerability to fibrillation.[14]

## ROLE OF BETA RECEPTORS

Pharmacologic studies also indicate a major role of adrenergic factors in arrhythmogenesis during acute myocardial ischemia. Specifically, beta-adrenergic blocking drugs such as propranolol,[15,16] practolol,[17,18] and metoprolol[19] afford significant protection against VF during acute coronary artery occlusion in the experimental animal. The salutary influence of these agents appears to be due primarily to their adrenoreceptor-blocking properties rather than to their membrane-stabilizing actions.[17,18] Recently, practolol has been shown to be superior to propranolol in protecting against VF during coronary artery ligation.[20] Pearle and coworkers suggested that part of the beneficial effect of beta-adrenergic blockade of a noncardioselective agent such as propranolol may be negated by its potential vasoconstrictor effect, which is due to its inhibition of beta$_2$-receptor–mediated vascular smooth muscle relaxation. Indeed, there have been a number of patients with Prinzmetal's variant angina in whom aggravation of symptoms resulted from the use of propranolol.[21] Presumably in these cases, the propranolol prompted vasoconstriction; such an effect would not be anticipated in response to cardioselective agents. This consideration introduces difficulties in selecting appropriate pharmacologic therapy inasmuch as it is uncertain whether sudden death in man is due to acute myocardial ischemia or to reperfusion. In the latter case, beta-adrenergic blockade might prove without avail because it is ineffectual in preventing VF following release of coronary artery occlusion (Fig. 5).[15,18,19]

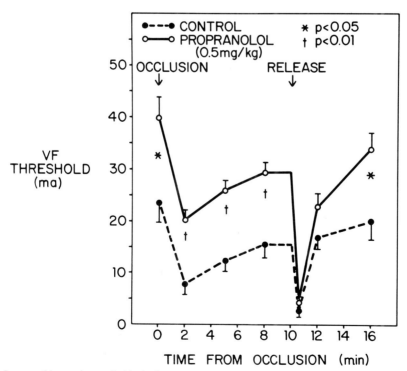

**Figure 5.** Influence of beta-adrenergic blockade on vulnerability to ventricular fibrillation (VF) during acute coronary artery occlusion and release-reperfusion.

## ROLE OF ALPHA RECEPTORS

The influence of alpha-adrenergic blockade on vulnerability to VF is of particular interest in the setting of acute coronary occlusion. Recent clinical evidence suggests that coronary vasospasm may be present during the early phases of acute myocardial infarction.[22-24] Thus, following coronary artery obstruction, alpha-adrenergic blockade may influence vulnerability not only through a possible effect on myocardial receptors but also through an action on vascular receptors. Indeed, it has been demonstrated that coronary vascular diameter depends on tonic alpha-adrenergically mediated vasoconstriction as well as upon metabolic regulation.[11,13,23-25] Alpha-adrenergic blockade with phentolamine decreases susceptibility to VF during myocardial ischemia.[15] It remains uncertain, however, whether the drug exerts its antifibrillatory influence through an action on myocardial alpha receptors or by an indirect effect of blocking coronary artery vasospasm.

An antifibrillatory influence of alpha-adrenergic blocking agents during release-reperfusion has been demonstrated by Sheridan and coworkers[26] and Stewart and colleagues.[27] It remains to be determined whether the drugs employed, namely phentolamine and prazosin, exerted their effects solely through an action on alpha-adrenergic receptors. The possibility that extra-adrenergic influences may play a role is suggested by the fact that both drugs alter the vulnerable period threshold beyond the level achieved by surgical removal of adrenergic inputs, implicating an extra-adrenergic effect of the drugs. In addition, administration of the alpha agonist phenylephrine[28] or methoxamine[29] is without effect on the vulnerable period threshold when the pressor response to the agonist is controlled. Alpha-blocking drugs also exert other effects that possibly influence ventricular vulnerability, namely, enhanced insulin secretion[30,31] and alteration in platelet function.[32] Thus the precise role of alpha-adrenergic receptors during myocardial ischemia and reperfusion awaits further clarification.

## ROLE OF CYCLIC NUCLEOTIDES

Cyclic nucleotides have been increasingly implicated as mediating factors in the arrhythmogenic influence of catecholamines.[33-36] Opie and coworkers have studied various factors that increased tissue cyclic adenosine monophosphate (AMP) and simultaneously decreased the VF threshold in the isolated perfused rat heart. The fibrillation threshold decreased as the tissue cyclic AMP content increased. The effects of beta$_1$ stimulation and of phosphodiesterase inhibition could both be related to alterations in the intracellular level of cyclic AMP. The effect of exogenous dibutyryl cyclic AMP in decreasing the VF threshold was not due to activation of adenyl cyclase because (1) the effect was still evident in the presence of a beta$_1$-specific blocker, atenolol,[37] and (2) the effect of exogenous dibutyryl cyclic AMP was greatly enhanced by the addition of a phosphodiesterase inhibitor, theophylline[34] (Fig. 6).

Although these observations do suggest that cyclic AMP is capable of influencing vulnerability to VF, its role in this regard as the second messenger of the effects of catecholamines on vulnerability will require further substantiation.

## VAGUS NERVE INFLUENCES

The prevailing view had been that vagal innervation did not extend to the ventricular myocardium. Clinical teaching had been in accord with this perception. If a tachycardia responded to cholinergic measures, the site of impulse formation was judged to be supraventricular. However, considerable data have now been amassed indicating that parasympathetic neural influences directly affect the inotropic, chronotropic, and electrophysiologic properties of the ventricles.[38-41] Kent and coworkers[38] demonstrated that vagus nerve stimulation

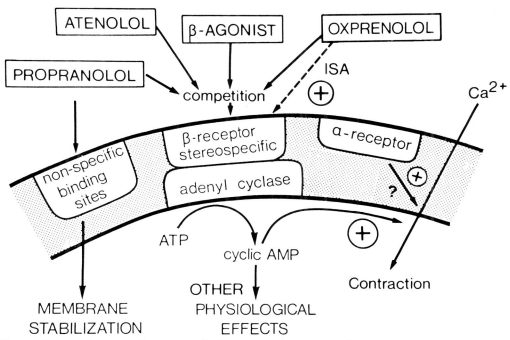

**Figure 6.** Beta-agonists act on the stereospecific beta-receptor in the heart cell membrane. Beta-blockade by propranolol is partly a specific competitive antagonism and partly a non-specific binding ("membrane stabilization") action. Alpha-agonists act through the recently isolated alpha-receptor and may inhibit adenyl cyclase. (From Opie,[34] with permission.)

increased the VF threshold in both the normal and ischemic canine ventricle. They demonstrated, moreover, the cholinergic innervation of the specialized conducting system through which the antifibrillatory action of the vagus is thought to occur. Our understanding has been enhanced by the studies of Zipes and coworkers[40,41] who utilized phenol to delineate the anatomic pathways mediating vagal influences on excitability of the normal and ischemic heart.

## SYMPATHETIC-PARASYMPATHETIC INTERACTIONS

Our view has been that the effect of the vagus on ventricular vulnerability is contingent on the level of pre-existing cardiac sympathetic tone.[42–45] This viewpoint is based on the observation that when sympathetic tone to the heart is augmented by thoracotomy,[45] sympathetic nerve stimulation,[45] or catecholamine infusion,[43,44] simultaneous vagal activation exerts a protective effect on ventricular vulnerability. Vagus nerve stimulation is without effect on ventricular vulnerability when adrenergic input to the heart is ablated by beta-adrenergic blockade (Fig. 7).[45]

The influence of the vagus on ventricular vulnerability appears to be due to activation of muscarinic receptors because vagally mediated changes in vulnerability are prevented by atropine administration.[44] The diminution of adrenergic effects by muscarinic activation has a physiologic and cellular basis. Muscarinic agents have been shown both to inhibit the release of norepinephrine from sympathetic nerve endings[46] and to attenuate the response to norepinephrine at receptor sites by cyclic nucleotide interactions (Fig. 8).[36,47]

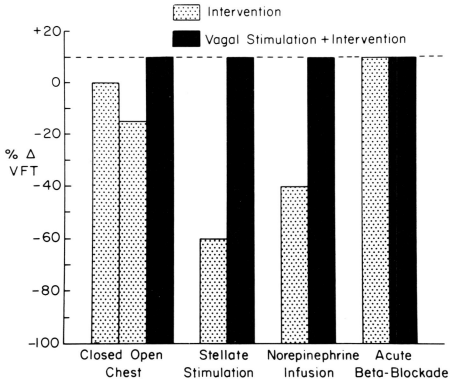

**Figure 7.** Influence of vagal stimulation in the presence of various levels of adrenergic tone. The vagal effect on ventricular fibrillation threshold (VFT) is demonstrable only when neural or humoral activity is increased. (From Lown and Verrier,[42] with permission.)

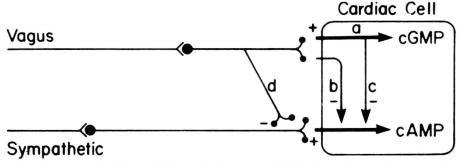

**Figure 8.** The interneuronal and intracellular mechanisms responsible for the vagal-sympathetic interactions. This accentuated antagonism between the parasympathetic and sympathetic systems may be accomplished in three different ways. First, the acetylcholine released at the vagal endings causes a direct reduction in the intracellular levels of cyclic AMP (arrow b). As stated in the text, cyclic AMP probably mediates the enhancement of contractility produced by sympathetic neural activity. Second, increased vagal activity raises intracellular levels of cyclic GMP. This nucleotide accelerates the hydrolysis of cyclic AMP (arrow c), thereby lowering its concentration in the myocardial cell. The third mechanism responsible for the accentuated antagonism between the two divisions of the autonomic nervous system involves extracellular processes. Some postganglionic vagal terminals (d) end near the postganglionic sympathetic terminals in the heart. The acetylcholine released at these vagal endings inhibits the release of norepinephrine from the sympathetic fibers. (From Berne and Levy,[142] with permission.)

## DIRECT VAGAL INFLUENCES

Muscarinic stimulation may also decrease susceptibility to ventricular arrhythmias by a direct action of acetylcholine on automaticity of conducting tissue. Tse and associates[48] have demonstrated that in isolated Purkinje fiber preparations, injection of acetylcholine suppresses automaticity and increases maximum diastolic potential. These actions of muscarinic stimulation on ventricular vulnerability are believed to be mediated mainly by an increase in $K^+$ conductance.[48] This mechanism differs from that of catecholamines, which alter automaticity by a change in slow, inward current.[49]

These direct actions of the vagus may explain certain clinical observations. For example, it has been found that increasing cardiac vagal drive by phenylephrine administration[50,51] or by carotid massage may terminate ventricular tachycardia. These maneuvers are more effective when the patients are pretreated with the cholinesterase inhibitor edrophonium and are ineffective following atropine administration. Inasmuch as these tachycardias were not prevented by propranolol administration, the vagal action may be due to a direct effect on the ventricles rather than to muscarinic antagonism of beta-adrenergic influences. A third possibility is that vagal influences on ventricular arrhythmias may be mediated by the attendant changes in heart rate.[52]

Direct actions of the vagus on ventricular electrophysiologic properties may, in part, explain why in certain patients sleep suppresses ventricular arrhythmias that are not controlled by propranolol therapy.[53] It is, indeed, established that certain stages of sleep are accompanied by substantial augmentation of cardiac vagal drive.[54]

## VAGUS NERVE ACTIVITY IN THE ISCHEMIC AND INFARCTED HEART

Yet unresolved is the issue of whether enhanced vagal activity alters cardiac predisposition to VF during acute coronary artery occlusion. Kent and Epstein[55,56] found that vagus nerve stimulation significantly increased the VF threshold and decreased susceptibility to fibrillation in the ischemic canine heart. Subsequently, Corr, Gillis, and their coworkers[57,58] observed that the presence of intact vagi protected against VF in chloralose-anesthetized cats during left anterior descending coronary artery ligation, but was not beneficial during right coronary artery obstruction. Yoon,[59] James,[60] and their associates were unable to demonstrate any effect of vagus nerve stimulation on VF threshold during left anterior descending coronary artery occlusion in the canine heart. Corr and coworkers[35] have even found that cholinergic stimulation may exacerbate rather than ameliorate the arrhythmias that ensue upon release of occlusion, with attendant reperfusion of the ischemic myocardium.

We have found that intense cholinergic stimulation by electrical stimulation of the decentralized vagi or by direct muscarinic enhancement with methacholine affords only partial protection during myocardial ischemia in dogs in which heart rate was maintained constant by pacing.[61,62] No salutary influence of cholinergic stimulation, however, was noted during reperfusion[62] (Fig. 9). However, additional countervailing factors come into play when myocardial perfusion is impaired. Thus, vagal stimulation does not completely suppress the arrhythmias that result from myocardial infarction.[63] In fact, it has been found that enhanced vagus activity or acetylcholine infusion consistently elicited ventricular tachycardia during the quiescent arrhythmia-free phase of myocardial infarction in dogs. This effect was completely rate-dependent because preventing the vagally induced bradycardia abolished the arrhythmias. Thus, the antiarrhythmic effects of the vagus may be augmented or reversed by its profound influence on heart rate in the setting of acute myocardial infarction.[63,64]

Vagal tone enhancement may be beneficial in preventing excessive elevations in heart rate associated with increased sympathetic drive to the heart and thereby conserving malperfused tissue from advancing ischemia. On the other hand, if profound bradycardia ensues, this may

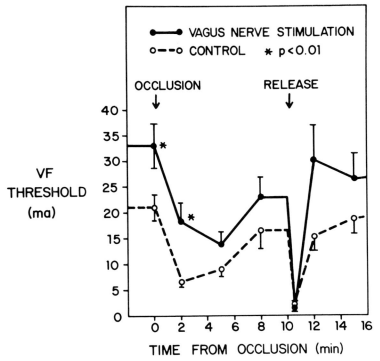

**Figure 9.** Influence of vagal stimulation on VF threshold during a 10-minute period of left anterior descending coronary artery occlusion followed by abrupt release. Vagal stimulation provided partial protection against vulnerability to VF during occlusion. No protection was afforded by vagal stimulation, however, during reperfusion. The results were obtained from 8 dogs with and 10 dogs without vagal stimulation. (From Verrier and Lown,[62] with permission.)

expose rate-sensitive ventricular ectopy, produce hypotension, and reduce coronary flow to jeopardized myocardial segments, which may in turn precipitate VF.

Clinical experience indicates that at the onset of acute myocardial infarction there is a tendency to bradycardia, believed to be mediated by enhanced vagal activity. As mentioned earlier, this was first brought to light by the Belfast group.[65] Among patients who came under intensive care within 4 hours of onset of the attack, bradycardia was found to be a remarkably frequent manifestation. With diaphragmatic infarction, 61 percent of patients who were seen within 1 hour of onset of symptoms exhibited some bradycardia. These arrhythmias were transient. When patients were seen within 30 minutes of acute myocardial infarction, signs of autonomic imbalance were detected in 92 percent of 68 patients.[1] In 41 of these (55 percent), there was excessive vagal activity, whereas in 27 (36 percent) there was sympathetic overactivity. Augmented parasympathetic activity was judged by heart rates of 60 beats per min or less, presence of atrioventricular block, or transient hypotension not caused by undue bradycardia.

There is little if any information on the level of vagal tone at the very inception of a heart attack, at the very time when the heart is most susceptible to VF. The case report by Biorck and Erhardt[66] is pertinent. They monitored a woman while she developed a heart attack. Within 1 minute of onset of symptoms, her heart rate receded from 65 to 40 beats per min, with progression to AV dissociation and nodal rhythm over the ensuing few minutes. Ventricular premature beats made their appearance only 41 minutes later, at a time when vagotonia was no longer in evidence.

The full clinical implication of vagal modulation of sympathetic tone during myocardial ischemia, especially as it relates to sudden cardiac death, is largely an unexplored area.

## ROLE OF CHANGES IN CORONARY VASOMOTOR TONE IN NEURALLY INDUCED ARRHYTHMIAS

Coronary artery spasm has been increasingly implicated in the provocation of transient myocardial ischemia. Primary decreases in coronary blood flow independent of systemic hemodynamic effects have been observed not only in variant angina[67-69] but also in classic and unstable angina.[69-73] Deanfield and coworkers[70] reported recurrent episodes of ST segment depression during ambulatory monitoring in patients with stable angina. These were not correlated with changes in heart rate and were shown to be associated with myocardial ischemia. They concluded that transient primary impairment in coronary artery blood flow rather than increased myocardial metabolic demand was a common stimulus for myocardial ischemia. It has been established that diverse events or stimuli can lead to coronary vasoconstriction, including cold exposure,[25,74-77] exercise,[69,70,73,78] myocardial infarction,[22,23] and verbal conditioning.[79] Whereas the precise mechanisms responsible for excessive and sustained coronary vasomotion are unclear, several studies indicate a central role for the sympathetic nervous system.[11,12,80-88]

The cold pressor test has been employed as a nonpharmacologic means for provoking coronary artery spasm.[25,74-77] Mudge and coworkers[74] have found that hand immersion in cold water produces coronary vasoconstriction, ST segment elevation, and chest pain in patients with coronary disease but not in normal individuals. The constrictor response is prevented by alpha-adrenergic blockade with phentolamine[74] and augmented by beta-adrenergic blockade with propranolol.[76] Potentiation of the coronary vasoconstrictor response by propranolol is thought to be mediated by unopposed alpha-adrenergic vasomotor tone.[76]

What is the basis for the differing coronary vasomotor responses to the cold pressor challenge in normal subjects versus those with ischemic heart disease? Mudge and colleagues[74] have proposed the following hypothesis to explain this finding. In the normal heart, constriction of large coronary vessels in response to a neurogenic stimulus can be compensated for by metabolically mediated vasodilation of small coronary vessels. However, in the diseased coronary vascular bed, coronary vasodilation downstream to the occlusion is already maximal to maintain resting flow at normal levels. Under these conditions, a vasoconstrictor stimulus cannot be offset and results in increased vascular resistance. The results of our recent study support this hypothesis. Whereas behavioral stress produces vasodilation in the normal dog's coronary circulation, profound vasoconstriction results in animals with prior coronary stenosis.[88]

## ROLE OF ALTERATIONS IN PLATELET FUNCTION

Intracoronary platelet aggregation may provide an important mechanism whereby neural factors predispose to cardiac arrhythmias. The induction of platelet aggregation with adenosine diphosphate causes both myocardial infarction and lethal arrhythmias in animals.[89] Pathologic studies in patients who have died suddenly have shown platelet microthrombi and platelet aggregates in numbers far greater than in those whose death was not sudden.[90-92]

Recent methodologic advances have made possible a detailed study of the effects of platelet aggregation on ventricular electrical stability. Folts and colleagues[93] have demonstrated that a critical coronary artery stenosis may induce a gradual decline of coronary blood flow over 5 to 10 minutes, which is followed by an abrupt (usually < 5 second) recovery of flow to the initial level. These changes may lead to ST segment elevation and may reduce the vulnerable period threshold for VF.[94] Considerable evidence implicates aggregation and disaggregation of platelets in these phenomena.[93-95] Various antiplatelet drugs such as aspirin, sulfinpyrazone, and prostacyclin have been shown to prevent the cyclical changes in coronary blood flow and the concomitant electrophysiologic alterations.[94,95] Furthermore, Folts and coworkers[93,96] have been able to capture platelet plugs distal to the stenosis. It has been observed that infused catecholamines frequently induce the flow changes in unresponsive animals.[97] It was uncertain, however, whether spontaneous fluctuations in autonomic nervous system activity can alter the pattern of cyclic coronary blood flow (CBF) changes during partial stenosis.

To help resolve this issue, we performed a study in chloralose-anesthetized dogs in which the effects of bilateral vagotomy and stellectomy were examined during partial stenosis of the left circumflex coronary artery.[98] Vagotomy reduced the frequency of CBF oscillations but not the magnitude of the flow changes. Bilateral cervical stellectomy reduced both the frequency of CBF changes and their magnitude. In five dogs in which cyclical CBF changes were reduced or abolished by decentralizing the stellate ganglia, electrical stimulation of the main body of the left ganglion evoked or enhanced the oscillation in two dogs, had no distinct effect in two dogs, and elicited no response in one dog (Figs. 10 and 11). A 5-minute infusion of epinephrine provoked the CBF changes in all animals for a period of 5 to 10 minutes. Blockade of muscarinic receptors by atropine resulted in a significant attenuation of flow changes, which may at least in part have been due to a direct effect of atropine on platelets. The conclusion was that cardiac sympathetic tone significantly influences the CBF pattern during critical coronary stenosis.

Alterations in platelet function may also provide an important mechanism whereby behavioral stress predisposes to cardiac arrhythmias. Haft and Fani[99] demonstrated that stress induces intracoronary aggregation of platelets in rats following heat and electric shock stress. Pathologic examination of the hearts revealed partial or total occlusion of coronary vessels by platelet thrombi and fibrin deposits. Examination of the hearts of monkeys following shock

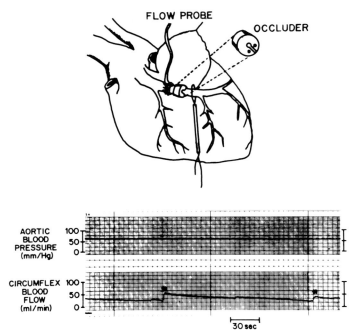

**Figure 10.** Schematic representation of the partial coronary occlusion model (upper panel). The cyclic changes in blood flow induced by aggregation and disaggregation of platelets are also depicted (lower panel). Note that blood pressure remains unchanged despite significant oscillations in coronary blood flow. (From Raeder, Verrier, and Lown,[98] with permission.)

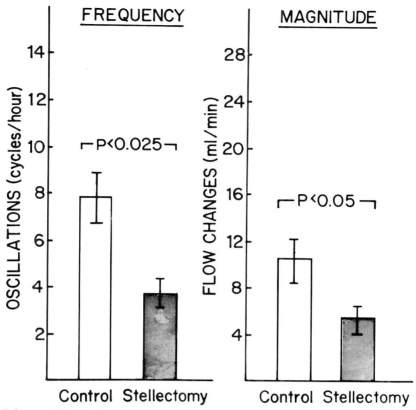

**Figure 11.** Influence of bilateral stellectomy on spontaneous oscillations in coronary blood flow during partial stenosis in nine dogs. (From Raeder, Verrier, and Lown,[98] with permission.)

avoidance stress by Corley and coworkers[100] revealed myofibrillar degeneration, myocytolysis, and fuchsinophilia. Similar cardiac pathology has resulted from electric shock, intense light and sound, and audiopresentation to rats of a rat-cat fight.[101]

## PSYCHOLOGIC FACTORS AND VF

An essential question is whether psychophysiologic stimuli can significantly affect cardiac vulnerability. More specifically, do behavioral stresses alter susceptibility to VF? To study this question, we examined the influence of mild aversive conditioning stimuli on ventricular vulnerability using the RE threshold method.[102] We compared the influence of two different environments on the vulnerable period threshold in conscious dogs. The first setting was a cage in which the animals were left undisturbed, whereas the second was a Pavlovian sling in which the animals received a mild transthoracic shock at the end of each conditioning session. The influence of the two environments was compared on days 4 and 5, at which time no shocks were administered. In the stressful environment, the dogs were restless, exhibited somatic tremor, and had elevated heart rate and arterial blood pressure. The RE threshold was reduced by 40 percent in the stressful environment. When acute left anterior descending coronary artery occlusion and release were carried out in the stressful setting, the incidence of VF was more than 3 times greater (14 percent versus 46 percent) than that observed in the nonstressful environment (Fig. 12).[103] Elevation of plasma catecholamine levels, particularly of epinephrine, closely correlates with the alteration in the vulnerable period threshold.[104]

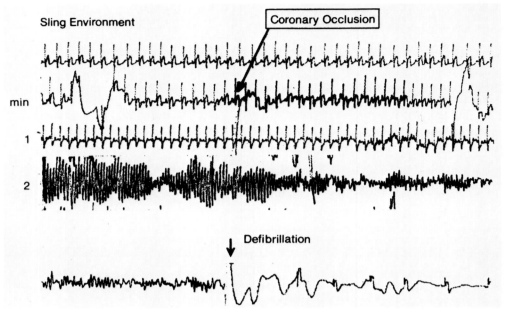

**Figure 12.** Coronary occlusion while the animal was in a sling environment resulted within 2 minutes in ventricular fibrillation. Note the instability of the baseline related to restlessness when the animal was merely standing quietly. When coronary occlusion was carried out while the animal was in the nonaversive cage environment, ventricular fibrillation did not occur. (From Verrier,[143] with permission.)

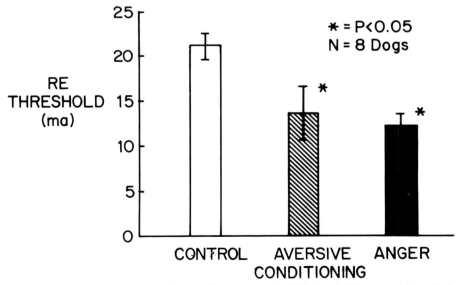

**Figure 13.** Effects of behavioral stress on the repetitive extrasystole (RE) threshold in normal dogs. Both passive aversive conditioning using a mild electric shock and induction of an anger-like state by food-access-denial produced significant reductions in the vulnerable-period threshold. Heart rate was maintained constant during cardiac electrical testing by ventricular pacing. (From Verrier and Lown,[86] with permission.)

The type of stress is not critical to the effects on vulnerability since diverse stresses[86] substantially lower the vulnerable period threshold (Fig. 13).[105] Moreover, beta-adrenergic blockade completely prevented stress-induced alterations in cardiac vulnerability, indicating that the decrease in threshold was mediated by the sympathetic limb of the autonomic nervous system.[103,105,106] Left or right stellectomy, however, did not prevent the reduction in vulnerable period threshold during psychologic stress, and only partial protection was conferred by bilateral stellectomy.[106] These results suggest that adrenergic inputs in addition to those derived from the stellate ganglia impinge upon the heart during stress to alter vulnerability. These inputs appear to derive mainly from the adrenal medulla.

## EFFECT OF VAGAL STIMULATION DURING STRESS

Vagal influences also appear to play a role in modulating vulnerability during psychologic stress. This view is based on the observations of DeSilva and colleagues[107] in our laboratory that enhancing cardiac vagal tone by administration of morphine to dogs in a stressful environment increases the vulnerable period threshold to the value observed in a nonstressful setting. When vagal efferent activity was blocked by atropine, a major portion of morphine's protective effect was abolished. Administration of morphine in the nonstressful setting, where cardiac adrenergic input was presumed to be low, failed to alter the vulnerable period threshold. These findings indicate that central activation of the vagi by morphine protects against vulnerability during stress and that this beneficial action is due to antagonism of the fibrillatory influence of enhanced adrenergic input to the heart.

## HUMAN STUDIES OF THE ROLE OF PSYCHOPHYSIOLOGIC FACTORS IN SUDDEN DEATH

Although it has been possible to design experiments in animals that demonstrate that stress is capable of significantly increasing vulnerability to VF, extrapolation of these results to the clinical problem of sudden death must be made with caution. Direct investigation of the human condition unfortunately has been extremely difficult for a number of ethical and conceptual reasons. Among the major considerations are the difficulty of replicating and quantifying behavioral stress in human subjects and the problems relating to the clinical endpoint. Notwithstanding these impediments, there is growing evidence suggesting a link between behavioral stress and the occurrence of fatal arrhythmias (Table 1).[108]

This significant progress has been the result of widespread community instruction in cardiopulmonary resuscitation and the introduction of DC defibrillation and cardioversion. Increasing numbers of patients experiencing sudden death are being successfully resuscitated and are contributing to our understanding of sudden death in man.[109] Over the past few years, 117 patients with recurring life-threatening ventricular arrhythmias were closely evaluated and followed by a "higher nervous activity" task force consisting of a psychiatrist, a psychologist, and members of the cardiovascular group.[110] Based on independent psychiatric assess-

**Table 1.** Prevalence of acute psychologic stress preceding sudden death[108]

| Investigators | Population sample | Time frame* | Total no. of cases | No. of cases with acute stress | Prevalence of acute stress |
|---|---|---|---|---|---|
| Myers and Dewar[121] | Postmortem | 30 min | 100 | 23 | 23% |
| | | 24 hr | 100 | 40 | 40% |
| Rissanen et al[122] | Portmortem | 2 hr | 118 | 23 | 19% |
| Reich et al[110] | Clinical | 24 hr | 117 | 25 | 21% |

*Refers to time period during which acute stresses occurred.

ment by members of the task force, 25 of the 117 patients (21 percent) were found to have had identifiable psychologic affective disorders immediately preceding the catastrophic arrhythmic event. In the majority of such patients (15 of the 25), the psychologic episode occurred within less than 1 hour before the onset of the malignant arrhythmia. The most common affective state was anger, which was observed in 17 of 25 (68 percent) of these individuals. These studies and others[53,111-115] thus point to a strong association between psychologic variables and the genesis of life-threatening ventricular arrhythmias.

## BETA-ADRENERGIC BLOCKADE AND VENTRICULAR ARRHYTHMIAS

The use of beta-adrenergic blocking agents also supports the foregoing view. Taggart and colleagues studied the effects of naturally occurring stressful situations on the incidence of cardiac arrhythmias in patients with ischemic heart disease.[116,117] In five of 24 subjects, multiple ventricular premature beats and ventricular tachycardia were precipitated while the subjects were driving in busy London traffic. The arrhythmias subsided when the drive ended. Among healthy race-drivers, no ventricular premature beats were noted despite markedly elevated catecholamine levels, which in the case of norepinephrine were found to be as much as 20 times above the levels observed following recovery from the race.[117] Public speaking also evoked frequent ventricular premature beats.[116] Beta-adrenergic blockade with a single 40-mg oral dose of oxprenolol prevented the cardiac rhythm abnormalities associated with the stress-related ventricular arrhythmias.[116]

Beta-adrenergic blockade has not, however, been invariably effective in suppressing stress-related ventricular arrhythmias in human subjects.[53] For example, Lown and associates have found that in certain patients sleep suppresses ventricular arrhythmias that are not controlled by propranolol therapy.[53] The basis for the superiority of sleep over beta-adrenergic blockade in reducing arrhythmias in these individuals is uncertain. Inasmuch as sleep results in major alterations in both cardiac sympathetic and vagal tone, a complex interplay of factors may be involved.

## BETA-BLOCKADE AND SUDDEN DEATH

To date, no direct information is available regarding the effectiveness of beta-blockade in preventing fatal arrhythmias during emotional stress. Some insights nevertheless can be derived from a natural biologic model of human sudden death, namely, the long Q–T syndrome.[115,118] Marked susceptibility to recurrent VF has been recorded in a series of syndromes characterized by an increased duration of cardiac repolarization and a prolonged Q–T interval. Schwartz and coworkers have suggested that the sympathetic nervous system is primarily involved in this clinical entity.[118] Their view is based on the following evidence: (1) syncopal attacks, which represent nonsustained episodes of VF, are triggered by exertion and intense

**Table 2.** Treatment and mortality in the long Q–T syndrome[118]

|  | Total | Outcome unknown | Deaths | Mortality |
|---|---|---|---|---|
| Asymptomatics | 196 | — | — | — |
| Treatment unknown | 93 | 83 | 10 | — |
| No treatment | 157 | 18 | 98 | 71% |
| Miscellaneous treatment | 50 | 5 | 13 | 35% |
| Beta-blockers | 216 | 2 | 12 | 6% |
| Left sympathectomy | 49 | — | 3 | 6% |
| Total LQ–TS patients | 754 |  |  |  |

emotions; (2) the T wave alterations that precede syncopal episodes can be reproduced by asymmetric stellate ganglion stimulation; and (3) in many patients, beta-adrenergic blockade or stellectomy is capable of reducing Q–T interval duration and preventing recurrent attacks[118] (Table 2).

## ALPHA-ADRENERGIC BLOCKADE AND VENTRICULAR ARRHYTHMIAS

There is a paucity of information regarding the influence of alpha-adrenergic blockade in the prevention of ventricular arrhythmias and sudden death in man. Most of the available data derive from the studies of Gould and coworkers, who found that oral phentolamine in small, well-tolerated doses abolished the premature ventricular beats associated with digitalis toxicity and chronic ischemic heart disease.[119] The drug also reduced the ventricular ectopic beat frequency in patients in the first 24 hours of acute myocardial infarction.[120] These studies involved a small number of patients and lacked appropriate control data, however, so the influence of alpha-adrenergic blockade in preventing malignant arrhythmias clearly merits more intensive investigation.

## FINAL COMMENTS

The aforementioned studies underscore the importance of neural factors in the genesis of cardiac arrhythmias. It is evident, moreover, that multiple intermediary mechanisms are involved. These include direct effects on myocardial excitable properties and indirect influences mediated through alterations in coronary vasomotor tone and platelet aggregability. The parasympathetic nervous system exerts its effect largely by opposing the action of the adrenergic inputs to the heart (Fig. 14).

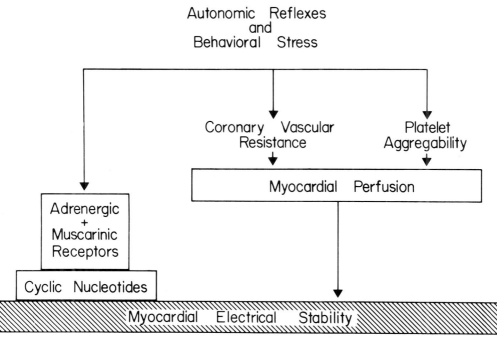

**Figure 14.** Summary of the mechanisms mediating the effects of the autonomic nervous system on ventricular electrical stability.

**Table 3.** Current approaches for containment of neural triggers for malignant ventricular arrhythmias[86]

---

CENTRAL
    Decreasing cardiac sympathetic tone
    —Neurochemical agents[123-127]
    —Dietary "precursor therapy"[127]
    Increasing vagal tone
    —Digitalis drugs[128]
    —Exercise conditioning[129,130]

PERIPHERAL
    —Adrenergic receptor blockade[126,131-134]
    —Stellectomy[118,130,135-137]
    —Calcium channel blockade[87,138-140]

---

These observations suggest that an important strategy for clinical management of malignant ventricular arrhythmias will require lessening cardiac sympathetic drive while enhancing vagal tone. We and others have initiated studies to determine whether neurochemical agents that induce such a pattern of autonomic neural outflow may thereby protect against ventricular arrhythmias[86] (Table 3). To date, the results have been most encouraging and provide support for the concept that containment of neurophysiologic triggers may provide a powerful therapeutic tool.

## ACKNOWLEDGMENTS

The authors express their appreciation to Sandra S. Verrier for her editorial assistance and to Marian Cordaro for typing the manuscript.

## REFERENCES

1. WEBB, SW, ADGEY, AAJ, AND PANTRIDGE, JF: *Autonomic disturbance at onset of acute myocardial infarction.* Br Med J 3:89, 1972.

2. PANTRIDGE, JF: *Autonomic disturbance at the onset of acute myocardial infarction.* In SCHWARTZ, PJ, BROWN, AM, MALLIANI, A, ET AL (EDS): *Neural Mechanisms in Cardiac Arrhythmias.* Raven Press, New York, 1978.

3. MALLIANI, A AND LOMBARDI, F: *Neural reflexes associated with myocardial ischemia.* In SCHWARTZ, PJ, BROWN, AM, MALLIANI, A, ET AL (EDS): *Neural Mechanisms in Cardiac Arrhythmias.* Raven Press, New York, 1978.

4. LOMBARDI, F, PATTON, CP, DELLA BELLA, P, ET AL: *Cardiovascular and sympathetic responses reflexly elicited through the excitation with bradykinin of sympathetic and vagal cardiac sensory endings in the cat.* Cardiovasc Res 16:57, 1982.

5. SCHWARTZ, PJ, PAGANI, M, LOMBARDI, F, ET AL: *A cardiocardiac sympathovagal reflex in the cat.* Circ Res 32:215, 1973.

6. BISHOP, VS, MALLIANI, A, AND THORÉN, P: *Cardiac mechanoreceptors.* In *Handbook of Physiology: The Cardiovascular System III.* The American Physiological Society, Bethesda, MD, 1980.

7. BEZOLD, A AND HIRT, L: *Über die physiologischen Wirkungen des essigsauren Veratrins.* Unters Physiol Lab Würzburg 1:75, 1867.

8. KRAYER, O: *The history of the Bezold-Jarisch effect.* Arch Exp Pathol Pharmakol 240:361, 1961.

9. CORR, PB, PEARLE, DL, HINTON, JR, ET AL: *Site of myocardial infarction: A determinant of the cardiovascular changes induced in the cat by coronary occlusion.* Circ Res 39:840, 1976.

10. LOMBARDI, F, VERRIER, RL, AND LOWN, B: *Relationship between sympathetic neural activity, coronary dynamics and vulnerability to ventricular fibrillation during myocardial ischemia and reperfusion.* Am Heart J 105:958, 1983.

11. MOHRMAN, DE AND FEIGL, EO: *Competition between sympathetic vasoconstriction and metabolic vasodilation in the canine coronary circulation.* Circ Res 42:79, 1978.

12. BUFFINGTON, CW AND FEIGL, EO: *Adrenergic coronary vasoconstriction in the presence of coronary stenosis in the dog.* Circ Res 48:416, 1981.

13. SCHWARTZ, PJ AND STONE, HL: *Tonic influence of the sympathetic nervous system on myocardial reactive hyperemia and on coronary blood flow distribution in dogs.* Circ Res 41:51, 1977.

14. SHEEHAN, FH AND EPSTEIN, SE: *Determinants of arrhythmic death due to coronary spasm: Effect of preexisting coronary artery stenosis on the incidence of reperfusion arrhythmia.* Circulation 65:259, 1982.

15. CORBALAN, R, VERRIER, RL, AND LOWN, B: *Differing mechanisms for ventricular vulnerability during coronary artery occlusion and release.* Am Heart J 92:223, 1976.

16. KHAN, MI, HAMILTON, JT, AND MANNING, GW: *Protective effect of beta adrenoceptor blockade in experimental coronary occlusion in conscious dogs.* Am J Cardiol 30:832, 1972.

17. FITZGERALD, JD: *The role of beta-adrenergic blockade in acute myocardial ischaemia.* In OLIVER, MF, JULIAN, DG, AND DONALD, KW (EDS): *Effects of Acute Ischaemia on Myocardial Function.* Williams & Wilkins, Baltimore, 1972.

18. HAI, HA, TEMTE, JV, AND LOWN, B: *Changes in ventricular fibrillation threshold during coronary artery occlusion and release induced by beta-adrenergic blockade.* Am J Cardiol 37:140, 1976.

19. BRODSKY, MA, VERRIER, RL, AND LOWN, B: *Effects of beta blockade with and without coronary dilators on vulnerability to ventricular fibrillation during coronary occlusion and reperfusion.* Circulation 66:II-33, 1982.

20. PEARLE, DL, WILLIFORD, D, AND GILLIS, RA: *Superiority of practolol versus propranolol in protection against ventricular fibrillation induced by coronary occlusion.* Am J Cardiol 42:960, 1978.

21. YASUE, H: *Beta-adrenergic blockade and coronary arterial spasm.* In SANDØE, E, JULIAN, DG, AND BELL, JW (EDS): *Management of Ventricular Tachycardia—Role of Mexiletine.* Excerpta Medica, Amsterdam, 1978.

22. OLIVA, PB AND BRECKINRIDGE, JC: *Arteriographic evidence of coronary arterial spasm in acute myocardial infarction.* Circulation 56:366, 1977.

23. MASERI, A, L'ABBATE, A, BAROLDI, G, ET AL: *Coronary vasospasm as a possible cause of myocardial infarction: A conclusion derived from the study of "preinfarction" angina.* N Engl J Med 299:1271, 1978.

24. BRAUNWALD, E: *Coronary spasm and acute myocardial infarction—new possibility for treatment and prevention.* N Engl J Med 299:1301, 1978.

25. MUDGE, GH, JR, GOLDBERG, S, GUNTHER, S, ET AL: *Comparison of metabolic and vasoconstrictor stimuli on coronary vascular resistance in man.* Circulation 59:544, 1979.

26. SHERIDAN, DJ, PENKOSKE, PA, SOBEL, BE, ET AL: *Alpha adrenergic contributions to dysrhythmia during myocardial ischemia and reperfusion in cats.* J Clin Invest 65:161, 1980.

27. STEWART, JR, BURMEISTER, WE, BURMEISTER, J, ET AL: *Electrophysiologic and antiarrhythmic effects of phentolamine in experimental coronary artery occlusion and reperfusion in the dog.* J Cardiovasc Pharmacol 2:77, 1980.

28. VERRIER, RL, CALVERT, A, LOWN, B, ET AL: *Effect of acute blood pressure elevation on the ventricular fibrillation threshold.* Am J Physiol 226:893, 1974.

29. KOWEY, PR, VERRIER, RL, AND LOWN, B: *Effect of alpha-adrenergic receptor stimulation on ventricular electrical properties in the normal canine heart.* Physiologist 23:160, 1980.

30. MAJID, PA, SAXTON, C, DYKES, JRW, ET AL: *Autonomic control of insulin secretion and the treatment of heart failure.* Br Med J 4:328, 1970.

31. OBEID, AI, VERRIER, RL, AND LOWN, B: *Influence of glucose, insulin, and potassium on vulnerability to ventricular fibrillation in the canine heart.* Circ Res 43:601, 1978.

32. PFISTER, B AND IMHOF, PR: *Inhibition of adrenaline-induced platelet aggregation by the orally administered alpha-adrenergic receptor blocker phentolamine (Regitine®).* Eur J Clin Pharmacol 11:7, 1977.

33. OPIE, LH, MULLER, CA, AND LUBBE, WF: *Cyclic AMP and arrhythmias revisited.* Lancet 2:921, 1978.

34. OPIE, LH: *Basis for cardiovascular therapy with beta-blocking agents.* Am J Cardiol 52:2D, 1983.

35. CORR, PB, PENKOSKE, PA, AND SOBEL, BE: *Adrenergic influences on arrhythmias due to coronary occlusion and reperfusion.* Br Heart J 40:62, 1978.

36. WATANABE, AM, LINDEMANN, JP, JONES, LR, ET AL: *Biochemical mechanisms mediating neural control of the heart.* In ABBOUD, FM, FOZZARD, HA, GILMORE, JP, ET AL (EDS): *Disturbances in Neurogenic Control of the Circulation.* American Physiological Society, Bethesda, MD, 1981.

37. LUBBE, WF, PODZUWEIT, T, DARIES, PS, ET AL: *The role of cyclic adenosine monophosphate in adrenergic effects on ventricular vulnerability to fibrillation in the isolated perfused rat heart.* J Clin Invest 61:1260, 1978.

38. KENT, KM, SMITH, ER, REDWOOD, DR, ET AL: *Beneficial electrophysiologic effects of nitroglycerin during acute myocardial infarction.* Am J Cardiol 33:513, 1974.

39. LEVY, MN: *Sympathetic-parasympathetic interactions in the heart.* Circ Res 29:437, 1971.

40. MARTINS, JB AND ZIPES, DP: *Epicardial phenol interrupts refractory period responses to sympathetic but not vagal stimulation in canine left ventricular epicardium and endocardium.* Circ Res 47:33, 1980.

41. PRYSTOWSKY, EN, JACKMAN, WM, RINKENBERGER, RL, ET AL: *Effect of autonomic blockade on ventricular refractoriness and atrioventricular nodal conduction in humans: Evidence supporting a direct cholinergic action on ventricular muscle refractoriness.* Circ Res 49:511, 1981.

42. LOWN, B AND VERRIER, RL: *Neural activity and ventricular fibrillation.* N Engl J Med 294:1165, 1976.

43. MATTA, RJ, VERRIER, RL, AND LOWN, B: *Repetitive extrasystole as an index of vulnerability to ventricular fibrillation.* Am J Physiol 230:1469, 1976.

44. RABINOWITZ, SH, VERRIER, RL, AND LOWN, B: *Muscarinic effects of vagosympathetic trunk stimulation on the repetitive extrasystole (RE) threshold.* Circulation 53:622, 1976.

45. KOLMAN, BS, VERRIER, RL, AND LOWN, B: *The effect of vagus nerve stimulation upon vulnerability of the canine ventricle: Role of sympathetic-parasympathetic interactions.* Circulation 52:578, 1975.

46. LEVY, MN AND BLATTBERG, B: *Effect of vagal stimulation on the overflow of norepinephrine into the coronary sinus during cardiac sympathetic nerve stimulation in the dog.* Circ Res 38:81, 1976.

47. WATANABE, AM AND BESCH, HR, JR: *Interaction between cyclic adenosine monophosphate and cyclic guanosine monophosphate in guinea pig ventricular myocardium.* Circ Res 37:309, 1975.

48. TSE, WW, HAN, J, AND YOON, MS: *Effect of acetylcholine on automaticity of canine Purkinje fibers.* Am J Physiol 230:116, 1976.

49. VASSALLE, M: *Cardiac automaticity and its control.* Am J Physiol 233:H625, 1977.

50. WEISS, T, LATTIN, GM, AND ENGELMAN, K: *Vagally mediated suppression of premature ventricular contractions in man.* Am Heart J 89:700, 1975.

51. WAXMAN, MB AND WALD, RW: *Termination of ventricular tachycardia by an increase in cardiac vagal drive.* Circulation 56:385, 1977.

52. WEISS, T, MANCIA, G, DELBO, A, ET AL: *The role of heart rate in the phenylephrine-induced suppression of premature ventricular beats.* Eur J Clin Invest 9:39, 1979.

53. LOWN, B, TYKOCINSKI, M, GARFEIN, A, ET AL: *Sleep and ventricular premature beats.* Circulation 48:691, 1973.

54. BAUST, W AND BOHNERT, B: *The regulation of heart rate during sleep.* Exp Brain Res 7:169, 1969.

55. KENT, KM, EPSTEIN, SE, COOPER, T, ET AL: *Cholinergic innervation of the canine and human ventricular conducting system: Anatomic and electrophysiologic correlation.* Circulation 50:948, 1974.

56. KENT, KM, SMITH, ER, REDWOOD, DR, ET AL: *Electrical stability of acutely ischemic myocardium: Influences of heart rate and vagal stimulation.* Circulation 47:291, 1973.

57. CORR, PB AND GILLIS, RA: *Role of the vagus nerves in the cardiovascular changes induced by coronary occlusion.* Circulation 49:86, 1974.

58. CORR, PB, PEARLE, DL, AND GILLIS, RA: *Coronary occlusion site as a determinant of the cardiac rhythm effects of atropine and vagotomy.* Am Heart J 92:741, 1976.

59. YOON, MS, HAN, J, TSE, WW, ET AL: *Effects of vagal stimulation, atropine, and propranolol on fibrillation threshold of normal and ischemic ventricles.* Am Heart J 93:60, 1977.

60. JAMES, RGG, ARNOLD, JMO, ALLEN, JD, ET AL: *The effects of heart rate, myocardial ischemia and vagal stimulation on the threshold for ventricular fibrillation.* Circulation 55:311, 1977.

61. VERRIER, RL, BROOKS, WW, AND LOWN, B: *Effect of cholinergic stimulation on vulnerability to ventricular fibrillation during myocardial ischemia and reperfusion.* Am J Cardiol 41:366, 1978.

62. VERRIER, RL AND LOWN B: *Sympathetic-parasympathetic interactions and ventricular electrical stability.* In SCHWARTZ, PJ, BROWN, AM, MALLIANI, A ET AL (EDS): *Neural Mechanisms in Cardiac Arrhythmias.* Raven Press, New York, 1978.

63. KERZNER, J, WOLF, M, KOSOWSKY, BD, ET AL: *Ventricular ectopic rhythms following vagal stimulation in dogs with acute myocardial infarction.* Circulation 47:44, 1973.

64. EL-SHERIF, N: *Reentrant ventricular arrhythmias in the late myocardial infarction period: 6. Effect of the autonomic system.* Circulation 58:103, 1978.

65. PANTRIDGE, JF, ADGEY, AAJ, GEDDES, JS, ET AL: *The Acute Coronary Attack.* Grune & Stratton, New York, 1975.

66. BIORCK, G AND ERHARDT, LF: *The earliest phase of acute myocardial infarction in man.* Acta Med Scand 193:251, 1973.

67. OLIVA, PB, POTTS, DE, AND PLUSS, RG: *Coronary arterial spasm in Prinzmetal angina: Documentation by coronary arteriography.* N Engl J Med 288:745, 1973.

68. CHIERCHIA, S, BRUNELLI, C, SIMONETTI, I, ET AL: *Sequence of events in angina at rest: Primary reduction in coronary flow.* Circulation 61:759, 1980.

69. HILLIS, LD AND BRAUNWALD, E: *Coronary-artery spasm.* N Engl J Med 299:695, 1978.

70. DEANFELD, JE, MASERI, A, SELWYN, AP, ET AL: *Myocardial ischaemia during daily life in patients with stable angina: Its relation to symptoms and heart rate changes.* Lancet 2:753, 1983.

71. MASERI, A, L'ABBATE, A, CHIERCHIA, S, ET AL: *Significance of spasm in the pathogenesis of ischemic heart disease.* Am J Cardiol 44:788, 1979.

72. MASERI, A, SEVERI, S, DENES, M, ET AL: *"Variant" angina: One aspect of a continuous spectrum of vaso-spastic myocardial ischemia. Pathogenetic mechanisms, estimated incidence and clinical and coronary arteriographic findings in 138 patients.* Am J Cardiol 42:1019, 1978.

73. LUCHI, RJ, CHAHINE, RA, AND RAIZNER, AE: *Coronary artery spasm.* Ann Intern Med 91:441, 1979.

74. MUDGE, GH, JR, GROSSMAN, W, MILLS, RM, JR, ET AL: *Reflex increase in coronary vascular resistance in patients with ischemic heart disease.* N Engl J Med 295:1333, 1976.

75. RICCI, DR, ORLICK, AE, CIPRIANO, PR, ET AL: *Altered adrenergic activity in coronary arterial spasm: Insight into mechanism based on study of coronary hemodynamics and the electrocardiogram.* Am J Cardiol 43:1073, 1979.

76. KERN, MJ, GANZ, P, HOROWITZ, JD, ET AL: *Potentiation of coronary vasoconstriction by beta-adrenergic blockade in patients with coronary artery disease.* Circulation 67:1178, 1983.

77. RAIZNER, AE, CHAHINE, RA, ISHIMORI, T, ET AL: *Provocation of coronary artery spasm by the cold pressor test: Hemodynamic, arteriographic and quantitative angiographic observations.* Circulation 62:925, 1980.

78. YASUE, H, OMOTE, S, TAKIZAWA, A, ET AL: *Exertional angina pectoris caused by coronary arterial spasm: Effects of various drugs.* Am J Cardiol 43:647, 1979.

79. LOWN, B: *Verbal conditioning of angina pectoris during exercise testing.* Am J Cardiol 40:630, 1977.

80. FEIGL, EO: *Coronary physiology.* Physiol Rev 63:1, 1983.

81. MARK, AL, ABBOUD, FM, SCHMID, PG, ET AL: *Differences in direct effects of adrenergic stimuli on coronary, cutaneous, and muscular vessels.* J Clin Invest 51:279, 1972.

82. PITT, B, ELLIOTT, EC, AND GREGG, DE: *Adrenergic receptor activity in the coronary arteries of the unanesthetized dog.* Circ Res 21:75, 1967.

83. ORLICK, AE, RICCI, DR, ALDERMAN, EL, ET AL: *Effects of alpha adrenergic blockade upon coronary hemodynamics.* J Clin Invest 62:459, 1978.

84. VATNER, SF, HIGGINS, CB, AND BRAUNWALD, E: *Effects of norepinephrine on coronary circulation and left ventricular dynamics in the conscious dog.* Circ Res 34:812, 1974.

85. ROSS, G: *Adrenergic responses of the coronary vessels.* Circ Res 39:461, 1976.

86. VERRIER, RL AND LOWN, B: *Behavioral stress and cardiac arrhythmias.* Annu Rev Physiol 46:155, 1984.

87. VERRIER, RL, RAEDER, E, AND LOWN, B: *Use of calcium channel blockers after myocardial infarction: Potential cardioprotective mechanisms.* In KULBERTUS, HE AND WELLENS, HJJ: *The First Year After a Myocardial Infarction.* Futura, Mount Kisco, NY, 1983.

88. VERRIER, RL, HAGESTAD, EL, AND LOWN, B: *Behaviorally induced coronary vasoconstriction in dogs with critical coronary artery stenosis.* Fed Proc 43:1003, 1984.

89. HAFT, JI, GERSHENGORN, K, KRANZ, PD, ET AL: *Protection against epinephrine-induced myocardial necrosis by drugs that inhibit platelet aggregation.* Am J Cardiol 30:838, 1972.

90. SCHWARTZ, C AND GERRITY, R: *Anatomical pathology of sudden unexpected cardiac death.* Circulation 52:III-18, 1975.

91. JORGENSEN, L, HAEREM, J, AND CHANDLER, A: *The pathology of acute coronary death.* Acta Anesthesiol Scand (Suppl) 29:193, 1968.

92. HAEREM, J: *Platelet aggregates and mural microthrombi in early stages of acute, fatal coronary disease.* Thromb Res 5:243, 1974.

93. FOLTS, JD, CROWELL, EB, AND ROWE, GG: *Platelet aggregation in partially obstructed vessels and its elimination with aspirin.* Circulation 54:365,1976.

94. KOWEY, PR, VERRIER, RL, LOWN, B, ET AL: *The effects of nitroglycerin on intracoronary platelet aggregation and ventricular vulnerability during partial coronary stenosis.* Am J Cardiol 47:489, 1981.

95. FOLTS, JD AND ROWE, GG: *Letter.* Circulation 56:333, 1977.

96. FOLTS, JD, GALLAGHER, K, AND ROWE, GG: *Blood flow reductions in stenosed canine coronary arteries: Vasospasm or platelet aggregation?* Circulation 65:248, 1982.

97. FOLTS, JD AND ROWE, GG: *Platelet aggregation in stenosed coronary arteries: Mechanism of sudden death?* Am J Cardiol 41:425, 1978.

98. RAEDER, EA, VERRIER, RL, AND LOWN, B: *Influence of the autonomic nervous system on coronary blood flow during partial stenosis.* Am Heart J 104:249, 1982.

99. HAFT, JI AND FANI, K: *Intravascular platelet aggregation in the heart induced by stress.* Circulation 47:353, 1973.

100. CORLEY, KC, SHIEL, FO, MAUCK, HP, ET AL: *Myocardial degeneration and cardiac arrest in squirrel monkey: Physiological and psychological correlates.* Psychophysiology 14:322, 1977.

101. RAAB, W: *Emotional and sensory stress factors in myocardial pathology.* Am Heart J 72:538, 1966.

102. LOWN, B, VERRIER, RL, AND CORBALAN, R: *Psychologic stress and threshold for repetitive ventricular response.* Science 182:834, 1973.

103. VERRIER, RL AND LOWN, B: *Influence of neural activity on ventricular electrical stability during acute myocardial ischemia and infarction.* In SANDØE, E, JULIAN, DG, AND BELL, JW (EDS): *Management of Ventricular Tachycardia: Role of Mexiletine.* Excerpta Medica (International Congress Series #458), Amsterdam, 1978.

104. LIANG, B, VERRIER, RL, MELMAN, J, ET AL: *Correlation between circulating catecholamine levels and ventricular vulnerability during psychological stress in conscious dogs.* Proc Soc Exp Biol Med 161:266, 1979.

105. MATTA, RJ, LAWLER, JE, AND LOWN, B: *Ventricular electrical instability in the conscious dog: Effects of psychologic stress and beta adrenergic blockade.* Am J Cardiol 38:594, 1976.

106. VERRIER, RL AND LOWN, B: *Effects of left stellectomy on enhanced cardiac vulnerability induced by psychologic stress.* Circulation 55,56:III-80, 1977.

107. DeSILVA, RA, VERRIER, RL, AND LOWN, B: *The effects of psychological stress and vagal stimulation with morphine on vulnerability to ventricular fibrillation (VF) in the conscious dog.* Am Heart J 95:197, 1978.

108. DeSILVA, RA: *Central nervous system risk factors for sudden cardiac death.* Ann NY Acad Sci 382:143, 1982.

109. SCHAFFER, WA AND COBB, LA: *Recurrent ventricular fibrillation and modes of death in survivors of out-of-hospital ventricular fibrillation.* N Engl J Med 293:259, 1975.

110. REICH, P, DeSILVA, RA, LOWN, B, ET AL: *Acute psychological disturbances preceding life-threatening ventricular arrhythmias.* JAMA 246:233, 1981.

111. ENGEL, GL: *Sudden and rapid death during psychological stress: Folklore or folk wisdom?* Ann Intern Med 74:771, 1971.

112. LOWN, B AND DeSILVA, RA: *Roles of psychologic stress and autonomic nervous system changes in provocation of ventricular premature complexes.* Am J Cardiol 41:979, 1978.

113. SCHWARTZ, PJ, BROWN, AM, MALLIANI, A, ET AL: *Neural Mechanisms in Cardiac Arrhythmias.* Raven Press, New York, 1978.

114. WOLF, S: *Psychosocial forces in myocardial infarction and sudden death.* Circulation 39,40:IV-74, 1969.

115. MOSS, AJ AND SCHWARTZ, PJ: *Sudden death and the idiopathic long Q–T syndrome.* Am J Med 66:6, 1979.

116. TAGGART, P, CARRUTHERS, M, AND SOMERVILLE, W: *Electrocardiogram, plasma catecholamines and lipids, and their modification by oxprenolol when speaking before an audience.* Lancet 2:341, 1973.

117. TAGGART, P, GIBBONS, D, AND SOMERVILLE, W: *Some effects of motor-car driving on the normal and abnormal heart.* Br Med J 4:130, 1969.

118. SCHWARTZ, PJ: *Prevention of the arrhythmias in the long QT syndrome.* In KULBERTUS, HE (ED): *Medical Management of Cardiac Arrhythmias.* Churchill Livingstone, Edinburgh (in press).

119. GOULD, L, GOMPRECHT, RF, AND ZAHIR, M: *Oral phentolamine for treatment of ventricular premature contractions.* Br Heart J 33:101, 1971.

120. GOULD, L, REDDY, CVR, WEINSTEIN, T, ET AL: *Antiarrhythmic prophylaxis with phentolamine in acute myocardial infarction.* J Clin Pharmacol 15:191, 1975.

121. MYERS, A AND DEWAR, HA: *Circumstances attending 100 sudden deaths from coronary artery disease with coroners' necropsies.* Br Heart J 37:1133, 1975.

122. RISSANEN, V, ROMO, M, AND SILTANEN, P: *Premonitory symptoms and stress factors preceding sudden death from ischaemic heart disease.* Acta Med Scand 204:389, 1978.

123. FALK, RH, DeSILVA, RA, AND LOWN, B: *Reduction in vulnerability to ventricular fibrillation by bromocriptine, a dopamine agonist.* Cardiovasc Res 15:175, 1981.

124. GILLIS, RA: *Neurotransmitters involved in the central nervous system control of cardiovascular function.* In SMITH, OA, GALOSY, RA, AND WEISS, SM (EDS): *Circulation, Neurobiology, and Behavior.* Elsevier Science, New York, 1982.

125. RABINOWITZ, SH AND LOWN, B: *Central neurochemical factors related to serotonin metabolism and cardiac ventricular vulnerability for repetitive electrical activity.* Am J Cardiol 41:516, 1978.

126. SKINNER, JE AND VERRIER, RL: *Task force report on sudden cardiac death and arrhythmias.* In SMITH, OA, GALOSY, RA, AND WEISS, SM (EDS): *Circulation, Neurobiology, and Behavior.* Elsevier Science, New York, 1982.

127. WURTMAN, RJ AND FERNSTROM, JD: *Control of brain monoamine synthesis by diet and plasma amino acids.* Am J Clin Nutr 28:638, 1975.

128. BROOKS, WW, VERRIER, RL, AND LOWN, B: *Digitalis drugs and vulnerability to ventricular fibrillation.* Eur J Pharmacol 57:69, 1979.

129. BILLMAN, GE, SCHWARTZ, PJ, AND STONE, HL: *The effects of daily exercise on susceptibility to sudden cardiac death: Protection from ventricular fibrillation.* Fed Proc 42:586, 1983.

130. STONE, HL, BILLMAN, GE, AND SCHWARTZ, PJ: *Exercise and sudden death.* In KULBERTUS, HE AND WELLENS, HJJ (EDS): *The First Year after a Myocardial Infarction.* Futura, New York, 1983.

131. BETA-BLOCKER HEART ATTACK STUDY GROUP: *The beta-blocker heart attack trial.* JAMA 246:2073, 1981.

132. CORR, PB AND SHARMA, AD: *Alpha- versus beta-adrenergic influences on dysrhythmias induced by myocardial ischaemia and reperfusion.* In ZANCHETTI, A (ED): *Advances in Beta-blocker Therapy II.* Excerpta Medica, Amsterdam, 1982.

133. HJALMARSON, Å, ELMFELDT, D, HERLITZ, J, ET AL: *Effect on mortality of metoprolol in acute myocardial infarction.* Lancet 2:823, 1981.

134. NORWEGIAN MULTICENTER STUDY GROUP: *The timolol-induced reduction in mortality and reinfarction in patients surviving acute myocardial infarction.* N Engl J Med 304:801, 1981.

135. SCHWARTZ, PJ: *Unilateral stellectomy and dysrhythmias.* Circ Res 43:939, 1978.

136. SCHWARTZ, PJ, SNEBOLD, NG, AND BROWN, AM: *Effects of unilateral cardiac sympathetic denervation on the ventricular fibrillation threshold.* Am J Cardiol 37:1034, 1976.

137. SCHWARTZ, PJ, STONE, HL, AND BROWN, AM: *Effects of unilateral stellate ganglion blockade on the arrhythmias associated with coronary occlusion.* Am Heart J 92:589, 1976.

138. STONE, PH AND ANTMAN, EM: *Calcium Channel Blocking Agents in the Treatment of Cardiovascular Disorders.* Futura, New York, 1983.

139. STONE, PH, ANTMAN, EM, MULLER, JE, ET AL: *Calcium channel blocking agents in the treatment of cardiovascular disorders. Part 2: Hemodynamic effects and clinical applications.* Ann Intern Med 93:886, 1980.

140. ZIPES, DP AND GILMOUR, RJ, JR: *Calcium antagonists and their potential role in the prevention of sudden coronary death.* Ann NY Acad Sci 382:258, 1982.

141. VERRIER, RL AND LOWN, B: *Vagal tone and ventricular vulnerability during psychological stress.* Circulation 62:III-176, 1980.

142. BERNE, RM AND LEVY, MN: *Cardiovascular Physiology.* CV Mosby, St Louis, 1981.

143. VERRIER, RL, LOMBARDI, F, AND LOWN, B: *Neural factors and ventricular electrical instability.* In KULBERTUS, HE AND WELLENS, HJJ (EDS): *Sudden Death.* Martinus Nijhoff, The Hague, 1980.

# Platelets and Prostaglandins in Sudden Death: Therapeutic Implications

*John S. Gelman, M.B., F.R.A.C.P., and*
*Jawahar Mehta, M.D.*

Sudden death is responsible for 15 to 20 percent of all natural fatalities in the industrially developed world. During the past decade, much has been learned about the epidemiology, pathology, and electrophysiology of sudden cardiac death.

Coronary angiography in successfully resuscitated patients and autopsy findings confirm extensive coronary atherosclerosis as the most frequent underlying pathology; it is present in about 75 percent of victims. However, in only a minority of cases can acute myocardial infarction be incriminated as the precipitating factor. Based on experience in patients resuscitated from ventricular fibrillation, new Q waves indicative of myocardial infarction develop in only 19 percent and lactic dehydrogenase elevation characteristic of myocardial infarction in 38 percent of patients.[1] It is generally accepted that most sudden deaths are due to ventricular fibrillation and that this arrhythmia reflects a state of electrical instability. Electrophysiologic studies have contributed significantly to the identification and treatment of patients at risk of sudden death. However, little is known regarding the immediate events triggering the electrical instability.

Studies in experimental animals and in man have directed attention to the role of platelets and prostaglandins in transient myocardial ischemia and electrical instability.

## THEORETICAL CONSIDERATIONS

Ventricular fibrillation may occur during myocardial ischemia and during early or late phases of myocardial infarction. It is now believed that acute spontaneous reduction in coronary blood flow may be due to dynamic factors, namely, platelet thrombosis and coronary vasospasm. Restoration of blood flow may also precipitate ventricular fibrillation. This reperfusion arrhythmia may follow lysis of platelet thrombus occluding the coronary artery or release of coronary artery spasm. These mechanisms may be operative in sudden death victims with or without coronary atherosclerosis.

There are two major mechanisms by which platelets may produce myocardial injury and electrical instability (Fig. 1). First, physical obstruction of the coronary lumen may result from *thrombosis* of large epicardial coronary arteries or of the small intramyocardial branches. Occlusive thrombus in a major epicardial artery may lead to myocardial infarction. The degree of myocardial ischemia resulting from partial obstruction would depend on the severity of the obstruction and the collateral blood supply to the ischemic region. The severity of the obstruction would clearly be aggravated by underlying coronary atherosclerosis as well as associated vasospasm. Platelet aggregates in the coronary microcirculation could be derived from the proximal coronary artery thrombus (embolism) or from circulating platelet

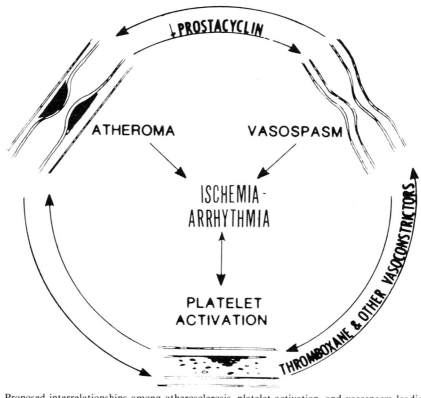

**Figure 1.** Proposed interrelationships among atherosclerosis, platelet activation, and vasospasm leading to myocardial ischemia and electrical instability. Alterations in prostacyclin and thromboxane may play key mediating role. (From Mehta, J: *Platelets and prostaglandins in coronary artery disease: Rationale for use of platelet-suppressive drugs.* JAMA 249:2818, 1983, with permission.)

aggregates, or could be formed in situ owing to local vascular injury and release of platelet-aggregating substances. Second, platelets may increase *humoral factors* that are capable of altering coronary vascular tone or causing tissue injury directly. Thromboxane $A_2$, serotonin, and epinephrine from activated platelets could cause coronary vasoconstriction with secondary myocardial ischemia. Myocardial injury and alteration of transmembrane ionic potentials could follow release of lysosomal enzymes and cationic proteins.

Following a review of platelet structure and physiology, we will consider the contribution of platelets and prostaglandins to thrombosis and atherogenesis. Their role in ischemia, myocardial infarction, vasospasm and reperfusion arrhythmias with special reference to sudden cardiac death will then be discussed.

## PLATELET STRUCTURE AND FUNCTION

Platelets are small, non-nucleated disks formed in the bone marrow from megakaryocytes. They are released into the circulation, have a life span of 7 to 10 days, and are then removed by the reticuloendothelial system.

Ultrastructural studies reveal three zones, each with a distinct function. (1) A peripheral zone comprises an exterior coat of acid mucopolysaccharides (glycocalyx), the trilaminar unit membrane, and a submembranous area. This zone is mainly concerned with platelet adhesion.

The outer coat provides a framework for attachment of factors V, VIII, and XI. The membrane possesses specific receptors for epinephrine, adenosine diphosphate (ADP), thrombin, collagen, fibrinogen, platelet-activating factor, and probably thromboxane $A_2$ and prostacyclin. In addition, membrane phospholipids release arachidonic acid, the substrate for prostaglandin synthesis. Numerous invaginations of the membrane provide a surface-connected canalicular system for extrusion of platelet contents and uptake of plasma substances. In the submembranous area, encircling microtubules form a cytoskeleton that maintains the shape of the platelet. (2) A cytoplasmic zone and submembranous area contain the contractile protein thromboesthenin, which is involved in platelet contraction. (3) The organelle zone includes alpha granules, dense bodies, and mitochondria. The alpha granules contain platelet-derived growth factor, coagulant proteins, fibrinogen, factors V and VIII, platelet factor 4, beta-thromboglobulin, and lysosomal enzymes. Dense bodies contain ADP, adenosine triphosphate (ATP), serotonin, calcium, and epinephrine.

## HEMOSTASIS AND THROMBOSIS

The major physiologic role of platelets is hemostasis. Arterial thrombosis may be considered an inappropriate or uncontrolled form of hemostatic process.

Vascular injury results in exposure of subendothelial structures to circulating platelets. Collagen is a potent stimulus for the attachment of circulating platelets. This process of *adhesion* is regulated by several factors; von Willebrand factor and its receptor glycoprotein on the platelet surface are necessary for adhesion of platelets to the subendothelial structures.[2] Hereditary absence of either of these produces abnormal platelet adhesion and a serious bleeding disorder.[3] Blood flow characteristics, in particular shear rates and hematocrit, also influence the rate and degree of attachment of circulating platelets to the injured blood vessel.

During adhesion to the damaged vascular wall, platelets secrete their granular contents. This process, *release reaction,* may be induced by the interaction of subendothelial collagen, ADP, epinephrine, and thrombin with specific platelet membrane receptors. Mobilization of calcium from the cell membrane to the cytoplasm appears to be important for both platelet release and aggregation. Phosphorylation of platelet myosin by calcium-activated kinases promotes platelet contraction and leads to release of platelet granules. Elevated cytoplasmic calcium results in platelet "stickiness" and hence *aggregation,* where unbound platelets attach to the adherent platelets with enlargement of the hemostatic plug.

There are three major mechanisms of platelet aggregation. The first involves extracellular release of ADP from the dense granules. Injured red cells or endothelial cells may also be a source of free ADP. ADP bound to its specific membrane receptor promotes aggregation by stimulating fibrinogen bridges between platelets, decrease in cyclic AMP, and synthesis of thromboxane $A_2$.[4] The second mechanism involves synthesis of thromboxane $A_2$ ($TXA_2$). ADP, collagen, and calcium can activate phospholipases that catalyze the release of arachidonic acid from platelet membrane phospholipid. Arachidonic acid is subsequently converted to $TXA_2$ by thromboxane synthetase. $TXA_2$ is the most potent platelet-aggregating agent yet described; it causes an active transport of calcium from platelet membranes to the cytoplasm and reduction in platelet cyclic adenosine monophosphate (AMP). The proaggregatory effects of ADP, epinephrine, collagen, and low-dose thrombin are mediated in part by conversion of arachidonic acid to $TXA_2$. Other mechanisms, such as high-dose thrombin- and platelet-activating factor–induced aggregation, are independent of ADP or $TXA_2$.

Platelets are intimately involved with the *coagulation* system. Activated platelet membrane (platelet factor 3) accelerates the formation of activated factor X. Specific platelet membrane receptors for coagulation factors V and Xa allow rapid interaction with prothrombin to form thrombin at sites of platelet aggregation. Direct activation of coagulation factors XI and X by platelets in vitro has been described.[5] Thrombin converts fibrinogen to fibrin, which stabilizes and strengthens the platelet thrombus.

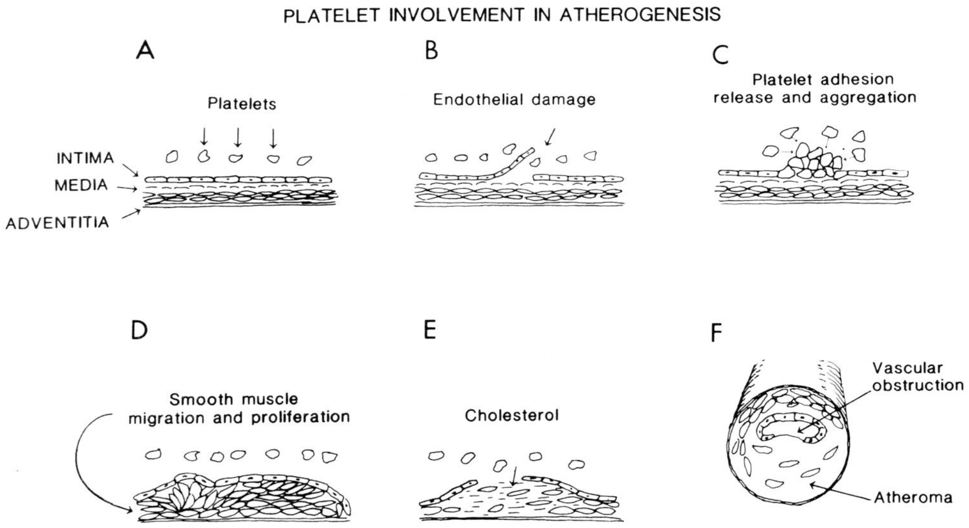

PLATELET INVOLVEMENT IN ATHEROGENESIS

**Figure 2.** Platelet involvement in atherogenesis. See text for explanation.

## ATHEROSCLEROSIS

Traditionally, there have been two major theories for the pathogenesis of atherosclerosis. The "incrustation" theory proposes that a white thrombus is deposited in the area of damaged intima.[6,7] Organization of the thrombus by smooth muscle cells and fibroblasts, together with lipid accumulation, leads to intimal thickening. The "insudation" or "imbibition" theory involves the filtration of blood lipids from the arterial lumen into the intima.[8]

During the last several years, an important role of platelets in atherogenesis has been recognized. Current concept holds that following endothelial injury, platelet adherence, release reaction, and aggregation occur at the site of future atherosclerosis. Platelet-derived factors cause vascular damage and spasm, and increase vascular permeability. It is not known whether these factors participate in the primary intimal injury or are involved in the propagation of injury. Following abnormal platelet–vessel wall interaction, platelet-derived growth factor stimulates and promotes the proliferation and migration of smooth muscle cells and fibroblasts. This is the nidus for atherosclerosis. Lipids accumulate in this lesion. Perhaps a defective lipid removal mechanism leads to growth of the atherosclerotic plaque. These events are illustrated in Figure 2.

This platelet–vascular injury hypothesis is based on considerable epidemiologic and experimental evidence, which can be briefly summarized as follows: (1) Platelet clumps are often encountered in areas of atherosclerosis in animals and man;[9] (2) platelet-release products can promote vascular permeability and induce endothelial injury and vasospasm;[10–13] (3) platelet adhesion and degranulation occur before smooth muscle cell migration and proliferation;[14] (4) platelets release smooth muscle growth factor;[15] (5) platelet-released products are increased in atherosclerosis-susceptible pigeons;[16] (6) atherosclerosis is absent in animals with deficient platelet number or function;[17–20] and (7) the incidence of atherosclerosis is low in patients with von Willebrand's disease (defective platelet function) and in Greenland Eskimos with inactive $TXA_3$.

## PROSTAGLANDINS AND PLATELET–VESSEL WALL INTERACTION

Most prostaglandins in man are derived from arachidonic acid, a constituent of the cell membrane phospholipid. In the past, prostaglandins of D, E, and F series were considered important in platelet homeostasis and vasomotor control. Discovery of novel pathways of arachidonic acid metabolism in various body tissues has enhanced immensely our understanding of platelet-vessel wall interaction (Fig. 3). By action of enzyme cyclo-oxygenase, arachidonic acid is converted to labile cyclic endoperoxides ($PGG_2$ and $PGH_2$) that are metabolized to $PGE_2$, $PGF_{2\alpha}$, and $TXA_2$ in the platelets. $TXA_2$ plays a major role in promoting platelet release reaction and aggregation and is a potent vasoconstrictor. It may, therefore, contribute to the development of atherosclerosis and tissue ischemia.

The effects on $TXA_2$ generation of hypercholesterolemia, a major risk factor for atherosclerosis, are of particular relevance. $TXA_2$ synthesis from arachidonic acid is greater in cholesterol-rich platelets than in cholesterol-depleted platelets in vitro.[21] Increased platelet $TXA_2$ production has also been reported in diet-induced hypercholesterolemia in rabbits[22] and in patients with type IIa hyperlipidemia.[23]

Prostacyclin ($PGI_2$) is the major product of arachidonic acid metabolism in blood vessels.[24] It is synthesized predominantly in the vascular endothelium by action of prostacyclin synthetase on cyclic endoperoxides derived from arachidonic acid. Endoperoxides released from platelets may also act as a substrate for $PGI_2$ synthesis. $PGI_2$ is the most potent endogenous inhibitor of platelet aggregation and is a vasodilator. It is, therefore, of great interest that levels of $PGI_2$ are decreased in experimental and human atherosclerosis.[22,25] In addition, animals with diet-induced hypercholesterolemia show impaired $PGI_2$ production, possibly because of lipid peroxide inhibition of prostacyclin synthetase.[22]

Besides the cyclo-oxygenase pathway, arachidonic acid is also metabolized via the lipoxygenase pathway, resulting in formation of hydroxy and hydroperoxy derivatives, and leukotrienes. This pathway was initially observed in leukocytes.[26,27] Leukotrienes are involved in leukocyte chemotaxis and chemokinesis, vasoconstriction, and vascular permeability.[28] It has been proposed that leukotrienes may modulate release of $TXA_2$ and $PGI_2$, and thus influence the platelet–vessel wall interaction and the course of acute ischemic events.[29]

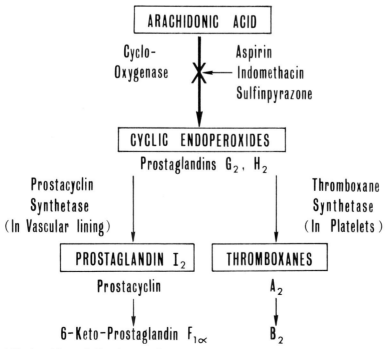

**Figure 3.** Arachidonic acid metabolism in man. See text for details.

# PLATELETS AND ISCHEMIC HEART DISEASE

## Sudden Cardiac Death

### Experimental Animal Studies

Hughes and Tonks[30] first demonstrated that diffuse myocardial necrosis could result from platelet aggregates in the microcirculation of the rabbit heart.

Jorgensen and coworkers[31] infused ADP directly into the coronary arteries of pigs. Platelet aggregates were noted in the coronary microcirculation of all animals sacrificed or dying during the first 5 minutes of infusion. It is also of interest that in animals that survived longer, there was a 30 to 40 percent decrease in frequency of platelet aggregates, even though myocardial necrosis was present in nearly all animals. This finding may be explained by disaggregation and disappearance of platelet aggregates after causing the ischemic damage, but before pathologic examination.

The primary role of platelets in myocardial injury was supported by two other experiments: (1) ADP infusion preceded by $^{32}$P-induced thrombocytopenia was not accompanied by myocardial necrosis, and (2) the frequency of myocardial necrosis was significantly less common among pigs given intracoronary infusions of AMP, which, unlike ADP, does not induce platelet aggregation.

Intravascular aggregation of platelets in the small vessels of the heart has also been demonstrated following the intravenous administration of catecholamines to dogs.[32] This finding was associated with diffuse myocardial necrosis. In subsequent studies, Haft and associates found that pretreatment with aspirin,[33] dipyridamole,[33] or clofibrate[34] prevented catecholamine-induced myocardial necrosis. These findings would appear to support an etiologic role for platelet aggregation in the genesis of these lesions. They may have particular relevance to the association between emotional stress and myocardial infarction and sudden death in humans.

A canine model of partial coronary stenosis developed by Uchida, Aiken, Folts, and coworkers has facilitated investigation of the role of platelet aggregation in myocardial ischemia. A plastic cylinder placed around a major coronary artery and adjusted to produce a 60 to 80 percent diameter reduction results in periodic decreases in coronary blood flow over a 5- to 10-minute period in about 60 percent of animals.[35] Gradual decrease in flow is usually followed by a sudden return to control flow. On occasion, however, coronary blood flow totally ceases, leading to ventricular fibrillation and sudden death. These workers have also described ventricular fibrillation following abrupt restoration of coronary blood flow, perhaps related to the reperfusion phenomenon. The cyclic changes in coronary blood flow can be inhibited by antiplatelet agents, suggesting that platelet thrombus formation at the site of narrowing is the cause of these cyclic changes.[36] In 40 percent of animals that do not show these blood flow changes spontaneously, administration of small amounts of platelet aggregants can precipitate the cyclic variations (Fig. 4).

Recently, Kowey and associates[37] have utilized this model in assessing the effects of platelet aggregation on ventricular electrical instability. Reductions in coronary blood flow were accompanied by significant decreases in the repetitive extrasystole and ventricular fibrillation thresholds. The reduction of coronary blood flow and vulnerable period thresholds were prevented by $PGI_2$. Indomethacin, an inhibitor of cyclo-oxygenase, and hence $TXA_2$ synthesis, also prevented these changes. A marked increase in vulnerability of ventricular fibrillation was noted during reperfusion that occurs with platelet dislodgment.

After induction of an experimental platelet thrombus in a major coronary artery, Moschos and colleagues[38] consistently observed microcirculatory thrombosis in the ischemic area, especially in the periphery. Pretreatment of the animals with aspirin or dipyridamole minimized the extent of microcirculatory thrombosis without affecting the proximal epicardial coronary

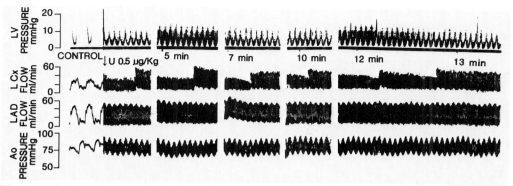

**Figure 4.** Effects of intravenous (IV) infusion of a platelet aggregant (epoxymethanodienoic acid [U]) in dog with narrowed left circumflex coronary artery (LCx). Note appearance of decrease in coronary flow with abrupt return to supernormal levels. Pattern was repeated every 2 to 4 minutes. Prostacyclin given IV abolished this phenomenon. There were no changes in left ventricular (LV) diastolic pressure or aortic (Ao) pressure. Left anterior descending (LAD) coronary blood flow was normal. (From Mehta, J: *Platelets and prostaglandins in coronary artery disease: Rationale for use of platelet-suppressive drugs.* JAMA 249:2818, 1983, with permission.)

thrombus. A decrease in the incidence of arrhythmias and mortality in the treated animals was also noted. These workers have speculated that the microcirculatory thrombosis may be secondary to embolism from the proximal platelet thrombus, and that small vessel obstruction may influence the extent of myocardial infarction by impairment of collateral blood flow. It is tempting to attribute the beneficial effects of aspirin and dipyridamole to their anti–platelet aggregation properties. However, the same investigators have also demonstrated reduction of fatal arrhythmias during nonthrombotic coronary occlusion in animals treated with aspirin[39] or sulfinpyrazone.[40] The authors have postulated a direct effect of these agents on cell membrane, unrelated to platelet inhibition.

## Pathology

Anatomic abnormalities are present in virtually all cases of sudden cardiac death.[41] However, there is no single anatomic feature that is pathognomonic of sudden death. As indicated earlier, although the vast majority of patients with sudden cardiac death have extensive coronary atherosclerosis, completely normal coronary arteries are also encountered (Fig. 5). Transmural myocardial infarction is usually associated with thrombotic occlusion of the coronary artery proximal to the area of infarction. DeWood and associates[42] found complete occlusion of the infarct-related coronary artery in 86 percent of patients studied by arteriography during the first 6 hours of an acute myocardial infarction. Pathologic studies during the first 6 hours after infarction have often not demonstrated such a thrombus. Several factors may account for this apparent discrepancy. The transient nature of platelet aggregates has been demonstrated by experimental animal studies, and the negative postmortem findings may reflect disaggregation of platelet plugs prior to the pathologic examination. Secondly, platelet plugs may be stabilized by local vasospasm that may also be evanescent. Finally, postmortem autolysis of platelet thrombi and fixative artifacts may predispose to underestimation of the incidence of platelet thrombi.

Haerem[43] reported a significantly greater frequency of platelet microthrombi in patients with coronary artery disease who died suddenly than in those who died from other causes. He observed the predominance of "chronic inflammatory microlesions" among sudden cardiac death victims.[44] Platelet thrombi in the coronary microcirculation were also seen by Frink and coworkers[45] in four of six patients less than 45 years old who died suddenly. These were associated with nonobstructive thrombi in the proximal coronary arteries.

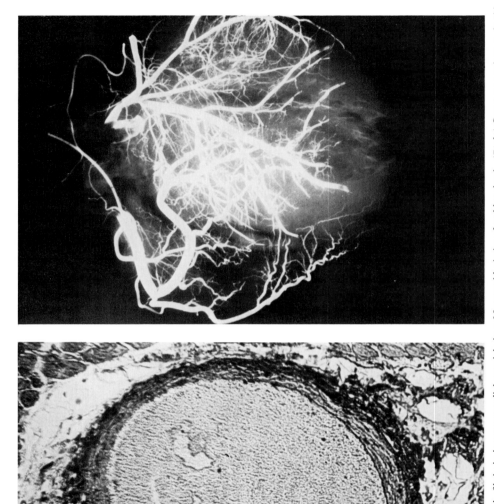

**Figure 5.** *(Left)* Platelet thrombus with little fibrin in intramyocardial arteriole in a 25-year-old victim of sudden death. *(Right)* Coronary angiogram in this patient showed nonocclusive thrombosis of the LAD coronary artery. No evidence of atherosclerosis is present. (From El-Maraghi and Genton,[46] with permission.)

Other workers have noted conflicting findings regarding the frequency of platelet aggregates in the coronary microcirculation. El-Maraghi and Genton[46] found no difference in the incidence of microthrombi in sudden cardiac death patients with ischemic heart disease (10 of 50 patients or 20 percent) compared with patients who survived longer (9 of 93 patients or 10 percent). However, when sudden death cases were analyzed by age, an important difference emerged. Platelet microthrombi were more common in patients less than 45 years old, compared with those older (8 of 14 versus 2 of 36 patients, p = 0.0002). In 5 of the 10 sudden death cases, the presence of microthrombi was related to thrombosis in a major coronary artery supplying the area. This finding is suggestive of an embolic mechanism. In the other five cases, microcirculatory involvement was diffuse and not related to a thrombosed epicardial coronary artery. The authors postulated that the initial myocardial ischemia may release chemical inducers of platelet aggregation and induce myocardial damage in areas remote from the initial injury.

## Clinical Studies

The Framingham Study demonstrated that the risk factors for coronary atherosclerosis, such as smoking, hypertension, hyperlipidemia, and diabetes mellitus, were the same for sudden cardiac death. No specific risk factor profile was identified in subjects at increased risk of dying suddenly as opposed to other coronary events. Certain population subsets, however, appear to have a higher likelihood of sudden death, for example, white women who smoked heavily had a fourfold risk.[47] The clinical importance of risk factor modification is underlined by the evidence that cessation of smoking may reduce the risk of sudden cardiac death following myocardial infarction.[48] Platelet function abnormalities have been found in all the classic risk factors. It may well be that the predisposition to atherosclerosis is, in part at least, mediated through platelet "hyperactivity."

An increased number of circulating platelet aggregates has been reported in smokers. Platelet hyperactivity may reflect mobilization of catecholamines or thrombin generation associated with cigarette smoking. Although patients with hypertension have enhanced platelet adhesion and elevated beta-thromboglobulin levels,[49] the major effects of hypertension are related to hemodynamic stress on blood vessels. Hyperlipidemia is associated with enhanced platelet reactivity and shortened platelet survival. Carvalho and associates[50] have shown that patients with type IIa hyperlipoproteinemia have a markedly increased sensitivity to the aggregatory effects of epinephrine. Increased platelet aggregation has been reported in diabetics, especially those with complications. In diabetics with retinopathy, plasma beta-thromboglobulin is elevated. This finding implies in vivo platelet activation and release of alpha-granule contents.[51] Platelet microthrombi have been observed in diabetic microangiopathy.[52]

## Myocardial Ischemia

In our laboratory, we have examined platelet function in patients undergoing cardiac catheterization.[53] In patients with angiographically significant coronary artery disease, a 10 to 40 percent reduction in platelet counts is observed between aortic and coronary venous blood. No such gradient is found in patients with normal coronary arteries. This difference may relate to adhesion of platelets at sites of coronary atherosclerosis. During coronary sinus pacing–induced tachycardia, we found marked activation of platelets exiting in the coronary sinus but not in the aortic blood of subjects with coronary atherosclerosis.[54] No such activation occurred in patients with normal coronary arteries. This platelet activation must have occurred in the atherosclerotic coronary vascular bed. The increased platelet aggregation during pacing-induced stress may be related to turbulence or to release of catecholamines or metabolic products of ischemia.

During exercise-provoked ischemia, Green and colleagues[55] reported a significant increase in plasma platelet factor 4 (PF-4) in 11 of 20 patients with coronary artery disease. No such increase was found in 18 of 20 patients with normal exercise tests. We have observed an increase in beta-thromboglobulin in plasma during exercise in patients with angina pectoris. The secretion of PF-4 and beta-thromboglobulin during exercise-induced ischemia implies concomitant activation of platelets. The inability of other workers to duplicate these findings may be partly explained by methodologic differences.[56] Activation of platelets and their release have been implicated in unstable angina. In a study of 19 patients with unstable angina at rest, plasma levels of platelet-derived beta-thromboglobulin and PF-4 were significantly elevated during or within 4 hours after episodes of angina, but were usually normal during pain-free intervals.[57]

### Myocardial Infarction

ADP-induced platelet aggregation is usually increased within a few hours to 2 weeks after infarction[58] and returns to normal within 6 weeks.[59] Most studies have shown increased circulating platelet aggregates within 48 hours of acute transmural myocardial infarction. The number of circulating platelet aggregates usually returns to normal by the seventh day after infarction, unless extension of infarction has occurred.[60] Increased levels of PF-4 have also been reported following infarction.[61] In a British study, platelet release of serotonin correlated with mortality at 1 year after myocardial infarction.[62]

### Coronary Artery Spasm

Robertson and coworkers[63] have found increased numbers of platelet aggregates in coronary sinus blood, but not in arterial blood during vasospastic angina. This was not the case during ischemia-free periods. However, lack of benefit in reducing ischemic events with antiplatelet drugs did not suggest a primary role for platelets in these patients.

### PROSTAGLANDINS AND ISCHEMIC HEART DISEASE

The opposite biologic effects of $TXA_2$ and $PGI_2$ on platelet aggregation and vascular tone have led to the concept of a balance between these two prostanoids. Thus, a deficiency of $PGI_2$ relative to $TXA_2$ would favor platelet aggregation and dynamic vasoconstriction. This concept has stimulated intensive investigation of $PGI_2$, agents that promote $PGI_2$ activity, and selective pharmacologic $TXA_2$ inhibitors in ischemic heart disease.

Several investigators have found enhanced synthesis of $TXA_2$ in patients with coronary artery disease. This increase in platelet prostaglandin generation has been observed in patients during pacing-induced myocardial ischemia,[64] during unstable angina pectoris,[65] during and following acute myocardial infarction,[66] and during variant angina.[67] On the other hand, it is now evident that $PGI_2$ release is significantly decreased in these subjects. In addition, platelets from patients with unstable angina and acute myocardial infarction have markedly decreased sensitivity to the antiaggregatory effects of $PGI_2$ and increased sensitivity to the proaggregatory actions to $TXA_2$.[65] These mechanisms may lead to platelet clot formation and coronary vasoconstriction. The consequent reduction in blood flow to the myocardium could result in angina, infarction, and arrhythmias (see Fig. 1).

### ANTIPLATELET DRUGS AND SUDDEN DEATH

The effect of antiplatelet drugs on sudden cardiac death has been evaluated in patients with myocardial infarction and in others with unstable angina. The rationale for their use is based on the recognized role of platelet hyperactivity in the development and complications of coronary atherosclerosis. It should be pointed out that any protective effect against sudden death may not necessarily be mediated by inhibition of platelet function. As mentioned earlier, aspirin and sulfinpyrazone have direct antiarrhythmic effects on a cellular basis and beneficial effects on collateral blood flow that may be independent of platelets.

Whatever the underlying mechanism, the value of antiplatelet agents in reducing sudden cardiac death can be assessed only by large, well-designed clinical trials. There have been several such trials in patients surviving myocardial infarction (Table 1). No studies using antiplatelet drugs, however, have been reported in the primary prevention of myocardial infarction. The major antiplatelet drugs used have been cyclo-oxygenase inhibitors (aspirin and sulfinpyrazone) and a phosphodiesterase inhibitor (dipyridamole).

In five of the six studies evaluating *aspirin,* there was an apparent reduction in mortality with use of aspirin. Considering the data from each individual trial, the observed differences in mortality were not statistically significant. When the results of these studies are pooled, aspirin reduces the risk of cardiovascular death by 16 percent. This statistical approach, however, may be criticized for several reasons, including the variable doses of aspirin used, the different entry times after myocardial infarction, and unmatched study populations. These inconclusive results may relate to the patient population studied and inadequate platelet inhibition due to the antiplatelet drug regimens used.

Platelet activation may not play a primary role in the pathogenesis of sudden cardiac death or reinfarction in this population of patients. It is perhaps not surprising that antiplatelet agents have not shown a dramatic effect on short-term prognosis in patients with previous myocardial infarction. The major determinant of survival is the extent of myocardial damage. Electrical instability in these patients may be a manifestation of a scarred ventricle rather than transient ischemia mediated by platelets. A more appropriate assessment of efficacy of antiplatelet agents may require a long-term study in younger patients, particularly those with demonstrable platelet function abnormalities.

The dose regimen of aspirin has been criticized on theoretical grounds. Aspirin inhibits synthesis of cyclic endoperoxides by acetylation of platelet as well as vessel wall cyclo-oxygenase. As a result, both platelet $TXA_2$ and vascular $PGI_2$ synthesis are inhibited. Small doses of aspirin (325 mg every 3 or 4 days) may selectively inhibit $TXA_2$ while sparing $PGI_2$ synthesis.[68] In experimental animal studies, very high doses of aspirin have augmented thrombogenesis.[69] Thus, high doses may negate the beneficial effects derived from suppression of $TXA_2$. The clinical efficacy of a low-dose regimen has been recently demonstrated in a cooperative study in patients with unstable angina. Lewis and coworkers[70] found that aspirin in a dosage of 324 mg daily reduced the incidence of death and nonfatal myocardial infarction by 51 percent and 53 percent, respectively.

The time of entry to the study may be of critical importance. Mortality following myocardial infarction is highest in the first 6 months. Late entry to such a trial may account for variable efficacy of drugs on mortality.

Finally, the platelet-suppressive agents used may be limited in their ability to effectively inhibit platelet activation. Cyclo-oxygenase inhibitors, aspirin and sulfinpyrazone, will inhibit $TXA_2$ synthesis. However, thrombin-mediated aggregation is not prevented by these agents, and aspirin does not inhibit platelet adhesion.

In the Anturane Reinfarction Trial, *sulfinpyrazone* reduced the incidence of sudden cardiac death by 74 percent during the first 2 to 7 months following infarction and by 43 percent at 24 months. This was achieved with few side reactions. No effects on fatal or nonfatal myocardial reinfarction rates were found. The authors concluded that sulfinpyrazone prevents sudden cardiac death during the high-risk period shortly after an acute myocardial infarction, but there is no further apparent benefit beyond the seventh month after infarction. Major controversy has arisen over the methodology of the study and the classification of sudden death. Methodology criticisms have been directed at exclusion of patients after randomization to sulfinpyrazone or placebo treatment, and failure to analyze the results on an "intention to

**Table 1.** Platelet-suppressive drugs in secondary prevention after myocardial infarction (MI)

| Study | Drug, daily dosage | Time between MI and entry | Number of patients | % Reduction (drug vs placebo) | | | Conclusion |
|---|---|---|---|---|---|---|---|
| | | | | Mortality | Sudden death | Nonfatal MI | |
| Elwood et al, 1974 | Aspirin 300 mg | 10 weeks (average) | 1239 | 25 | — | — | Favorable trend |
| Coronary Drug Project Aspirin Study, 1976 | Aspirin 972 mg | 7 years (average) | 1529 | 30 | 19 | 5 | Favorable trend |
| German-Austrian Multicenter Trial, 1977, 1979 | Aspirin 1.5 g | 30–42 days | 626 | 18 | 36 | 28 | Favorable trend |
| Elwood and Sweetnam, 1979 | Aspirin 900 mg | 50% within 7 days | 1682 | 17 | — | 34* | Favorable trend |
| Anturane Reinfarction Trial, 1980 | Sulfinpyrazone 800 mg | 25–35 days | 1558 | 30 | 43* | 25 | Reduction of sudden death in first 6 months |
| Aspirin Myocardial Infarction Study, 1980 | Aspirin 1 g | 25 months (average) 85% after 6 months | 4524 | +11† | +35 | 22 | Aspirin not recommended for routine use |
| Persantine Aspirin Reinfarction Study, 1980 | Aspirin 972 mg or Aspirin 972 mg + dipyridamole 225 mg | 2 months–5 years 80% after 6 months | 2026 | 18 16 | +27 16 | 29 19 | Favorable trend for aspirin or combination on total mortality and coronary incidence |

*Statistically significant by study criteria.
†Plus sign (+) indicates increase.

treat" basis. The second area of debate is the possible misclassification of deaths in the study. Inappropriate inclusion of patients in the sudden death category as opposed to the myocardial infarction group may have overestimated the drug's beneficial effect on sudden death. Until these matters are clarified, no definite conclusions can be reached regarding the efficacy of sulfinpyrazone in survivors of myocardial infarction.

One study has reported the effects of *dipyridamole* alone in patients with myocardial infarction.[71] Unfortunately, the number of patients is relatively small, and data from long-term followup are not provided. The Persantine-Aspirin Reinfarction Study (PARIS) showed a similar mortality (total and coronary) and similar incidence of coronary events in patients treated with aspirin alone compared to those treated with aspirin and dipyridamole. In view of the different sites of action as well as the increased plasma concentration of dipyridamole with concomitant aspirin administration, one might have expected this drug combination to be synergistic. On the other hand, aspirin may reduce the availability of $PGI_2$ precursor and thereby limit the beneficial effects of dipyridamole.[72] Awareness of this potentially adverse interaction provides a basis for the drug regimen used in a recent Mayo Clinic study.[73] Dipyridamole was used alone for 2 days before coronary artery bypass surgery and then aspirin was added, resulting in significantly improved bypass graft patency.

Several *beta-adrenergic blocking drugs* have been shown to exert a beneficial effect on mortality in survivors of myocardial infarction. There appears to be no common denominator in terms of cardioselectivity, lipid solubility, membrane-stabilizing activity, or intrinsic sympathomimetic activity. Beta blockers suppress resting and exercise-induced platelet aggregation and inhibit $TXA_2$ synthesis by direct action on the platelet membrane, possibly by reducing calcium availability.[74] Although the precise mechanism by which these agents are useful in reducing mortality is not known, it is possible that their antiplatelet function is the common underlying mechanism.

In summary, a favorable trend for the use of antiplatelet agents in most trials support their clinical use in patients at high risk. Doses should be kept small, for example, aspirin 325 mg every 2 to 4 days, and treatment should be initiated early. The potential for adverse drug interactions (e.g., aspirin and dipyridamole) and drug side effects (e.g., gastrointestinal hemorrhage and gout) must be recognized.

## CONCLUSIONS

Sudden cardiac death has multiple pathogenetic mechanisms. Transient myocardial ischemia leading to electrical instability is likely to account for at least some cases of sudden death. Whether or not platelets actually initiate thrombosis, atherosclerosis, or coronary spasm, they appear to play a major role in the development of these ischemic processes.

Future research should be directed at identification of patients in whom platelet-suppressive therapy may be most beneficial. Such patients may include those with abnormal platelet function or younger patients in whom atherosclerosis is detected at an early stage.

Finally, further investigation is needed for new drugs acting at specific sites of platelet and prostaglandin pathways. This approach may lead to improved understanding of the pathogenesis of coronary artery disease and better management of its complications.

## ACKNOWLEDGMENT

We wish to thank Kelly Greetham for her assistance in the preparation of this manuscript.

## REFERENCES

1. COBB, LA, WERNER, JA, AND TROBAUGH, GB: *Sudden cardiac death: 1. A decade's experience with out-of-hospital resuscitation.* Mod Concepts Cardiovasc Dis 49:31, 1980.

2. JENKINS, CSD, PHILLIPS, DR, CLEMETSON, KJ, ET AL: *Platelet membrane glycoproteins implicated in ristocetin-induced aggregation.* J Clin Invest 57:112, 1976.

3. WEISS, HJ, TSCHOPP, TB, BAUMGARTNER, HR, ET AL: *Decreased adhesion of giant (Bernard-Soulier) platelets to subendothelium: Further implications on the role of von Willebrand's factor in hemostasis.* Am J Med 57:920, 1974.

4. HARLEN, J AND HARKER, LA: *Hemostasis, thrombosis and thromboembolic disorders: The role of arachidonic acid metabolites in platelet–vessel wall interactions.* Med Clin North Am 65:863, 1981.

5. DE GAETANO, G: *Platelets, prostaglandins and thrombotic disorders.* Clinics in Hematology 10:303, 1981.

6. VON ROKITANSKY, C: *A Manual of Pathological Anatomy,* Vol 4. Sydenham Society, London, 1852, pp 261–269.

7. DUGUID, JB AND ROBERTSON, WB: *Mechanical factors in atherosclerosis.* Lancet 1:1205, 1957.

8. VIRCHOW, R: *Cellular Pathology: As Based Upon Physiological and Pathological Histology.* Dober Publications, New York, 1977.

9. JORGENSEN, L, PACKHAM, MA, ROWSELL, HC, ET AL: *Deposition of formed elements of blood on the intima and signs of intimal injury in the aorta of rabbit, pig and man.* Lab Invest 27:341, 1972.

10. HUGHES, A AND TONKS, RS: *Intravascular platelet clumping in rabbits.* J Pathol Bacteriol 84:379, 1962.

11. NACHMAN, RL, WEKSLER, B, AND FERNS, B: *Increased vascular permeability produced by human platelet granule cationic extract.* J Clin Invest 49:274, 1970.

12. GOLDBERG, ID, STEMERMAN, MB, AND HANDIN, RI: *Vascular permeation of platelet factor-4 after endothelial injury.* Science 209:611, 1980.

13. GERTZ, SD: *Vascular damage and thrombosis from spasm.* N Engl J Med 300:197, 1979.

14. SPAET, TH, STEMERMAN, MB, VEITH, FJ, ET AL: *Intimal injury and regrowth in the rabbit aorta: Medial smooth muscle cells as a source of neo-intima.* Circ Res 36:58, 1975.

15. ROSS, R, GLOMSET, J, KAZIYA, B, ET AL: *A platelet dependent serum factor that stimulates the proliferation of arterial smooth muscle cells in vitro.* Proc Natl Acad Sci USA 71:1207, 1974.

16. FUSTER, V, LEWIS, JC, KOTTKE, BA, ET AL: *Platelet factor 4–like activity in the initial stages of atherosclerosis in pigeons.* Thromb Res 10:169, 1977.

17. COHEN, P AND MCCOMBS, HL: *Platelets and atherogenesis: Part 2. Amelioration of cholesterol atherogenesis in rabbits with reduced platelet counts as a result of $^{32}P$ administration.* J Atheroscler Res 8:389, 1968.

18. FRIEDMAN, RJ, STEMERMAN, MB, WENZ, B, ET AL: *The effect of thrombocytopenia on experimental atherosclerotic lesion formation in rabbits.* J Clin Invest 60:119, 1977.

19. FUSTER, V, DEWANJEE, MK, KAYE, MP, ET AL: *Evaluation of platelet deposition following selective endothelial injury of the carotid artery in normal and von Willebrand pigs.* Circulation 62(Suppl):III-98, 1980.

20. FUSTER, V, BOWIE, EJW, FASS, BN, ET AL: *Arteriosclerosis in von Willebrand and normal pigs: Spontaneous and high cholesterol diet–induced.* J Clin Invest 61:722, 1978.

21. STUART, MG, GERRARD, JM, AND WHITE, JG: *Effect of cholesterol on production of thromboxane $B_2$ by platelets in vitro.* N Engl J Med 302:5, 1980.

22. GRYGLEWSKI, RJ, DEMBINSKA-KIEC, A, ZMUDA, A, ET AL: *Prostacyclin and thromboxane $A_2$ biosynthesis capacities of heart, arteries and platelets at various stages of experimental atherosclerosis in rabbits.* Atherosclerosis 31:358, 1978.

23. TREMOLI, E, FOLCO, G, AGRADI, E, ET AL: *Platelet thromboxanes and serum cholesterol.* Lancet 1:107, 1979.

24. MONCADA, S AND VANE, JR: *Arachidonic acid metabolites and the interactions between platelets and blood vessels.* N Engl J Med 300:1142, 1979.

25. SINZINGER, H, WINTER, M, FEIGL, W, ET AL: *Prostacyclin (PGI$_2$)-generation by different types of human atherosclerosis lesions.* Lancet 2:469, 1979.

26. SAMUELSSON, B, BORGEAT, P, HAMMARSTROM, S, ET AL: *Leukotrienes in a new group of biologically active compounds.* In SAMUELSSON, B, RAMWELL, P, AND PAOLETTI, R (EDS): *Advances in Prostaglandin and Thromboxane Research.* Raven Press, New York, 1980, pp 1–18.

27. BORGEAT, P AND SAMUELSSON, B: *Arachidonic acid metabolism in polymorphonuclear leukocytes: Effect of ionophore A 23187.* Proc Natl Acad Sci USA 76:2148, 1979.

28. PIPER, PJ: *Pharmacology of leukotrienes.* Br Med Bull 39:255, 1983.

29. AIKEN, JW: *Arachidonic acid metabolism and the cardiovascular system.* In MEHTA, J AND MEHTA, P (EDS): *Platelets and Prostaglandins in Cardiovascular Disease.* Futura, New York, 1981, p 23.

30. HUGHES, A AND TONKS, RS: *Experimental embolic carditis.* J Pathol Bacteriol 72:497, 1956.

31. JORGENSEN, L, ROSWELL, HC, HOVIG, T, ET AL: *Adenosine diphosphate–induced platelet aggregation and myocardial infarction in swine.* Lab Invest 17:616, 1967.

32. HAFT, JI, KRANZ, PD, ALBERT, FJ, ET AL: *Intravascular platelet aggregation in the heart induced by norepinephrine.* Circulation 46:698, 1972.

33. HAFT, JI, GERSHENGORN, K, KRANZ, PD, ET AL: *Protection against epinephrine-induced myocardial necrosis by drugs that inhibit platelet aggregation.* Am J Cardiol 30:838, 1972.

34. HAFT, JI, KRANZ, PD, ALBERT, F, ET AL: *Protection against epinephrine-induced myocardial necrosis with clofibrate.* Am Heart J 86:805, 1973.

35. FOLTS, JD, GALLAGHER, K, AND ROWE, GG: *Phasic coronary blood flow changes with partial coronary artery obstruction.* Physiologist 17:223, 1974.

36. FOLTS, JD, GALLAGHER, K, AND ROWE GG: *Blood flow reductions in stenosed canine coronary arteries: Vasospasm or platelet aggregation?* Circulation 65:248, 1982.

37. KOWEY, PR, VERRIER, RL, LOWN, B, ET AL: *Influence of intracoronary platelet aggregation on ventricular electrical properties during partial coronary artery stenosis.* Am J Cardiol 51:596, 1983.

38. MOSCHOS, CB, LAHIRI, K, LYONS, M, ET AL: *Relation of microcirculatory thrombosis to thrombus in the proximal coronary artery: Effect of aspirin, dipyridamole and thrombolysis.* Am Heart J 86:61, 1973.

39. MOSCHOS, CB, HAIDER, B, DE LA CRUZ, C, JR, ET AL: *Anti-arrhythmic effects of aspirin during nonthrombotic coronary occlusion.* Circulation 57:681, 1978.

40. MOSCHOS, CB, ESCOBINAS, AJ, AND JORGENSEN, OB, JR: *Effect of sulfinpyrazone on ischemic myocardium.* In MCGREGOR, M, MUSTARD, JF, OLIVER, O, ET AL (EDS): *Cardiovascular Actions of Sulfinpyrazone.* Symposia Specialists, Miami, 1980, p 175.

41. JAMES, TN: *Chance and sudden death.* J Am Coll Cardiol 1:164, 1983.

42. DEWOOD, MA, SPORES, J, NOTSKE, R, ET AL: *Prevalence of total coronary occlusion during the early hours of transmural myocardial infarction.* N Engl J Med 303:897, 1980.

43. HAEREM, JW: *Sudden coronary death: The occurrence of platelet aggregates in the epicardial arteries of man.* Atherosclerosis 14:514, 1971.

44. HAEREM, JW: *Myocardial lesions in sudden unexpected coronary death.* Am Heart J 90:562, 1975.

45. FRINK, RJ, TROWBRIDGE, JO, AND ROONEY, PA, JR: *Nonobstructive coronary thrombosis in sudden cardiac death.* Am J Cardiol 42:48, 1978.

46. EL-MARAGHI, N AND GENTON, E: *The relevance of platelet and fibrin thromboembolism of the coronary microcirculation with special reference to sudden cardiac death.* Circulation 62:936, 1980.

47. KULLER, LH, PERPER, J, AND COOPER, M: *Demographic characteristics and trends in arteriosclerotic heart disease mortality: Sudden death and myocardial infarction.* Circulation 52:III-1, 1975.

48. WILHELMSON, C, VEDIN, JA, ELMFELDT, E, ET AL: *Smoking and myocardial infarction.* Lancet 1:415, 1975.

49. MEHTA, J AND MEHTA, P: *Platelet function in hypertension and effect of therapy.* Am J Cardiol 47:231, 1981.

50. CARVALHO, AC, COLMAN, RW, AND LEES, RS: *Platelet function in hyperlipoproteinemia.* N Engl J Med 290:434, 1974.

51. PRESTON, FE, WARD, JD, MARCALA, BM, ET AL: *Elevated β-thromboglobulin levels and circulating platelet aggregates in diabetic microangiopathy.* Lancet 1:238, 1978.

52. BLOODWORTH, JM, JR AND MOLITOR, DL: *Ultrastructural aspects of human and canine diabetic retinopathy.* Invest Ophthalmol 4:1037, 1965.

53. MEHTA, P, MEHTA, J, AND PEPINE, CJ: *Platelet aggregation across the myocardial vascular bed in man: I. Normal versus diseased coronary arteries.* Thromb Res 14:623, 1979.

54. MEHTA, J, MEHTA, P, AND PEPINE, CJ: *Platelet aggregation in aortic and coronary venous blood in patients with and without coronary disease: III. Role of tachycardia stress and propranolol.* Circulation 58:881, 1978.

55. GREEN, LH, SEROPPIAN, E, AND HANDIN, RI: *Platelet activation during exercise-induced myocardial ischemia.* N Engl J Med 302:193, 1980.

56. MATHIS, PC, WOHL, H, WALLACH, SR, ET AL: *Lack of release of platelet factor 4 during exercise-induced myocardial ischemia.* N Engl J Med 304:1275, 1981.

57. SOBEL, M, SALZMAN, EW, DAVIES, GC, ET AL: *Circulating platelet products in unstable angina pectoris.* Circulation 63:300, 1981.

58. DREYFUSS, F AND ZAHAVI, J: *Adenosine diphosphate induced platelet aggregation in myocardial infarction and ischemic heart disease.* Atherosclerosis 17:107, 1973.

59. ENTICKNAP, JB, GOODING, PG, LANSLEY, TS, ET AL: *Platelet size and function in ischemic heart disease.* J Ather Res 10:41, 1969.

60. MEHTA, P AND MEHTA, J: *Platelet function studies in coronary artery disease: V. Evidence for enhanced platelet microthrombus formation activity in acute myocardial infarction.* Am J Cardiol 43:757, 1979.

61. HANDIN, RI, MCDONOUGH M, AND LESCH, M: *Elevation of platelet factor-4 in acute myocardial infarction: Measurements by radioimmunoassay.* J Lab Clin Med 91:340, 1978.

62. HEPTINSTALL, S, MULLEY, GP, TAYLOR, PM, ET AL: *Platelet release reaction in myocardial infarction.* Br Med J 1:80, 1980.

63. ROBERTSON, RM, ROBERTSON, D, FRIESINGER, GC, ET AL: *Platelet aggregates in peripheral and coronary sinus blood in patients with spontaneous coronary artery spasm.* Lancet 2:829, 1980.

64. LEWY, RI, WEINER, L, WALINSKY, P, ET AL: *Thromboxane release during pacing-induced angina pectoris: Possible vasoconstrictor influence on the coronary vasculature.* Circulation 61:1165, 1980.

65. MEHTA, J, MEHTA, P, AND CONTI, CR: *Platelet function studies in coronary heart-disease: IX. Increased platelet prostaglandin generation and abnormal platelet sensitivity to prostacyclin and endoperoxide analog in patients with angina pectoris.* Am J Cardiol 46:945, 1980.

66. SZCZEKLIK, A, GRYGLEWSKI, RJ, MUSIAL, J, ET AL: *Thromboxane generation and platelet aggregation in survivals of myocardial infarction.* Thromb Haemostas 40:66, 1978.

67. LEWY, RI, SMITH, JB, SILVER, MJ, ET AL: *Detection of thromboxane $B_2$ in the peripheral blood of patients with Prinzmetal's angina.* Prostaglandins Med 2:243, 1979.

68. MASOTTI, G, GALANTI, G, POGGESI, L, ET AL: *Differential inhibition of prostacyclin introduction and platelet aggregation by aspirin.* Lancet 2:1213, 1979.

69. KELTON, JG, HIRSH, J, CARTER, CJ, ET AL: *Thrombogenic effect of high-dose aspirin in rabbits: Relationship to inhibition of vessel wall synthesis of prostaglandin $I_2$–like activity.* J Clin Invest 62:895, 1978.

70. LEWIS, HD, DAVIS, JW, ARCHIBALD, DG, ET AL: *Protective effects of 324 mg aspirin against acute myocardial infarction and death in men with unstable angina.* N Engl J Med 309:396, 1983.

71. GENT, AE, BROOK, CGD, FOLEY, TM, ET AL: *Dipyridamole: A controlled trial of its effect in myocardial infarction.* Br Med J 4:366, 1968.

72. MEHTA, J AND MEHTA, P: *Dipyridamole and aspirin relation to platelet aggregation and vessel wall prostaglandin generation.* J Cardiovasc Pharmacol 4:688, 1982.

73. CHESEBRO, JM, CLEMENTS, IP, FUSTER, V, ET AL: *A platelet-inhibitor drug trial in coronary artery bypass operations: Benefit of perioperative dipyridamole and aspirin therapy on early postoperative vein graft patency.* N Engl J Med 307:73, 1982.

74. MEHTA, J, MEHTA, P, HORALEK, C, ET AL: *Effects of propranolol therapy on platelet release and prostaglandin generation in patients with coronary heart disease.* Circulation 66:1294, 1982.

# Initiating Events of Sudden Cardiac Death

*Ioannis P. Panidis, M.D., and Joel Morganroth, M.D.*

A variety of cardiac and noncardiac diseases have been associated with sudden death (Table 1). Underlying cardiovascular disease is implicated in the majority of victims of sudden death, with coronary artery disease accounting for more than 75 percent.[1] Sudden death occurring within 24 hours after the onset of the final illness can be classified as "arrhythmic" when the victim collapses abruptly and the pulse ceases without prior circulatory collapse; death "in circulatory failure" occurs after the peripheral circulation collapses with later cessation of pulse.[2] In several cardiac and noncardiac conditions (e.g., cardiogenic shock, acute pulmonary embolism, rupture or dissection of aortic aneurysm, acute pericardial tamponade, cerebrovascular accidents), sudden death occurs as a consequence of generalized circulatory failure, hypoxia, or severe metabolic derangement. This mode of sudden death is usually preceded by characteristic clinical symptoms, the final illness usually lasts longer, and death usually occurs in the hospital.[3] However, in the majority of patients with cardiac disease, especially coronary artery disease, sudden death is usually arrhythmic in origin, and occurs rather instantaneously and most commonly out of the hospital. In fact, sudden death is the leading cause of death in patients with coronary artery disease, and approximately two thirds of the patients die before reaching medical care.[4] The understanding of the mechanisms leading to sudden arrhythmic death, the pathophysiologic events underlying its occurrence, and the means of preventing this catastrophic event are major concerns in modern cardiology. The available information regarding the pathophysiologic and clinical events immediately preceding sudden cardiac death will be reviewed in this chapter. In addition, the electrocardiographic events as recorded by ambulatory Holter monitoring immediately before and during the time of sudden death will be discussed.

## CLINICAL EVENTS PRECEDING SUDDEN CARDIAC DEATH

What precipitates the terminal event in sudden cardiac death may be impossible to know with certainty. Examining the activities and the clinical symptoms that victims of sudden death experience prior to the final event may be helpful in recognizing precipitating factors and possible clinical patterns immediately preceding sudden cardiac death. Because these data are usually obtained from relatives and other witnesses of the sudden death event and not directly from the patient, there may be some ambiguity about the symptoms. From a review of existing data, it appears that chest pain is a relatively infrequent prodromal symptom, occurring in only 11 to 35 percent of the patients.[5] Fatigue and dyspnea are probably the most frequent symptoms experienced by patients approaching a sudden cardiac demise. It is noteworthy that approximately one fourth to one third of patients who subsequently

**Table 1.** Conditions associated with sudden death*

A. Cardiac
  1. Coronary artery disease
    Acute myocardial infarction
    Myocardial rupture
  2. Cardiomyopathies
  3. Valvular heart disease
  4. Congenital anomalies
  5. Congenital Q–T syndrome
  6. Acute pericardial tamponade
  7. Cardiac tumors (e.g., myxoma)
  8. Wolff-Parkinson-White syndrome
  9. Drugs (e.g., digoxin, quinidine)
B. Noncardiac
  1. Cerebrovascular accidents
  2. Dissection or rupture of aortic aneurysm
  3. Malignant obesity and the Pickwickian syndrome
  4. Cor pulmonale and pulmonary hypertension
  5. Acute pulmonary embolism
  6. Acute or chronic alcoholism

*From Panidis and Morganroth,[36] with permission.

suffered sudden cardiac death had consulted their family physician within the 4 weeks preceding the final event.[5] Thus, although many patients have premonitory symptoms within 24 hours of the final episode, these symptoms are by no means specific and may have been present for several weeks, and even months prior to the sudden death event. A change in the pattern of previous symptoms (angina or dyspnea) may be observed in a few patients in the days prior to the sudden death.[6] The pathophysiologic background and the etiologic relation, if any, of these symptoms to the sudden death event are unknown.

There is even less information regarding the clinical symptoms experienced just before or during the sudden death episode. The dramatic occurrence of sudden death is most commonly observed during routine daily activities of an individual. A detailed description of the clinical events that took place immediately before and during a sudden cardiac death episode has been reported by Hinkle and associates.[7] A 61-year-old man with previous history of hypertension and myocardial infarction was wearing an ambulatory Holter monitor the day of his sudden death. The patient experienced no symptoms that day and walked, as was his custom, from his office to the train station. A few minutes after he entered the train and sat down, a passenger sitting nearby noticed that he had slumped against the window and appeared to be ill. He was then found to be unconscious and was making jerking movements with his arms. Resuscitation efforts were not successful, and the patient died of ventricular fibrillation, which was documented by the Holter monitoring.

Sudden death usually occurs during physical activity, standing, sitting, and less frequently during sleep.[8] Friedman and coworkers,[9] in their study of instantaneous cardiac death, found that about half of 59 patients died during or immediately after physical exertion. Based on the available data concerning the relation of physical activity to sudden death, it appears that there is some increased incidence of sudden death with exertion, particularly if it is severe and unusual.[3,9,10]

## PATHOPHYSIOLOGIC EVENTS INITIATING SUDDEN DEATH

Patients with coronary artery disease may die suddenly from acute myocardial infarction shortly after admission to the hospital or a few days after transfer from the coronary care

**Table 2.** Mechanisms of sudden cardiac death*

---

A. Generalized circulatory failure
B. Electromechanical dissociation
C. "Electrical" (arrhythmic) death
  1. Bradyarrhythmias
      Sinus arrest
      Complete heart block
      Cardiac standstill
  2. Ventricular arrhythmias
      Ventricular tachycardia
      Torsades de pointes
      Ventricular flutter/fibrillation

---

*From Panidis and Morganroth,[36] with permission.

unit when they were apparently stabilized. Mechanisms of sudden cardiac death in these patients most commonly include generalized circulatory failure or electromechanical dissociation (caused by cardiac rupture or massive myocardial infarction); bradyarrhythmias (usually associated with inferior myocardial infarction) and primary ventricular fibrillation may also account for these deaths[1] (Table 2). Most often, however, sudden cardiac death in patients with coronary artery disease occurs outside of the hospital, and in approximately 90 percent of the cases, it is caused by a primary electrical event (usually a ventricular tachyarrhythmia or ventricular fibrillation).[2] The exact pathophysiologic events leading to sudden death in these latter patients are not known. Only a minority experience chest pain before the fatal event, and pathologic evidence of acute myocardial infarction is found in only 20 to 30 percent.[2,11,12] Nonetheless, in patients in whom no acute myocardial infarction is found, there is usually evidence of extensive atherosclerotic heart disease, although many patients may have been completely asymptomatic prior to their sudden death.[13,14] Impaired left ventricular function and a history of congestive heart failure appear to be additional risk factors associated with an increased incidence of sudden cardiac death in patients with coronary artery disease.[15,16] In younger patients who had suffered a cardiac arrest, usually congestive or hypertrophic cardiomyopathy was found.[17] It happens only rarely after intensive investigation of patients who suffer cardiac arrest that there is no evidence of underlying heart disease.

The exact pathophysiologic sequence leading to electrical instability, ventricular fibrillation, and sudden death is not known. Acute coronary thombosis of a major coronary artery has been documented in a few cases.[7] It has been proposed that coronary spasm, platelet aggregation, or both may induce myocardial ischemia and trigger a ventricular arrhythmia in an electrically unstable heart; these arrhythmias may occur at the onset of impaired coronary flow or in the reperfusion stage and then degenerate into ventricular fibrillation.[18,19] This hypothesis is supported by the finding of ST–T changes (elevation or depression) recorded during Holter monitoring in patients suffering sudden cardiac death[7,20–24] (Fig. 1).

It appears that sudden cardiac death is usually an electrophysiologic phenomenon occurring in a chronically damaged heart with advanced coronary atherosclerosis. The structural and electrical instability may alter the electrophysiologic properties of the cell membranes and may produce fatal ventricular arrhythmias, in some cases under the influence of acute myocardial ischemia. The exact interrelation of these factors remains to be determined.

## ELECTROCARDIOGRAPHIC EVENTS DURING SUDDEN CARDIAC DEATH

Most of the information regarding the electrocardiographic events preceding sudden cardiac death are obtained from the continuous electrocardiographic monitoring done in coronary care units or done by mobile resuscitation teams treating out-of-hospital sudden

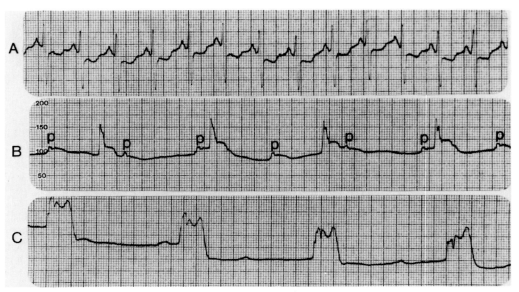

**Figure 1.** Sequential, but not continuous, Holter monitor recording from a patient who suffered acute inferior myocardial infarction and sudden death. *(A)* Sinus tachycardia with significant ST segment depression (1 to 2 mm) suggestive of ischemia is present. *(B)* Complete heart block develops with idioventricular rhythm; ST segment elevation is now present, consistent with an acute epicardial injury pattern. *(C)* Slowing of the idioventricular rhythm with further widening of QRS complex occurs, and the patient expired. P = P waves

deaths.[25,26] Inasmuch as there is generally some delay between the sudden collapse and the start of emergency care, documentation of the electrical event preceding sudden death is usually not feasible, and only the terminal rhythm is recorded. Adgey and colleagues[26] reported that when an electrocardiogram was obtained within 4 minutes from the onset of symptoms of cardiac arrest, the majority of patients (91 percent) exhibited ventricular fibrillation; when cardiac resuscitation was not possible within 4 minutes from the onset of cardiac arrest, 82 percent manifested cardiac standstill.

Recently, several reports detailed the electrocardiographic findings in patients with sudden cardiac death occurring in the hospital or outside of the hospital while they fortuitously were wearing a Holter monitor.[7,20–24,27–35] Review of the clinical and Holter monitoring data from 72 patients reported in these studies revealed some common characteristics.[36] The majority of these patients were males older than 50 years, and all but 2 of the 72 patients had a previous history of underlying heart disease. Coronary artery disease was present in the vast majority; valvular and hypertensive heart disease and congestive cardiomyopathy were other, less common etiologies. In the few cases in which the preceding activity was reported, sudden cardiac death occurred during routine daily activities (e.g., watching television at home, walking, or sitting in a chair).[7,21,22] The outcome was almost invariably fatal when sudden cardiac arrest occurred outside of the hospital; resuscitation was more successful in patients who were hospitalized.[36]

Review of the Holter monitoring findings showed that the terminal event was a bradyarrhythmia, expressed as sinus arrest, complete heart block, or ventricular asystole in 7 of the 72 patients (10 percent). In the remaining 65 patients, a ventricular tachyarrhythmia was recorded. In 54 of these 65 patients, ventricular fibrillation was the terminal rhythm, and it was always preceded by a variable duration of ventricular tachycardia or ventricular flutter.[36] Recent reports of Holter monitor recordings done at the time of sudden cardiac death have confirmed these findings.[37–39]

## Bradyarrhythmias

Emergency resuscitation teams have reported that 15 to 25 percent of patients with out-of-hospital cardiac arrest have bradycardia or asystole, whereas complete heart block is relatively uncommon.[40-42] The incidence of bradyarrhythmic or asystolic cardiac arrest found by Holter monitor recordings during sudden death episodes also ranges between 10 and 25 percent.[36,38] Bradyarrhythmias recorded during Holter monitoring include sinus arrest with slow junctional rhythm,[22,30] asystole with idioventricular rhythm,[27] sinus bradycardia followed by second-degree AV block and asystole,[24] and complete heart block[35] (see Fig. 1). Approximately 1 to 3 percent of patients with acute myocardial infarction, especially inferior infarction, develop cardiac asystole without any premonitory arrhythmias. Lown and Wolf[43] found that 61 percent of patients with inferior myocardial infarction who come under care within 1 hour exhibit some type of bradyarrhythmia. These observations, along with findings on Holter monitor studies,[22,24,27,30,38] suggest that bradycardic or asystolic cardiac arrest accounts for only a minority of the sudden cardiac deaths but is usually associated with a high mortality.[42] It is possible that the electrocardiographic changes observed during the bradyarrhythmia and the terminal event are not the cause of the sudden death; they may actually represent associated electrocardiographic findings during electromechanical dissociation and, if so, sudden cardiac death in these patients probably will not be prevented by antiarrhythmic drugs or pacemaker therapy.

The association between bradyarrhythmia-related sudden cardiac death and prior intraventricular or bundle branch block is not clear. Data from the Framingham study suggest that subjects with intraventricular conduction disturbances in the presence of underlying cardiac disease may have a higher incidence of sudden death, especially when ventricular premature contractions are also documented.[44] In addition, patients with acute myocardial infarction who develop bundle branch block, and even temporary complete heart block, appear to be at a higher risk for developing late sudden death.[45] Whether prophylactic permanent pacemaker therapy in these patients would prevent sudden cardiac death has not been clearly shown. Other studies[38] have found no evidence of prior atrioventricular or bundle branch block disturbances in patients dying of bradyarrhythmic sudden death.

## Ventricular Fibrillation

Ventricular fibrillation can be observed in patients with acute myocardial infarction complicated by overt congestive heart failure or cardiogenic shock and usually is associated with poor in-hospital and long-term prognoses.[46,47] Primary ventricular fibrillation occurs in 5 to 10 percent of patients admitted to coronary care units during an otherwise uncomplicated post–myocardial infarction course.[46,48] This terminal arrhythmia is also usually found in patients with coronary artery disease who suffer sudden cardiac death outside of the hospital. Data from the Seattle Heart Watch and other hospital medical emergency systems estimate that in at least three fourths of the victims of out-of-hospital cardiac arrest, ventricular fibrillation is the documented underlying rhythm disturbance.[49-52] Data from Holter monitor studies suggest that the prevalence of ventricular fibrillation during sudden death episodes ranges between 75 and 90 percent.[33-38]

A common finding in these Holter monitoring studies of victims of sudden cardiac death is the presence of frequent and complex ventricular arrhythmias recorded during the monitoring session.[33-38] Previous epidemiologic observations established that ventricular premature beats (VPBs) represent a risk factor for the development of sudden death in patients with chronic coronary artery disease and after myocardial infarction.[53-56] This association between increased VPB frequency and subsequent risk of sudden cardiac death is even higher in

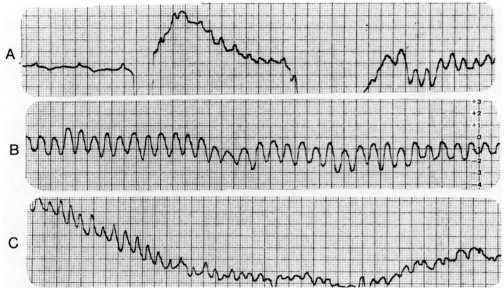

**Figure 2.** Sequential, but not continuous, Holter monitor recording from a patient with recent myocardial infarction who suffered sudden death in the hospital. *(A)* Normal sinus rhythm is followed by rapid ventricular tachycardia at a rate of 270 beats per min (ventricular flutter) *(B)*, which degenerates into ventricular fibrillation *(C)* after 72 seconds. Cardiac asystole occurred after 12 minutes of ventricular fibrillation, and the patient expired.

patients with clinical congestive heart failure and impaired left ventricular function (left ventricular ejection fraction less than 40 percent).[16,57] A period of increasingly frequent or complex ventricular arrhythmias has been reported to occur in the 1 to 2 hours prior to the ventricular fibrillation.[33,34] Review of the Holter monitor studies during sudden deaths also reveals that ventricular fibrillation almost always is preceded by a variable period of ventricular tachycardia or ventricular flutter[33,38] (Fig. 2). The ventricular tachycardia preceding ventricular fibrillation is usually characterized by a longer duration and more rapid rate.[34]

Previous studies have implicated long cycle lengths and repetitive ventricular stimuli as causes of temporal dispersion of ventricular refractoriness and tendency to ventricular fibrillation.[58] Other investigators suggest that acceleration of the heart rate is associated with an increased ventricular premature depolarization frequency or rate of ventricular tachycardia.[59] Several other studies, however, found no consistent patterns of cycle length or heart rate prior to the occurrence of ventricular fibrillation.[33,35]

The R-on-T phenomenon has been proposed as an important marker for identifying persons at high risk for sudden cardiac death from ventricular fibrillation in the setting of acute myocardial infarction or chronic coronary artery disease.[55,60,61] Recent Holter monitor studies, however, have shown that late coupling VPBs can also initiate ventricular tachycardia and ventricular fibrillation.[23,30,34,35,38] Thus, it appears that under different circumstances, both early and late VPBs can precipitate lethal ventricular arrhythmias and ventricular fibrillation, and that the incidence of prodromal R-on-T phenomenon is not as common as it was previously suggested. Ventricular fibrillation invariably leads to ventricular asystole and death unless electrical cardioversion is quickly applied. In two of our patients[35] with ventricular fibrillation during sudden cardiac death, successful resuscitation was achieved by electric cardioversion after 60 and 90 seconds, respectively, in ventricular fibrillation. Spontaneous termination of ventricular fibrillation has only rarely been reported.[32,34]

86

## Torsades de Pointes

Although ventricular fibrillation appears to be the most common terminal rhythm recorded on Holter monitor in patients with sudden death, in some patients ventricular tachycardia that does not progress to ventricular fibrillation may be the cause of syncope or cardiac arrest.[35-38] Polymorphous ventricular tachycardia associated with prolonged Q–T interval (torsades de pointes) is not uncommonly found in such patients[30,32-35] (Fig. 3). This distinct type of ventricular tachycardia most frequently results from Type I antiarrhythmic agents (usually quinidine, procainamide, or disopyramide). It often occurs in association with electrolyte abnormalities (such as hypokalemia and hypomagnesemia) and can be observed in patients with coronary artery disease and the congenital Q–T syndrome[62,63] (Fig. 4). Although this arrhythmia is often self-terminating, its outcome is unpredictable, and it may degenerate into ventricular fibrillation.

Denes and coworkers[32] reported five patients who were taking digoxin and quinidine and developed torsades de pointes and ventricular fibrillation during Holter monitoring. All five patients had clinical evidence of severe congestive heart failure. Similarly, Nikolic and associates[30] reported three patients (two were taking quinidine and one mexiletine) who had sudden cardiac death due to torsades de pointes. We[35] identified during Holter monitoring five hospitalized patients who had sudden cardiac arrest caused by torsades de pointes. Three of these five patients had a history of congestive heart failure and were taking either quinidine or procainamide (see Fig. 3). These findings suggest that significant left ventricular dysfunc-

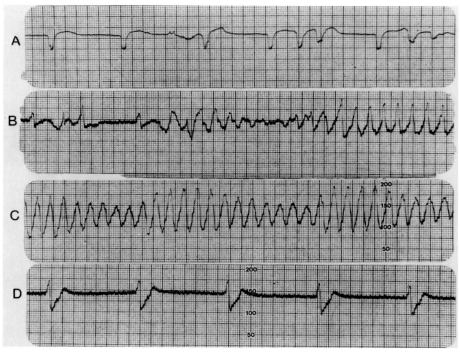

**Figure 3.** Sequential, but not continuous, Holter monitor recording from a patient with coronary artery disease, congestive heart failure, and prior ventricular arrhythmias for which he was receiving digoxin and quinidine. *(A)* Frequent ventricular premature complexes, occasionally in pairs, are present, and the Q–T interval is prolonged. *(B and C)* Sustained polymorphous ventricular tachycardia at a rate of 240 beats per min lasted for 3 minutes and 45 seconds, and was followed *(D)* by idioventricular rhythm. The patient expired.

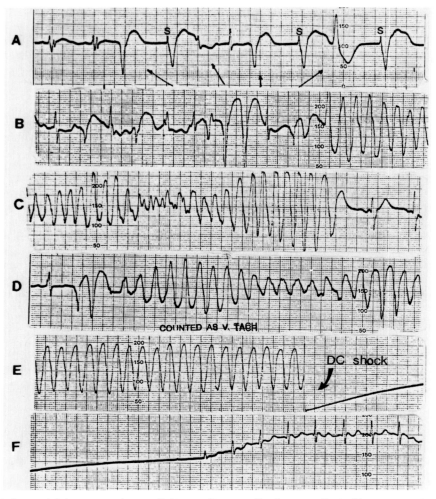

**Figure 4.** Sequential, but not continuous, Holter monitor recording from a patient with coronary artery disease who was admitted to the hospital for the evaluation of syncope. The only medication was digoxin, and the electrolytes were normal when she developed another syncopal episode while this Holter was recorded. *(A)* Normal sinus rhythm with intermittent pacing spikes (S) and occasional ventricular premature complexes (arrows) are evident; the Q–T interval is prolonged. *(B* and *C)* A sustained polymorphous ventricular tachycardia (torsades de pointes) at a rate of 270 beats per min resulted in syncope and resolved spontaneously after 4 minutes. *(D)* Another episode of torsades de pointes at a rate of 220 beats per min was followed by ventricular flutter *(E)* and resulted in syncope. *(F)* Direct current (DC) shock was applied 1 min later (arrow), and normal sinus rhythm was restored. Patient survived these syncopal episodes, but she died suddenly out of hospital a few months later while on procainamide and disopyramide.

tion may be a predisposing factor in the development of torsades de pointes in patients treated with Type I antiarrhythmic agents. Aggravation of ventricular arrhythmias may result from all antiarrhythmic drugs, and its incidence ranges between 6 and 16 percent of treated patients.[64] Ruskin and coworkers[65] recently reported six patients who suffered out-of-hospital cardiac arrest. All six patients had ventricular tachycardia or ventricular fibrillation while on antiarrhythmic drugs; these arrhythmias were also induced in the electrophysiologic laboratory. However, no ventricular arrhythmia could be induced in the latter patients when the antiarrhythmic drugs were discontinued. Such potentially fatal ventricular arrhythmias induced by antiarrhythmic drugs can occur even with therapeutic blood levels.[65] Thus, caution should be used when prescribing these agents, and only patients who meet strict indications should be treated.

## CLINICAL IMPLICATIONS

Several epidemiologic and clinical studies have attempted to identify high-risk groups of patients with underlying heart disease who are prone to sudden cardiac death. Patients with coronary artery disease or cardiomyopathy with significant left ventricular dysfunction, and patients with frequent and complex ventricular arrhythmias appear to be at particularly high risk. The exact pathophysiologic mechanisms leading to the terminal event are not known. It has been suggested that platelet aggregation and coronary spasm or myocardial ischemia of any cause may play a role in inducing lethal ventricular arrhythmias. In most patients, electrical instability in the presence of structural heart disease probably is the pathophysiologic substrate on which ventricular arrhythmias occur and lead to sudden cardiac death.

The increasing use of ambulatory Holter monitoring[66] has provided detailed information regarding the electrocardiographic abnormalities observed immediately before and during sudden cardiac death in patients who were fortuitously monitored during the final event.[36] Review of approximately 120 such patients who had sudden cardiac death during Holter monitoring revealed that ventricular tachycardia leading to ventricular fibrillation was the commonest terminal rhythm, recorded in approximately 75 to 90 percent of the patients.

Identification of high-risk patients and treatment of malignant ventricular arrhythmias by antiarrhythmic drugs may be helpful in decreasing the incidence and preventing sudden cardiac death.[67] Although successful suppression of malignant ventricular arrhythmias by antiarrhythmic drugs has not been shown definitely to protect patients from sudden cardiac death, initial results appear promising.[68]

Caution should be employed when prescribing an antiarrhythmic drug because all these agents have the potential of inducing lethal ventricular arrhythmias (torsades de pointes) and may actually cause cardiac arrest.[65] Careful selection of the patients and scrutiny of the indications should be applied when these agents are used, and their efficacy should be appropriately controlled. Invasive electrophysiologic testing appears to be helpful in identifying high-risk patients and in selecting appropriate antiarrhythmic therapy.[69,70] Effective suppression of ventricular arrhythmias in such patients, as demonstrated by electrophysiologic testing, has been shown to prevent recurrent sudden cardiac death in victims resuscitated from a first sudden death episode. Further studies of the clinical, pathophysiologic, and electrocardiographic events initiating sudden cardiac death are needed so that better means of prevention of this common, catastrophic event can be developed.

## REFERENCES

1. LOWN, B: *Cardiovascular collapse and sudden cardiac death.* In BRAUNWALD, E (ED): *Heart Disease: A Textbook of Cardiovascular Medicine.* WB Saunders, Philadelphia, 1980, pp 778–817.

2. HINKLE, LE AND THALER, HT: *Clinical classification of cardiac deaths.* Circulation 65:457, 1982.

3. WARREN, JV: *Critical issues in the sudden death syndrome.* In MCINTOSH, HD (ED): *Cardiology Series,* Baylor College of Medicine 5:5, 1982.

4. KANNEL, WB, DOYLE, JT, MCNAMARA, PM, ET AL: *Precursors of sudden coronary death: Factors related to the incidence of sudden death.* Circulation 51:606, 1975.

5. FEINLEIB, M, SIMON, AB, GILLUM, RF, ET AL: *Prodromal symptoms and signs of sudden death.* Circulation 51, 52(Suppl III):155, 1975.

6. RISSANEN, V: *Premonitory symptoms of sudden death.* Primary Cardiol Clinics 2:19, 1980.

7. HINKLE, LE, ARGYROS, DC, HAYES, JC, ET AL: *Pathogenesis of an unexpected sudden death: Role of early cycle ventricular premature contractions.* Am J Cardiol 39:873, 1977.

8. KLUGER, J: *Sudden death: Prediction and prevention.* Cardiovasc Reviews and Reports 3:106, 1982.

9. FRIEDMAN, M, MANWARING, JH, ROSENMAN, RH, ET AL: *Instantaneous and sudden deaths: Clinical and pathological differentiation in coronary artery disease.* JAMA 225:1319, 1973.

10. KALA, R, ROMO, M, SILTANEN, P, ET AL: *Physical activity and sudden cardiac death.* Adv Cardiol 25:27, 1978.

11. SCHWARTZ, CJ AND GERRITY, RG: *Anatomical pathology of sudden unexpected cardiac death.* Circulation 51,52(Suppl III):18, 1975.

12. LIBERTHSON, RR, NAGEL, EL, HIRSCHMAN, JC, ET AL: *Prehospital ventricular defibrillation: Prognosis and follow-up course.* N Engl J Med 291:317, 1974.

13. KULLER, LH: *Sudden death—definition and epidemiologic considerations.* Prog Cardiovasc Dis 23:1, 1980.

14. BASHE, WJ, JR, BABA, N, KELLER, MD, ET AL: *Pathology of atherosclerotic heart disease in sudden death: II. The significance of myocardial infarction.* Circulation 51, 52(Suppl III):63, 1975.

15. FOLLANSBEE, WB, MICHELSON, EL, AND MORGANROTH, J: *Nonsustained ventricular tachycardia in ambulatory patients: Characteristics and association with sudden cardiac death.* Ann Intern Med 92:741, 1980.

16. MARCHLINSKI, FE, BUXTON, AE, WAXMAN, HL, ET AL: *Identifying patients at risk of sudden death after myocardial infarction: Value of the response to programmed stimulation, degree of ventricular ectopic activity and severity of left ventricular dysfunction.* Am J Cardiol 52:1190, 1983.

17. BENSON, DW, BENDITT, DG, ANDERSON, RW, ET AL: *Cardiac arrest in young, ostensibly healthy patients: Clinical, hemodynamic, and electrophysiologic findings.* Am J Cardiol 52:65, 1983.

18. PREVITALI, M, KLERSY, C, SALERNO, JA, ET AL: *Ventricular tachyarrhythmias in Prinzmetal's variant angina: Clinical significance and relation to the degree and time course of ST segment elevation.* Am J Cardiol 52:19, 1983.

19. GOLDBERG, S, GREENSPON, AJ, URBAN, PL, ET AL: *Reperfusion arrhythmia: A marker of restoration of antegrade flow during intracoronary thrombolysis for acute myocardial infarction.* Am Heart J 105:26, 1983.

20. BLEIFER, SB, BLEIFER, DJ, HANSMANN, DR, ET AL: *Diagnosis of occult arrhythmias by Holter electrocardiography.* Prog Cardiovasc Dis 16:569, 1974.

21. GRADMAN, AH, BELL, PA, AND DEBUSK, RF: *Sudden death during ambulatory monitoring: Clinical and electrocardiographic correlations. Report of a case.* Circulation 55:210, 1977.

22. POOL, J, KUNST, K, AND VAN WERMESKERKEN, JL: *Two monitored cases of sudden death outside hospital.* Br Heart J 40:627, 1978.

23. BOUDOULAS, H, DERVENAGAS, S, SCHAAL, SF, ET AL: *Malignant premature ventricular beats in ambulatory patients.* Ann Intern Med 91:723, 1979.

24. SALERNO, D, HODGES, M, GRAHAM, E, ET AL: *Fatal cardiac arrest during continuous ambulatory monitoring.* N Engl J Med 305:700, 1981.

25. COBB, LA, BAUM, RS, ALVAREZ, H, ET AL: *Resuscitation from out of hospital ventricular fibrillation: 4 years follow-up.* Circulation 51,52(Suppl III):223, 1975.

26. ADGEY, AAJ, SCOTT, ME, ALLEN, JD, ET AL: *Management of ventricular fibrillation outside hospital.* Lancet 1:1169, 1969.

27. LAHIRI, A, BALASUBRAMANIAN, V, AND RAFTERY, EB: *Sudden death during ambulatory monitoring.* Br Med J 1:1676, 1979.

28. KLEIN, RC, VERA, Z, MASON, DT, ET AL: *Ambulatory Holter monitor documentation of ventricular tachyarrhythmias as mechanism of sudden death in patients with coronary artery disease.* Clin Res 27:7A, 1979.

29. BISSETT, JK, WATSON, JW, SCOVIL, JA, ET AL: *Sudden death in cardiomyopathy: Role of bradycardia-dependent repolarization changes.* Am Heart J 99:625, 1980.

30. NIKOLIC, G, BISHOP, RL, AND, SINGH, JB: *Sudden death recorded during Holter monitoring.* Circulation 66:218, 1982.

31. SAVAGE, DD, CASTELLI, WP, ANDERSON, SJ, ET AL: *Sudden unexpected death during ambulatory electrocardiographic monitoring: The Framingham study.* Am J Med 74:148, 1983.

32. DENES, P, GABSTER, A, AND HUANG, SK: *Clinical, electrocardiographic and follow-up observations in patients having ventricular fibrillation during Holter monitoring: Role of quinidine therapy.* Am J Cardiol 48:9, 1981.

33. LEWIS, BH, ANTMAN, EM, AND GRABOYS, TB: *Detailed analysis of 24 hour ambulatory electrocardiographic recordings during ventricular fibrillation or torsade de pointes.* J Am Coll Cardiol 2:426, 1983.

34. PRATT, CM, FRANCIS, MJ, LUCK, JC, ET AL: *Analysis of ambulatory electrocardiograms in 15 patients during spontaneous ventricular fibrillation with special reference to preceding arrhythmic events.* J Am Coll Cardiol 2:789, 1983.

35. PANIDIS, IP AND MORGANROTH, J: *Sudden death in hospitalized patients: Cardiac rhythm disturbances detected by ambulatory electrocardiographic monitoring.* J Am Coll Cardiol 2:798, 1983.

36. PANIDIS, IP AND MORGANROTH, J: *Holter monitoring and sudden cardiac death.* Cardiovasc Reviews and Reports 5:283, 1984.

37. MILNER, PG, PLATIA, EV, REID, PR, ET AL: *Holter monitoring recording at the time of sudden cardiac death.* Circulation 68(Suppl III):106, 1983.

38. KEMPF, FC, JR AND JOSEPHSON, ME: *Sudden cardiac death recorded on ambulatory electrocardiogram.* Circulation 68(Suppl III):355, 1983.

39. ROELANDT, J, KLOOTWIJK, P, AND LUBSEN, J: *Prodromal and lethal arrhythmias in sixteen sudden death patients documented with long term ambulatory electrocardiography (LAE).* Circulation 68(Suppl III):356, 1983.

40. LIBERTHSON, RR, NAGEL, EL, HIRSCHMAN, JC, ET AL: *Pathophysiologic observations in prehospital ventricular fibrillation and sudden cardiac death.* Circulation 49:790, 1974.

41. ISERI, LT, HUMPHREY, SB, AND SINER, EJ: *Prehospital bradyasystolic cardiac arrest.* Ann Intern Med 88:741, 1978.

42. MYERBURG, RJ, ZAMAN, L, LUCERI, R, ET AL: *Prehospital cardiac arrest with idioventricular rhythm.* Circulation 68(Suppl III):356, 1983.

43. LOWN, B AND WOLF, M: *Approaches to sudden death from coronary heart disease.* Circulation 44:130, 1971.

44. KANNEL, WB, KREGER, BE, AND McGEE, DL: *Sudden death in subjects with intraventricular conduction disturbance: The Framingham Study.* Circulation 68(Supp III):356, 1983.

45. ATKINS, JM, LESHIN, SJ, BLOMQVIST, G, ET AL: *Ventricular conduction blocks and sudden death in acute myocardial infarction: Potential indications for pacing.* N Engl J Med 288:281, 1973.

46. KILLIP, T AND KIMBALL, JT: *Survey of the coronary care unit: Concepts and results.* Prog Cardiovasc Dis 11:45, 1968.

47. LIE, KI, LIEM, KL, AND DURRER, D: *Management in hospital of ventricular fibrillation complicating acute myocardial infarction.* Br Heart J (Suppl) 40:78, 1978.

48. LAWRIE, DM, HIGGINS, MR, GODMAN, MG, ET AL: *Ventricular fibrillation complicating acute myocardial infarction.* Lancet 2:523, 1968.

49. COBB, LA, CONN, RD, AND SAMSON, WE: *Pre-hospital coronary care: The role of a rapid response, mobile intensive coronary care system.* Circulation 44(Suppl II):45, 1971.

50. WEAVER, WD, LORCH, GS, ALVAREX, HA, ET AL: *Angiographic findings and prognostic indicators in patients resuscitated from sudden cardiac deaths.* Circulation 54:895, 1976.

51. EISENBERG, MS, HALSTROM, A, AND BERGNER, L: *Long-term survival after out-of-hospital cardiac arrest.* N Engl J Med 306:1340, 1981.

52. MYERBURG, RJ, KEFFLER, KM, ZAMAN, L, ET AL: *Survivors of pre-hospital cardiac arrest.* JAMA 274:1485, 1982.

53. MOSS, AJ: *Clinical significance of ventricular arrhythmias in patients with and without coronary artery disease.* Prog Cardiovasc Dis 23:33, 1980.

54. RUBERMAN, W, WEINBLATT, E, GOLDBERG, JD, ET AL: *Ventricular premature beats and mortality after myocardial infarction.* N Engl J Med 297:750, 1977.

55. MOSS, AJ, DAVIS, HT, DeCAMILLA, J, ET AL: *Ventricular ectopic beats and their relation to sudden and nonsudden cardiac death after myocardial infarction.* Circulation 60:998, 1979.

56. KOTLER, MN, TABATZNIK, M, MAWER, M, ET AL: *Prognostic significance of ventricular ectopic beats with respect to sudden death in the late post infarction period.* Circulation 47:959, 1973.

57. SCHULZE, RA, STRAUSS, WH, AND PITT, B: *Sudden death in the year following myocardial infarction: Relation to ventricular premature contractions in the late hospital phase and left ventricular ejection fraction.* Am J Med 52:190, 1977.

58. HAN, J AND GOEL, BG: *Electrophysiologic precursors of ventricular tachyarrhythmias.* Arch Intern Med 129:749, 1977.

59. WINKLE, RA: *The relationship between ventricular ectopic beat frequency and heart rate.* Circulation 66:439, 1982.

60. EL-SHERIF, N, MYERBURG, RJ, SCHERLAG, BJ, ET AL: *Electrocardiographic antecedents of primary ventricular fibrillation: Value of the R-on-T phenomenon in myocardial infarction.* Br Heart J 38:415, 1976.

61. DHURANDHAR, R, MACMILLAN, R, AND BROWN, K: *Primary ventricular fibrillation complicating acute myocardial infarction.* Am J Cardiol 27:347, 1971.

62. KAY, GN, PLUMB, VJ, ARCINIEGAS, JG, ET AL: *Torsade de pointes: The long-short initiating sequence and other clinical features: Observations in 32 patients.* J Am Coll Cardiol 2:806, 1983.

63. HOROWITZ, LN, GREENSPAN, AM, SPIELMAN, SR, ET AL: *Torsades de pointes: Electrophysiologic studies in patients without transient pharmacologic or metabolic abnormalities.* Circulation 63:1120, 1981.

64. VELEBIT, V, PODRID, P, LOWN, B, ET AL: *Aggravation and provocation of ventricular arrhythmias by antiarrhythmic drugs.* Circulation 65:886, 1982.

65. RUSKIN, JN, MCGOVERN, B, GARAN, H, ET AL: *Antiarrhythmic drugs: A possible cause of out-of-hospital cardiac arrest.* N Engl J Med, 309:1302, 1983.

66. MORGANROTH, J: *Optimal use of long-term ambulatory electrocardiographic monitoring.* Cardiovasc Review and Reports 2:333, 1981.

67. HOROWITZ, LN AND MORGANROTH, J: *Can we prevent sudden cardiac death?* Am J Cardiol 50:535, 1982.

68. GRABOYS, TB, LOWN, B, PODRID, PJ, ET AL: *Long-term survival of patients with malignant ventricular arrhythmia treated with antiarrhythmic drugs.* Am J Cardiol 50:437, 1982.

69. ROY, D, WAXMAN, HL, KIENZLE, MG, ET AL: *Clinical characteristics and long-term follow-up in 119 survivors of cardiac arrest: Relation to inducibility at electrophysiologic testing.* Am J Cardiol 52:969, 1983.

70. RUSKIN, JN, DIMARCO, JP, AND, GARAN, H: *Out-of-hospital cardiac arrest: Electrophysiologic observations and selection of long-term antiarrhythmic therapy.* N Engl J Med 303:607, 1980.

# Epidemiology of Sudden Death:
# Insights from the Framingham Study*

*William B. Kannel, M.D., and Daniel L. McGee, Ph.D.*

Because sudden death is such a common feature of coronary disease, there is a growing interest in obtaining further insights into the way it evolves, both in the general population and in persons with clinically overt coronary heart disease. If preventive measures are to be devised, continued research is needed to further delineate the segment of the general population at especially high risk of sudden death and the pathogenetic mechanism(s) that precipitate the catastrophe.

The purpose of this chapter is to examine the way sudden coronary deaths evolve in a general population, to delineate those who are at high risk of sudden death, and to determine potentially modifiable predisposing factors. This will be done based on 26 years of followup of the Framingham Study cohort for development of coronary heart disease (CHD) including sudden death.

## The Framingham Study Sample

The cohort under observation is comprised of 5209 men and women aged 30 to 62 years on entry to the study. New CHD events were monitored at biennial intervals by re-examination, daily monitoring of hospitalizations in the only hospital in town, information from personal physicians, medical examiner reports, and death certificates. The circumstances surrounding each death were carefully ascertained from the medical examiners' reports, hospital records, death certificates, and interviews with the decedents' spouses and personal physicians.

At each routine biennial examination, information was routinely collected on lifestyles and personal attributes suspected of possibly being related to development of coronary heart disease. Information was included on coffee and cigarette use, physical activity, and diet, among others. Possible atherogenic traits examined included blood lipids, blood pressure, and blood glucose. Evidence of a possibly compromised coronary circulation was sought by electrocardiographic examination. Susceptibility to these influences was assessed by determining the family history for premature development of cardiovascular disease.

The sampling procedure, laboratory methods, specific criteria for disease endpoints, response rates, and completeness of followup have been published elsewhere.[1,2]

The experience from ambulatory and coronary care unit (CCU) monitoring indicates that the underlying mechanism in most sudden deaths is ventricular fibrillation.[3] How often this arrhythmia occurs in the course of an evolving myocardial infarction or a reversible ischemic episode is not clear. Data from patients resuscitated from cardiac arrest suggests that less

*Supported in part by contracts numbers NIH-NO1-HV-92922 and NIH-NO1-HV-52971.

than one third of cardiac arrests occurs in evolving myocardial infarctions, but this may only apply to resuscitatable events.[4] It is also not clear how often the pathogenesis of sudden death involves an acute coronary occlusion, severe stenosis without thrombus, or coronary artery spasm.

The linkage of sudden deaths to coronary artery disease is largely by inference, inasmuch as few other diseases can kill in a matter of minutes. Etiologic relationship to coronary disease is assumed when aortic dissection, ruptured aneurysm, and pulmonary embolism are excluded clinically or on postmortem examination. Thus, death within minutes in persons not ill at the time with a potentially lethal illness permits classification as *coronary* sudden deaths with reasonable certainty. However, the 24-hour definition advocated by the World Health Organization (WHO) is less specific.[2]

**Statistical Analysis**

Two types of analyses are presented in this report. In the first, subjects were classified according to level of suspected cardiovascular risk factors over the first four biennial examinations and those free of clinical evidence of CHD placed at risk of sudden death over the remaining 20 years of followup. For continuous variables, the average value of the four initial biennial examinations was used to place the subjects at risk. For discrete variables, the occurrence of the variable on any one examination was used. The second analysis involved a pooled cross-sectional approach. In this analysis, each individual is placed at risk according to his or her characteristics and each examination—this characterization being considered a single observation. A single individual may thus contribute multiple observations to the analysis.

For continuous variables, the logistic model was used to relate the level of a characteristic to the risk of sudden death. Coefficients of the logistic model were estimated using an iterative maximum likelihood approach.[5] For dichotomous variables, summary relative odds were calculated and the significance for departure from unity tested using the methods of Mantel-

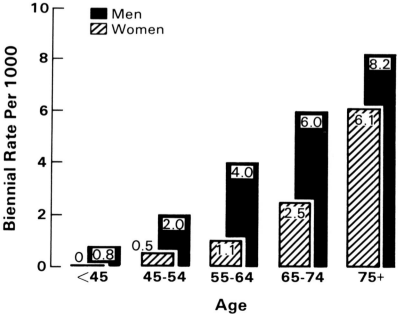

**Figure 1.** Incidence of sudden death by age and sex in persons free of coronary heart disease, 26-year followup, Framingham Study.

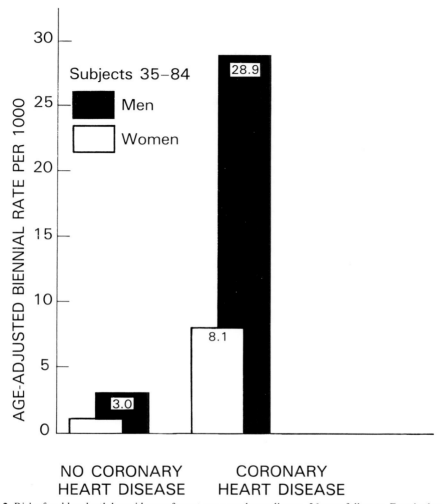

**Figure 2.** Risk of sudden death by evidence of overt coronary heart disease, 26-year followup, Framingham Study.

Haenszel.[6] All multivariate analyses were performed using the logistic model. Wherever age-adjusted rates are presented, they were calculated by the direct method using the sex-specific total population age distribution as the standard population.

## RESULTS

### Incidence

The incidence of sudden death increased steadily with age, with women lagging men in incidence by 20 years. Overall, sudden death incidence in women is only one third that in men (Fig. 1).

Among persons with known CHD, sudden deaths occur at about nine times the rate of those at the same age and free of overt coronary heart disease (Fig. 2). The excess risk of sudden death following a myocardial infarction or angina pectoris is comparable. Only half of sudden death victims have prior overt CHD, and half the annual toll of CHD mortality occurs suddenly.

## Atherogenic Cardiovascular Risk Factors

For descriptive purposes, 20-year age-adjusted rates are presented, by tertile of some continuous variables and also according to the presence of some dichotomous characteristics.

### Hypertension

Elevated blood pressure is a powerful independent predisposing factor for all clinical manifestations of CHD. This is true whether the systolic or the diastolic pressure is elevated and also whether the hypertension is labile or fixed. An excess risk can be demonstrated in elderly as well as in young persons and in women as well as men.

For sudden death in particular, the same relationship holds true (Table 1). Risk of sudden death in the Framingham cohort increased with the level of both systolic and diastolic pressures. There was no indication of a stronger relationship to diastolic than systolic pressure. Even a mild degree of hypertension doubled the risk of sudden death. Use of antihypertensive medications was also associated with higher rates of sudden death. This in all likelihood reflects higher pretreatment blood pressures. The impact of hypertension on sudden death incidence is no greater than on CHD in general (Fig. 3), and the fraction of CHD deaths that are sudden is no greater in hypertensive than normotensive persons.[2]

### Cholesterol

The serum total cholesterol is not as strongly related to sudden death incidence as it is to other clinical manifestations of coronary disease. The reason for this is unclear. In men, no significant relationship was noted in the Framingham Study (Table 2). In women, however, there is a distinct trend to higher incidence proportional to cholesterol level. Recent evidence indicates that the serum total cholesterol is related to CHD incidence because of its correlation with the atherogenic LDL-cholesterol fraction. The HDL-cholesterol component, however, is inversely related to CHD incidence.[7] Hence, it is possible that when data on cholesterol fractionated into these components becomes available for sudden death, the lipid–sudden death relationship may be clarified.

### Glucose Intolerance

Diabetes doubles the risk of atherosclerotic cardiovascular mortality. Its impact is greater in women than men, tends to diminish with advancing age, and varies substantially with the level of coexistent risk factors.[8] The cardiovascular risk is not entirely explicable in terms of the major cardiovascular risk factors. The morbid impact of diabetes is greatest for peripheral

**Table 1.** Risk of sudden death by blood pressure status over four biennial examinations, 26-year followup, subjects aged 35 to 84, Framingham Study

| Tertile of pressure distribution | 20-year age-adjusted rate per 1000 | | | |
| | Systolic pressure | | Diastolic pressure | |
| | Men* | Women† | Men* | Women |
|---|---|---|---|---|
| Low | 25.4 | 4.1 | 34.1 | 10.2 |
| Middle | 39.6 | 14.9 | 40.1 | 13.0 |
| High | 67.6 | 16.8 | 59.8 | 19.3 |

*p < .001
†p < .05

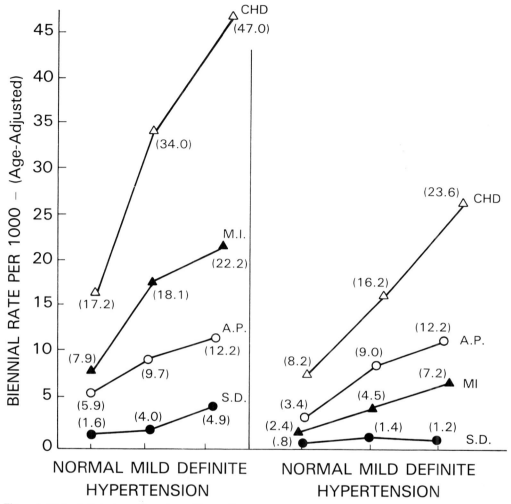

**Figure 3.** Risk of clinical manifestations of heart disease by hypertensive status at each biennial examination, 26-year followup, subjects aged 35 to 84, Framingham Study.

**Table 2.** Risk of sudden death by specified risk factors, 26-year followup, subjects aged 35 to 84, Framingham Study

| | 20-year age-adjusted rate per 1000 | | | | | |
|---|---|---|---|---|---|---|
| | Relative weight | | Serum cholesterol | | Heart rate | |
| Tertile of distribution‡ | Men* | Women | Men | Women† | Men† | Women |
| Low | 27 | 7 | 35 | 1 | 39 | 16 |
| Middle | 46 | 13 | 52 | 11 | 36 | 13 |
| High | 65 | 22 | 44 | 23 | 65 | 15 |

*P < .001
†P < .05
‡Av. over first 4 exams.

**Table 3.** Risk of sudden death by diabetic status, 26-year followup, subjects aged 35 to 84, Framingham Study

| Abnormality | 20-year age-adjusted rate per 1000 | | | |
| | Diabetic status* | | Glucosuria status† | |
| | Men | Women‡ | Men‡ | Women‡ |
|---|---|---|---|---|
| Absent | 45.6 | 13.6 | 30 | 10 |
| Present | 50.7 | 43.9 | 89 | 118 |

*First 4 exams
†Each biennial exam
‡P < .01

arterial disease, although coronary disease is still the most frequent sequela. Diabetes also directly damages the myocardium, thereby predisposing to cardiac failure.[8] The unique contribution of diabetes to atherogenesis may derive from its effects on blood clotting including diminished fibrinolytic activity or increased fibrinogen and factors VII or VIII.[9]

In the Framingham cohort, glucose intolerance or overt diabetes was associated with an increased risk of sudden death only in women (Table 3), although glucosuria was associated with increased occurrence of sudden death in both sexes. However, even the association of glucosuria and increased risk of sudden death was more pronounced in women than men.

## Hematocrit

There appears to be an excess of coronary heart disease in general and sudden death in particular in persons at the upper end of the normal distribution of hematocrit in the general population (Table 4). To a great extent, this relationship appears to derive from the greater prevalence of hypertension found in persons with high normal hematocrit values.

### Living Habits

## Exercise

It is suspected that the transformation of man by modern technology from a physically active agrarian person to a more sedentary industrial person has exacted a penalty in ill health. Most attention has been focused on possible cardiovascular consequences. Physical activity is believed to be important because it affects the operating efficiency of the cardiovascular system and because it influences the level of the major risk factors. However, evidence on both these points is incomplete.

**Table 4.** Risk of sudden death by hematocrit, 26-year followup, subjects aged 35 to 84, Framingham Study

| Tertile of hematocrit distribution | 20-year age-adjusted rate per 1000 | |
| | Men* | Women |
|---|---|---|
| Low | 37.4 | 11.5 |
| Middle | 35.1 | 18.9 |
| High | 65.9 | 22.3 |

*p < .05

Nevertheless, despite inherent self-selection of leisure activity and physically active jobs, and difficulties in quantitating physical activity, epidemiologic evidence strongly suggests that endurance exercise protects against coronary heart disease.[10,11] Thus far, the evidence suggests that the protection is confined to men and is modest compared with the major cardiovascular risk factors, but appears to persist even when these are taken into account.[11] The protection in men can be demonstrated into advanced age.[11]

Whereas the protection against coronary mortality in general has been demonstrated, the role of physical activity in sudden death specifically is more speculative. The Harvard College Alumni Study found no relationship of execise to sudden death.[12] Friedman and coworkers,[3] who found that most sudden death victims had a Type A time-urgent personality, also noted that a significant number of the victims had engaged in moderate or strenuous exercise shortly before collapsing. However, Siscovick and associates[13] concluded that vigorous exercise may be protective against sudden coronary death related to primary cardiac arrest, although the data were retrospective.

The data fall short of either proving or disproving that a high level of exercise is of benefit in reducing the risk of sudden death. Sound recommendations to indulge in more vigorous exercise for the purpose of avoiding sudden coronary death must await controlled trial evidence. To date, such data have been inconclusive owing to a high drop-out rate and difficulty in maintaining comparability with respect to other risk factors.

## Cigarette Smoking

Deaths from CHD related to cigarette smoking exceed those from lung cancer by a factor of three. Sizable excess risks have been noted for myocardial infarction, sudden death, and peripheral arterial disease.[14] Cigarette smoking transiently enhances the adhesiveness of platelets, raises the blood pressure, accelerates the heart rate, and lowers the ventricular fibrillation threshold of the heart. Additionally, the oxygen-carrying capacity of the blood is compromised by a buildup of carboxyhemoglobin, while tissue utilization of oxygen by myoglobin is impaired. These effects coupled with an acute rise in catecholamines could precipitate a myocardial infarction or sudden death in persons with a compromised coronary circulation.

In the Framingham Study, sudden death was strongly related to cigarette smoking in men but not in women, when examined in relation to cigarette smoking at *each biennial examination*. When analyzed in relation to cigarette smoking at the first four examinations, there was no significant relationship (Table 5). This finding very likely is a reflection of the fact that many cigarette smokers have quit the habit in recent years.[14] The effect of cigarette smoking appears to be transient, noncumulative, and reversible. Those who quit smoking in the Framingham Study promptly reverted to a risk only half that of those who continued to smoke, irrespective of the duration of their prior cigarette smoking.[14]

**Table 5.** Risk of sudden death by cigarette smoking status, 26-year followup, subjects aged 35 to 84, Framingham Study

| Cigarette smoking status | 20-year age-adjusted rate per 1000 | | | |
| --- | --- | --- | --- | --- |
| | Each exam | | First 4 exams | |
| | Men* | Women | Men | Women |
| Nonsmoker | 18 | 11 | 39 | 14 |
| Smoker | 41 | 11 | 48 | 14 |

*Difference significant at p < .001 level

## Obesity

Obesity is associated with an excessive occurrence of CHD, largely as a consequence of its association with atherogenic risk factors.[15–17] Because of its great prevalence in the United States and its adverse metabolic and physiologic concomitants, obesity is a powerful contributor to cardiovascular morbidity and mortality. Correction of obesity can simultaneously improve hypertension, glucose intolerance, the LDL/HDL ratio, and hyperuricemia, thereby favorably altering the cardiovascular risk profile.

In view of the aforementioned considerations, it is not surprising that obesity is a powerful contributor to sudden death incidence in men. Its impact is as great as that for hypertension (Tables 2 and 6). Risk of sudden death in the Framingham Study increased with the degree of adiposity in both sexes but was significant only for men (see Table 2). Furthermore, the proportion of CHD deaths that are sudden also appears to increase with the degree of overweight.[2]

## Other Considerations

### Heart Rate

Risk of CHD in general and of CHD mortality in particular has been noted to increase with the resting heart rate in men but not in women.[2] Whether this relationship reflects autonomic arousal or physical fitness is not clear. To some extent it could reflect the associated blood pressure with which heart rate is modestly correlated. As for CHD in general, sudden death incidence is greater with increased heart rate in men but not women (see Tables 2 and 6).

### Electrocardiographic Precursors

Persons free of overt CHD may nonetheless have a severely compromised coronary circulation manifested only by electrocardiographic abnormalities. Such asymptomatic coronary disease predisposes to sudden death. According to the Framingham Study data, electrocardiographic evidence of left ventricular hypertrophy (LVH) or intraventricular conduction disturbance is associated with an increased risk of all clinical manifestations of CHD.[18] Risk of sudden death in persons with such ECG abnormalities is increased (Table 6). Nonspecific ST and T wave abnormalities and even sinus tachycardia (see Table 2) appear to double the risk of sudden death.

**Table 6.** Comparison of strength of specified risk factors for sudden death, 26-year followup, subjects aged 35 to 84, Framingham Study

| | Bivariate* standardized logistic coefficients | |
| --- | --- | --- |
| *Average of measurements, exams 1–4* | *Men* | *Women* |
| Systolic pressure | .3468† | .2699‡ |
| Diastolic pressure | .3168† | .1935 |
| Serum cholesterol | .2153 | .4344‡ |
| Relative weight | .3692† | .2833 |
| Hematocrit | .2653‡ | .2964 |
| Heart rate | .2108‡ | −.0668 |

*Other variable in the logistic model is age at exam 4.
†$p < .001$
‡$p < .05$

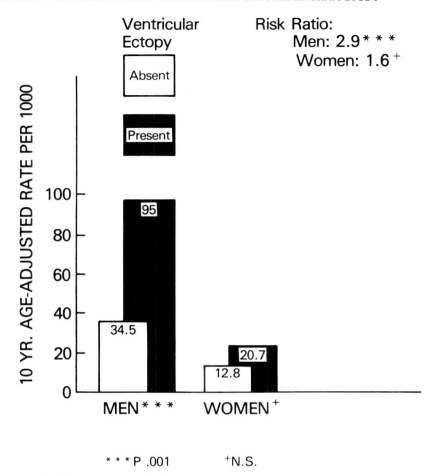

**Figure 4.** Risk of sudden death by ventricular ectopy status (ventricular ectopy at eighth biennial examination), Framingham Study, subjects 42 to 76 years of age.

Ventricular premature beats (VPBs) are widely acknowledged to be precursors of sudden death. In the Framingham Study, VPBs on a routine ECG were associated with an increased risk of sudden death (Fig. 4). However, ECG signs of LVH, intraventricular block, and non-specific ST–T abnormalities all carry as great a risk as ventricular premature beats. Moreover, in sudden death victims, VPBs often coexist with these ECG abnormalities.

In patients with established coronary heart disease, VPBs, tachycardia, ECG signs of LVH or intraventricular block, or persistence of ECG evidence of myocardial infarction are all associated with a substantial further escalation of risk. Frequent or multifocal VPBs on the resting ECG appear to be more specific for sudden death risk in patients with established CHD than in asymptomatic persons. Twice the expected number of CHD deaths occurred in the Coronary Drug Project placebo group that had VPBs as in those without them.[19] This excess risk of deaths included sudden death and was found to be independent of coexistent risk ractors.

Advanced grades of VPBs are often a sign of a diseased myocardium. Such VPBs are found most frequently in patients with ejection fractions less than 40 percent.[20] However, despite the frequent coexistence of coronary artery disease, those patients resuscitated from sudden death sometimes survive for long periods, suggesting that such VPBs do not invariably reflect extensive myocardial damage. Nonetheless, 30 percent of patients who experience primary ventricular fibrillation can expect a recurrence within 1 year.[21]

### Multivariate Risk Profiles

By incorporating risk factors into a multivariate logistic formulation. it is possible to arrive at a composite estimate of risk for the constellation of risk factors. Using the indicated set of variables, it is evident that risk varies over a wide range in relation to the multivariate risk (Fig. 5). About 42 percent of the sudden deaths in men and 52 percent of those in women arise from the segment of the population in the top decile of multivariate risk. This multivariate technique of combining risk factors has the advantage of including potential candidates at high risk of sudden death, because of multiple marginal abnormalities that would otherwise be overlooked by discrete categoric assessment according to number of "risk factors."

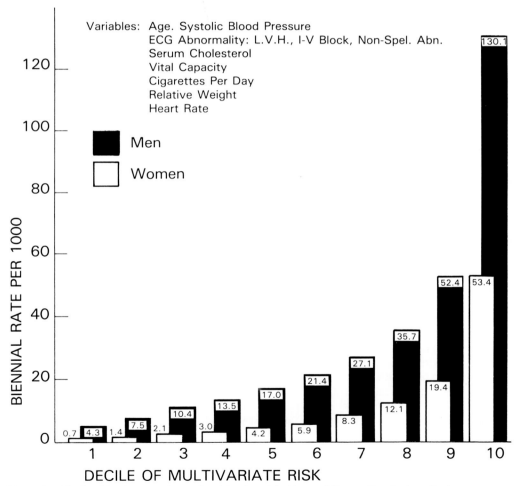

**Figure 5.** Risk of sudden death by decile of multivariate risk, 26-year followup, Framingham Study.

## Risk Factors in Overt CHD

Once overt coronary disease appears, sudden death risk escalates about ninefold. When the disease has reached this advanced stage, the standard atherogenic risk factors measured after onset of CHD no longer appear to have much predictive value. Only ECG abnormalities, arrhythmia, and evidence of poor cardiac function appear to be predictive.

## Clinical Implications

Prospective studies indicate that sudden death victims share most of the major risk factors for CHD. However, none of the factors thus far identified will distinguish sudden death victims from those predisposed to CHD in general. Because the same factors predispose to both conditions, the key to prevention of sudden death would appear to be the reduction of risk of coronary attacks, all of which are potentially lethal. The first prolonged attack of ischemic chest pain carries a 33 percent case fatality rate.

Many of the risk factors for CHD are correctable. It is possible to stop cigarette smoking, to reduce obesity, to lower serum cholesterol by dietary means, to lower elevated blood pressure with drugs or hygienic measures, and to get more exercise. Although rational, evidence that these measures will reduce the incidence of sudden death is meager. Those who quit smoking, however, have been shown to have only half the coronary mortality of those who continue to smoke. Use of beta blockers seems to reduce sudden death rates in high-risk coronary patients. Reduction of obesity has been shown to improve all elements of the cardiovascular risk profile including blood pressure, LDL/HDL cholesterol ratio, glucose tolerance, and uric acid values.[15-17] Unfortunately, no trial evidence exists that this will reduce incidence of sudden death or coronary attack rates.

Control of complex and frequent VPBs by drugs has thus far been disappointing. The association of ventricular premature beats with sudden death seems to apply mainly in persons with an ischemic, irritable myocardium. It may be that the underlying disease must be addressed rather than the VPBs.

Proponents of exercise to prevent CHD usually advocate vigorous, endurance exercise sufficient to produce a training effect. However, few data are available that prospectively test the relation of *physical fitness* to sudden death. Thus far, only physical *exercise* has been extensively examined. Although moderate noncompetitive exercise appears to be safe, sudden deaths have been reported in persons engaged in jogging, marathons, and other vigorous exercise.[3,11-13] Uncertainty prevails about the amount of exercise needed to achieve cardiovascular benefits. Some studies seem to show a substantial amount of protection at less than high-intensity leisure-time activity.[11,12]

Subgroups of convalescent myocardial infarction (MI) patients with a substantial risk of death within the first year can be identified. Those at low risk are usually asymptomatic, and have had a benign acute course, a normal creatinine, a normal post-MI ECG, no tachycardia, a normal exercise ECG prior to discharge, and few VPBs on ambulatory monitoring. They are usually normotensive, without a fall in blood pressure from premorbid values, and show no evidence of cardiac failure. For those at high risk of sudden death and reinfarction based on the aforementioned profile, therapeutic measures such as anticoagulants, platelet inhibitors, antiarrhythmic agents, and particularly beta blockers may be considered.

Attention to the standard CHD risk factors is of greater importance for the recovered MI patient once the early high mortality period has passed. At this point, consideration should be given to long-term preventive management designed to retard further progression of the underlying disease.

Prevention of sudden death requires the prevention of either initial or recurrent coronary attacks. This goal is best accomplished by a comprehensive multifactorial risk factor intervention. No single measure can be relied upon to prevent either coronary attacks or resultant sudden deaths, but for sudden death prevention, major emphasis on weight control and quitting cigarette smoking would seem justified.

## SUMMARY

Sudden death victims share most of the major risk factors for coronary disease in general; and the key to prevention is to reduce the risk of coronary attacks, especially by avoidance of cigarettes, correction of obesity, and reduction of blood pressure. The incidence increases with age, with sudden death incidence in women only a third that in men. By incorporating CHD risk factors into a multivariate logistic formulation, a composite estimate of risk is obtained over a wide range. A severely compromised coronary circulation manifested only by ECG abnormalities carries a high risk of sudden death. VPBs associated with sudden death often occur concurrently with ECG signs of LVH, intraventricular block, and nonspecific ST–T abnormalities. Convalescent MI patients with a low risk of sudden death are usually asymptomatic; have a normal creatinine, normal post-MI ECG, no tachycardia, a normal exercise ECG, few VPBs on monitoring, and normotension; and show no signs of cardiac failure.

## REFERENCES

1. DAWBER, TR, MEADORS, GF, AND MOORE, FE: *Epidemiologic approaches to heart disease: The Framingham Study.* Am J Public Health 41:279, 1951.
2. KANNEL, WB AND THOMAS, HE, JR: *Sudden coronary death: The Framingham Study.* Ann NY Acad Sci 382:3, 1982.
3. FRIEDMAN, M, MANWARING, JH, ROSENMAN, RH, ET AL: *Instantaneous and sudden deaths: Clinical and pathological differentiation in coronary artery disease.* JAMA 225:1319, 1973.
4. BAUM, RS, ALVAREZ, H, AND COBB, LA: *Survival after resuscitation from out-of-hospital ventricular fibrillation.* Circulation 50:1231, 1974.
5. WALKER, SH AND DUNCAN, DB: *Estimation of the probability of an event as a function of several independent variables.* Biometrika 54:167, 1967.
6. MANTEL, N AND HAENSZEL, W: *Statistical aspects of the analysis of data from retrospective studies of disease.* JNCI 22:719, 1959.
7. ABBOTT, RD, GARRISON, RJ, WILSON, PW, ET AL: *Coronary heart disease risk: The importance of joint relationships among cholesterol levels in individual lipoprotein classes.* Prev Med 2:131, 1982.
8. KANNEL, WB AND MCGEE, DL: *Diabetes and glucose tolerance as risk factors for cardiovascular disease: The Framingham Study.* Diabetes Care 2:120, 1979.
9. CHAKABARTI, R AND MEADE, TW: *Clotting factors, platelet function and fibrinolytic activity in diabetics and in a comparison group: WHO Multinational Group.* Diabetologia 12:383, 1976.
10. FROELICHER, VF AND BROWN, P: *Exercise and coronary heart disease.* J Cardiac Rehab 1:277, 1981.
11. KANNEL, WB AND SORLIE, PD: *Some health benefits of physical activity: The Framingham Study.* Arch Intern Med 139:857, 1979.
12. PAFFENBARGER, RS, WING, AL, AND HYDE, RT: *Physical activity as an index of heart attack risk in college alumni.* Am J Epidemiol 108:161, 1978.
13. SISCOVICK, DS, WEISS, NS, HALLSTROM, AP, ET AL: *Physical activity and primary cardiac arrest.* N Engl J Med 248:3113, 1982.
14. KANNEL, WB: *Update on the role of cigarette smoking in coronary heart disease.* Am Heart J 101:319, 1981.
15. GARRISON, RJ, WILSON, PW, CASTELLI, WP, ET AL: *Obesity and lipoprotein cholesterol in the Framingham Offspring Study.* Metabolism 29:1053, 1980.
16. KANNEL, WB, DAWBER, TR, AND MCGEE, DL: *Perspectives on systolic hypertension: The Framingham Study.* Circulation 61:1179, 1980.
17. KANNEL, WB, GORDON, T, AND CASTELLI, WP: *Obesity, lipids and glucose intolerance: The Framingham Study.* Am J Clin Nutr 32:1238, 1979.
18. KANNEL, WB: *Preclinical ECG precursors of cardiovascular disease.* Primary Cardiol 3:27, 1977.

19. CORONARY DRUG PROJECT RESEARCH GROUP: *Factors influencing long-term prognosis after recovery from myocardial infarction—3 year findings of the CDP*. J Chronic Dis 27:267, 1974.

20. CALVERT, A, LOWN, B, AND GORLIN, R: *Ventricular premature beats and anatomically defined coronary disease*. Am J Cardiol 39:627, 1977.

21. MARKIEWICZ, W, HOUSTON, N, AND DEBUSK, RF: *Exercise testing soon after myocardial infarction*. Circulation 56:26, 1978.

22. MULTICENTER INTERNATIONAL STUDY: *Reduction in mortality after myocardial infarction with long-term β-adrenergic blockade*. Br Med J 2:419, 1977.

# Clinical Characteristics of Sudden Death: Implications for Survival*

*Robert J. Myerburg, M.D., Liaqat Zaman, M.D., Richard M. Luceri, M.D., Kenneth M. Kessler, M.D., Daneil Estes, R.N., Richard Trohman, M.D., Joseph Horgan, M.D., and Agustin Castellanos, M.D.*

As recently as 25 years ago, cardiac arrest in any clinical setting was almost uniformly fatal. With the development of the coronary care unit, including continuous monitoring and acute interventions for potentially lethal arrhythmias, most primary cardiac arrests in the hospital setting can be either averted or successfully treated. These arrests occur primarily in patients with acute myocardial ischemia or infarction, but may also occur in other settings such as complex metabolic abnormalities, the postoperative state, and acute toxicities. An even larger population at risk for cardiac arrest occurs in the prehospital setting, however; and it was not until the late 1960s and early 1970s, with the development of community-based emergency rescue systems, that some impact was noted in this realm. During the past 10 years, further progress has been made, to the point now where significant numbers of patients who would have died in the prehospital setting in the recent past are now resuscitated, admitted to the hospital alive, ultimately discharged alive, and continue to live active lives.

## MECHANISMS OF PREHOSPITAL CARDIAC ARREST AND OUTCOME

Prior to the development of community-based emergency medical systems, with remote telemetry systems, there was a tendency to assume that all prehospital cardiac arrests were caused by the electrophysiologic mechanism of ventricular fibrillation and that the underlying etiology was almost always coronary artery disease with acute myocardial infarction. The development of an experience with prehospital cardiac arrest and its survivors modfied some of these thoughts. Prehospital cardiac arrest may occur by the mechanism of ventricular fibrillation, rapid ventricular tachycardia with a low-output state, or bradyarrhythmias or asystole. Though scattered information is available documenting the onset of prehospital cardiac arrest by each of these three mechanisms, the large studies on experiences with prehospital cardiac arrest do not allow us to assess the frequency with which each of these occurred as an *initiating* event. Ventricular tachycardia may degenerate into ventricular fibrillation or to asystole; and bradyarrhythmias may change to ventricular fibrillation. However, some idea may be obtained regarding the relative frequency and their implications from emergency rescue system data. Figure 1 demonstrates the Miami experience from the period 1975 to 1978.[1] Three hundred fifty-two consecutive patients were studied, in whom the onset of prehospital cardiac arrest was witnessed, emergency rescue personnel summoned without delay,

*Supported in part by a grant from the NHLBI, HL 28130, by an NHLBI Research Training Grant, HL 07436 (Drs. Horgan and Trohman), and a grant from the American Heart Association of Greater Miami (Dr. Kessler).

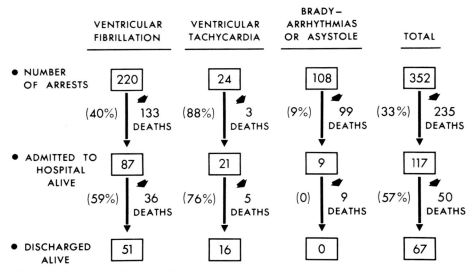

**Figure 1.** Survival patterns related to initial electrophysiologic mechanism recorded during prehospital cardiac arrest. The figures highlighted by the boxes indicate the number of patients in each of three categories—ventricular fibrillation, ventricular tachycardia, and bradyarrhythmia or asystole, plus totals. In each category, the data indicate the number of prehospital cardiac arrests (top), the number of patients successfully resuscitated in the field and transferred to the hospital alive (middle), and the number of patients who survived hospitalization and were discharged (bottom). The percentages in parentheses indicate survival at each level of care for each category. (From Myerburg et al,[1] with permission.)

and arrival at the scene with identification of the rhythm occurred within 4 minutes. Under these conditions, 220 of the 352 patients (62 percent) were in ventricular fibrillation at the time of the initial recording by emergency rescue personnel. Sustained ventricular tachycardia with hypotension was present in 24 of 352 victims (7 percent); and bradyarrhythmias of various types or asystole was present in 108 of 352 (31 percent). That some crossover between groups may occur is suggested by the data from the Seattle group, which showed that in the subgroup in which contact with emergency rescue system personnel is made within the first minute, more than 90 percent of the events are ventricular fibrillation. Regardless, the importance of the distribution of the mechanisms recorded at initial contact relates to the prognostic information contained in the initial mechanism telemetered. As indicated in Figure 1, the best outcome for both initial hospitalization and discharge alive occurs in the smallest group, those who present with ventricular tachycardia and hypotension. Of the 24 patients in this group, 21 were admitted to the hospital alive and 16 (67 percent) were ultimately discharged from the hospital alive. In contrast, the worst prognosis was observed in the bradyarrhythmic group, in which fewer than 10 percent of the patients are successfully resuscitated and admitted to the hospital alive, and the long-term outcome, even for this small group, is dismal. Intermediate between these two extremes is the population with ventricular fibrillation, in which 40 percent of the patients were successfully resuscitated and admitted to the hospital alive, and 51 of 220 (23 percent) were ultimately discharged alive. Subsequent data (see below) have shown continuing improvement in the outcome for ventricular fibrillation patients since 1978.

The importance of bradyarrhythmic events is shown from a different perspective in the data from Nagel and associates.[2] These investigators reported the relationship between the *initial heart rate after resuscitation from prehospital ventricular fibrillation* and early prognosis. Specifically, of those patients who were initially resuscitated from ventricular fibrillation to a bradycardic heart rate (defined as < 60 impulses per min regardless of mechanism),

73 percent died before hospitalization, 22 percent died during hospitalization, and only 5 percent were discharged alive. In contrast, among those who were defibrillated to a tachycardic rate, defined as a heart rate $> 100$ impulses per min, only 17 percent died before hospitalization, 40 percent died during hospitalization, and 43 percent were discharged alive. The figures for those defibrillated to a "normal" heart rate, defined as 60 to 100 impulses per min, were intermediate between the two extremes. Thus, bradycardia takes on an ominous prognostic perspective, not only as a primary event, but also in terms of the implications for a patient resuscitated from ventricular fibrillation to a bradyarrhythmia.

As more experience has been gained, there has been a clearly improving outcome in patients who suffer prehospital ventricular fibrillation and are promptly responded to by emergency medical rescue personnel. Comparing the experience in Miami from 1971 to 1973[3] with that from 1975 to 1978[1] (Fig. 2), the outcome in the earlier period was an overall rate of discharge alive of 14 percent, whereas in the later period the rate had improved to 23 percent ($p < .01$). These data are very similar to the outcome during the same time period in the Seattle, Washington, program,[4,5] in which the early survival rate during the early 1970s was less than 10 percent and improved to better than 25 percent by the end of the 1970s. Cur-

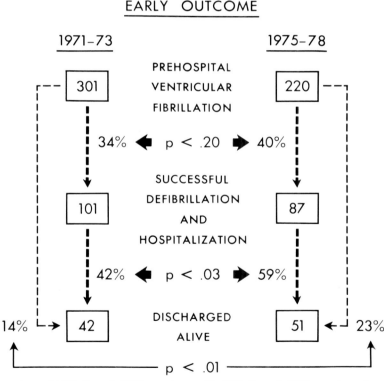

Figure 2. Comparison of 1971 through 1973 experience with 1975 through 1978 experience for early outcome. The difference between the two time periods for successful initial defibrillation and hospitalization was not significant, although the number of successful events was higher in the 1975 to 1978 period (40 percent versus 34 percent). Of those patients who reached the hospital alive, there was a significantly improved chance ($p < 0.03$) of being discharged alive in the 1975 to 1978 period. In addition, the overall chance for a prehospital ventricular fibrillation victim to be resuscitated, and later discharged form the hospital alive, had significantly improved (14 percent in 1971 to 1973 versus 23 percent in 1975 to 1978, $p < 0.01$). (From Myerburg et al,[1] with permission.)

rently, both Seattle and Miami are reporting long-term survival rates in the range of 30 to 35 percent for patients who have prehospital ventricular fibrillation with prompt community-based interventions.

## FACTORS THAT MAY BE IMPROVING SURVIVAL
## AFTER PREHOSPITAL CARDIAC ARREST

Activities in two different arenas may be influencing the early outcome in patients who suffer prehospital cardiac arrest and are responded to by emergency medical rescue systems. The first of these are the field activities themselves, and the second is the improvement of care once a resuscitated patient has arrived at the hospital. With regard to changes in pre-hospital events, two factors seem to stand out as major contributions to improving outcome. Eisenberg and coworkers[6] have reported data suggesting that immediate defibrillation significantly improves immediate and intermediate outcome. These investigators compared outcome during periods of time when emergency medical technicians were allowed to do only standard cardiopulmonary resuscitation (CPR), with defibrillation being delayed until arrival at a hospital emergency room, with settings in which the emergency medical technicians were trained and allowed to defibrillate at the scene of prehospital cardiac arrest. Their data demonstrate that only 23 percent of victims with prehospital ventricular fibrillation were successfully resuscitated and admitted to the hospital alive when standard CPR alone was used, whereas 53 percent (p < .05) were successfully admitted to the hospital alive when immediate defibrillation was carried out by the emergency medical technicians. Similarly, only 7 percent of the total population were subsequently discharged from the hospital alive after initial management by standard CPR techniques, in contrast to 26 percent (p < .05) when immediate defibrillation preceded transport to the hospital. Thus, early defibrillation appears to be influencing both the proportion of the patients arriving at the hospital alive, and the proportion in the hospital who are ultimately discharged alive. This factor may have a significant impact upon the improving outcome figures.

Bystander cardiopulmonary resuscitation by lay persons in the community is the second field factor that may be influencing outcome. Thompson and coworkers[7] reported observations on prehospital cardiac arrest victims, with and without bystander CPR, and demonstrated that there was no difference in the percentage of patients resuscitated at the scene and admitted alive (61 percent without and 67 percent with bystander CPR, Fig. 3); but those who had had bystander CPR had a 43 percent chance of surviving hospitalization and being discharged alive, in contrast to a 22 percent chance of being discharged alive among those patients who had not had bystander CPR (p < .001). The reasons for the improved outcome in those patients who had received bystander intervention appear to relate to protection of the central nervous system by this procedure. In the same study, Thompson and coworkers reported that only 6 percent of the patients without bystander intervention were conscious on admission to the hospital, and 9 percent had regained consciousness by the end of the first hospital day; 52 percent eventually regained consciousness. In contrast, 50 percent of the patients who had had bystander intervention were conscious on admission, 61 percent had regained consciousness by the end of the first hospital day, and 81 percent eventually regained consciousness. The differences were statistically significant in all three time periods, and suggest that bystander CPR does indeed protect the central nervous system from ischemic injury during cardiac arrest prior to arrival of emergency medical rescue personnel. The importance of this short-term protection of the central nervous system is further reflected in the *mechanisms of in-hospital death* that occur in patients who have been resuscitated from their cardiac arrhythmia but died during hospitalization. In the experience in Miami, of 48 in-hospital deaths in which adequate information is available, only 5 of the deaths (10 percent) were due to recurrent lethal arryhthmias, and 15 of the deaths (31 percent) were due to low-output states. The remaining 28 deaths (59 percent) were due to anoxic encephalopathy itself (18 deaths) or to infections in patients who had been respirator-dependent for long periods of

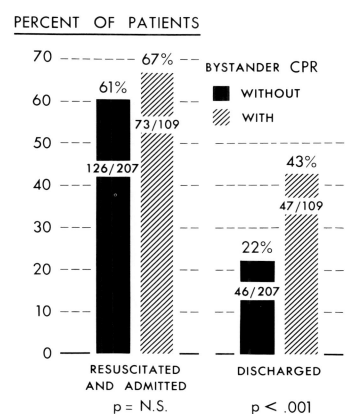

**Figure 3.** Influence of bystander cardiopulmonary resuscitation (CPR) on outcome. Of a total 319 emergency medical system (EMS) interventions, bystander CPR before arrival of EMS personnel had not been initiated in 207 events and had been initiated in 109. Solid bars represent events without bystander CPR; cross-hatched bars, those with bystander CPR. Bystander intervention had no significant influence on immediate resuscitation in the field, but did significantly improve chances of ultimate discharge from hospital. (Modified from Thompson et al.[7] From Myerburg et al,[22] with permission.)

time (10 deaths). Thus, the majority of deaths that occur in hospital after resuscitation from prehospital cardiac arrest occur as a direct or indirect consequence of central nervous system injury that occurs during the cardiac arrest; and thus it follows that any prehospital intervention that will tend to protect the central nervous system will improve in-hospital survival. The Thompson data[7] emphasize this point as well, demonstrating a low incidence of arrhythmic deaths in both the bystander CPR group and the group without bystander CPR, but a 50 percent reduction in deaths related to anoxic coma in the patients who had recieved bystander CPR. Thus, two factors that occur in the field seem to be exerting a beneficial effect on outcome in survivors of prehospital cardiac arrest. These include higher level of training of emergency medical technicians so that they are able to carry out immediate defibrillation, and community education programs targeted to teaching the lay population how to perform cardiopulmonary resuscitation in the event of a prehospital cardiac arrest.

## RECURRENT CARDIAC ARREST IN HOSPITAL

Recurrent cardiac arrest in hospital in survivors of prehospital cardiac arrest has been reported to have a high mortality.[2,8] We have subsequently observed that this is a relatively infrequent occurrence; but, when it does occur, it does indeed have a substantial (50 percent) mortality.[1] Of particular interest is a unique subpopulation that appears to be at risk for recurrent ventricular fibrillation in hospital. Figure 4 demonstrates our experience with 53 prehospital cardiac arrest victims who had been successfully resuscitated and hospitalized. After excluding 11 early hemodynamic deaths, 38 of 42 remaining patients had complex ventricular arrhythmias that did not respond to standard antiarrhythmic therapy, and 4 patients had infrequent ventricular ectopy. Ten of 11 recurrent cardiac arrests during hospitalization occurred among the 38 patients with complex ventricular arrhythmias, but the characteristics of the arrhythmias, their response to therapy, or their frequency did not discriminate the 10 who had recurrent cardiac arrests from the 28 who did not. Only one factor

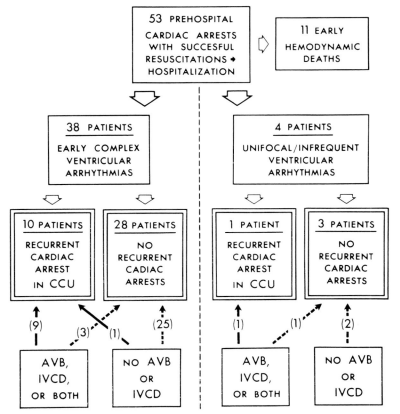

**Figure 4.** Relationship between early ventricular arrhythmias, conduction disturbances and recurrent ventricular fibrillation. Fifty-three consecutive patients had 72 hours of continuous Holter monitor recordings during early hospitalization after successful resuscitation in the field. Eleven of the 52 patients were never stabilized hemodynamically and died of low-output states. Of the remaining 42 patients, 38 had complex ventricular ectopic activity that was incompletely responsive to antiarrhythmic therapy during the early phase of hospitalization. In this subgroup, 10 patients had recurrent cardiac arrest (five of whom died) during the early phase of hospitalization. Among these same 38 patients, 12 patients had atrioventricular block, intraventricular conduction disturbances, or both, at the time of admission to the coronary care unit (CCU) or evolving during the first 72 hours. Nine of the 12 were among the 10 patients who had recurrent cardiac arrests in the CCU, and 25 of those without atrioventricular block or intraventricular conduction disturbances were among the 28 who did not have recurrent cardiac arrests. The severity of rhythm disturbances and their response to antiarrhythmic therapy were not different among those who did or did not have recurrent cardiac arrests. Hemodynamic and etiologic characteristics were similar. All recurrent cardiac arrests occurred by the mechanism of ventricular fibrillation, despite the relationship between atrioventricular block/intraventricular conduction defect and recurrent cardiac arrest (p < 0.001), and the absence of a relationship between the frequency or complexity of arrhythmias and recurrent ventricular fibrillation (p = NS). (From Myerburg et al,[1] with permission.)

112

appeared to discriminate between the two groups: the presence or absence of transient or permanent AV block or intraventricular conduction disturbances, or both. Specifically, of 12 patients who had AV block or intraventricular conduction disturbances, 9 developed recurrent cardiac arrest during hospitalization, and 3 did not. Only 1 of 10 recurrent cardiac arrests occurred in patients without AV block or intraventricular conduction disturbances. Furthermore, AV block was also present in the one patient who had recurrent cardiac arrest among the four patients without complex arrhythmias. Thus, the most sensitive and specific predictor of recurrent cardiac arrest in this patient population was the presence of conducting system abnormalities; but it is fascinating that the mechanism of arrest itself was not related directly to consequences of conduction abnormalities (i.e., bradyarrhythmias) but rather to recurrent ventricular fibrillation. The reason for the interaction between conduction disturbances and recurrent ventricular fibrillation remains unknown, but is reminiscent of a similar relationship in patients with acute anteroseptal myocardial infarction, bundle branch block, and late hospital ventricular fibrillation.[9]

## ETIOLOGY, CARDIAC ANATOMY, AND HEMODYNAMICS IN SURVIVORS OF PREHOSPITAL CARDIAC ARREST

Coronary artery disease is the most common etiologic factor underlying prehospital cardiac arrest. In our group of 117 survivors of prehospital cardiac arrest, in whom complete anatomic studies were available, 79 percent had coronary artery disease as the underlying etiology.[1] Among this group, acute myocardial *necrosis* had occurred at the time of cardiac arrest in 28 percent, but acute *transmural myocardial infarction* as a precipitating event occurred in only 20 percent of this subgroup (see below). Of the remaining survivors of prehospital cardiac arrest in our study, congestive cardiomyopathies were present in 10 percent of the patients. Conducting system disorders were identified in 7 percent of the patients, but these usually coexisted with other etiologic factors, and it was not possible to determine whether the conducting system disease or the other etiologic factor was the primary factor responsible for prehospital cardiac arrest. Valvular heart disease and hypertensive heart disease each were present in 5 percent of the population, and various other etiologies accounted for the remainder of the population. Only one patient in our study had no identifiable structural or functional abnormalities, and only one of the valvular heart disease patients had mitral valve prolapse.

We observed no unique coronary anatomic features in our survivors of prehospital cardiac arrest that would provide predictive value of prospective identification of long-term risk. Both the extent and distribution of coronary artery disease in this subgroup of the population were what would be expected in any general population of atherosclerotic heart disease patients with other clinical manifestations of their underlying disease. Nine percent of the patients had left main coronary disease, and the coronary lesions were otherwise equally distributed among the left anterior descending, circumflex, and right coronary arteries.[1] In terms of extent of disease, the majority of patients had two- or three-vessel disease, with only 13 percent of the patients having single-vessel disease. Discrete left ventricular aneurysms were present in 13 percent of the population studied; single or multiple segmental wall motion abnormalities were present in 40 percent of the population; and diffuse hypokinesis of the left ventricle was present in 33 percent of the population. The hemodynamic profile, however, was somewhat better than expected. Because many studies of risk of sudden death suggest that left ventricular dysfunction is a very powerful, if not the most powerful, risk factor, we expected a population of survivors of prehospital cardiac arrest to have very severe left ventricular functional abnormalities. In fact, more than 50 percent of the patients (see Fig. 5) had normal or near-normal indices of left ventricular function, including left ventricular end-diastolic pressure, cardiac index, and ejection fraction. This is consistent with similar data from Seattle.[10] Those with abnormal left ventricular function showed a distinct spectrum of

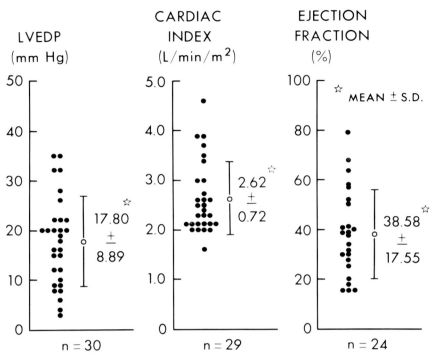

**Figure 5.** Hemodynamic data from 30 prehospital cardiac arrest victims studied during the initial hospitalization. These data indicate a broad range of cardiac function, with approximately one third of the group having normal or near-normal left ventricular function. (From Myerburg et al,[1] with permission.)

disease ranging from only mild dysfunction to severe left ventricular dysfunction. Thus, long-term survivors of prehospital cardiac arrest do not distinguish themselves as a group by the occurrence of extraordinarily poor left ventricular function, but the risk for long-term survival within the group may be considerably worse in that subgroup with significant left ventricular dysfunction. Finally, one must not confuse cardiac dysfunction rates in long-term survivors with the overall findings in the primary study group. Thirty-one percent of the early deaths in patients initially resuscitated were due to low-output states,[1] and these events are not included in the group of long-term survivors.

## ACUTE MYOCARDIAL INFARCTION: PRECIPITATING EVENT OR CONSEQUENCE?

Cobb and coworkers[11] have emphasized the importance of distinguishing whether or not acute transmural myocardial infarction is the precipitating event for prehospital cardiac arrest, for determining long-term prognosis. There are no true natural history studies available on the long-term consequences of prehospital cardiac arrest, inasmuch as all of the early studies had a variety of long-term interventions in their populations after a successful initial outcome.[3,5,8] Despite this, some reasonable assumptions can be derived from the early data. Both the Miami group[3] and the Seattle group[5] identified a 1-year recurrent cardiac arrest rate of approximately 30 percent in survivors of prehospital ventricular fibrillation, and a risk of 45 percent at 2 years. Cobb then analyzed the data according to the presence or absence of new transmural myocardial infarction at the time of prehospital cardiac arrest,[11] and pointed out that the presence of new Q waves on the electrocardiogram identified a patient population with a considerably lower 1- and 2-year cardiac arrest risk than the overall population. He also pointed out, later confirmed in our studies, that only about 20 percent of prehospital cardiac arrest survivors will have sufficient data to label them as primarily acute myocardial infarction with ventricular tachycardia or fibrillation secondary to that event, rather than the reverse. The patients who had prehospital cardiac arrest without evidence of acute transmural myocardial infarction constitute the very high-risk group (about 35 percent 1-year sudden death; about 50 percent 2 years), according to the early life table studies, and, therefore, it is important to take a conservative approach to distinguishing between those patients in whom myocardial infarction was primary, versus those in whom it may have been secondary to the cardiac arrest. For purposes of estimating future risk, we assume that patients who have *(1) a history compatible with cardiac pain prior to the onset of cardiac arrest, (2) new Q waves on the electrocardiogram, and (3) appropriate enzyme elevations* did in fact have ventricular fibrillation secondary to an acute myocardial infarction, and therefore, fall into a low risk group. They are no different than any group of acute myocardial infarction patients with early primary ventricular fibrillation, and should be evaluated and managed accordingly. In contrast, those patients in whom the history suggests that the potentially lethal arrhythmia is the primary event, or those patients in whom it is impossible to distinguish, are considered to be in the high-risk group, that is, cardiac arrest without myocardial infarction or with secondary myocardial infarction. This distinction is important because during long-term management for patient survival, it is better to err on the side of having a few extra low-risk patients added in with the high-risk group, rather than the converse. Patients who have not had an acute transmural myocardial infarction as the precipitating event must be treated as though they are at continuing risk for recurrent cardiac arrest, which involves intensive electrophysiologic evaluation and appropriate management.

## ELECTROPHYSIOLOGIC EVALUATION OF RISK IN SURVIVORS OF PREHOSPITAL CARDIAC ARREST AND APPROACHES TO THERAPY

Frequent and complex forms of ventricular arrhythmias have been demonstrated in > 75 percent of survivors of prehospital cardiac arrest.[12] As in other clinical settings, there is marked inter-patient and intrapatient variability in both frequency and complexity of arrhythmias on serial 24-hour tapes, such variability occuring both with and without drug therapy. Attempts to quantitatively suppress chronic premature ventricular contractions in these patients is usually unsuccessful,[13,14] although some advanced forms of these arrhythmias, specifically Lown Class 4-B (salvos) and Class 5 (R-on-T), may be selectively suppressed. Suppression of these forms may provide important predictive information regarding protection against recurrent cardiac arrest.[14,15] In contrast to claims for specific form suppression, overall frequency of premature ventricular contractions (PVCs) while on drug therapy has not proved useful in distinguishing patients who will or will not have recurrent prehospital cardiac arrest,[12,15] even though epidemiologic studies suggest that PVC frequency greater than an average of 10 ectopic beats per hour does constitute an increased risk. We have proposed the hypothesis that PVC suppression by antiarrhythmic drugs does not necessarily equate with protection against ventricular tachycardia or fibrillation.[16]

Invasive electrophysiologic studies, using programmed stimulation, for the purpose of identifying risk of recurrent cardiac arrest in survivors of prehospital cardiac arrest, have received considerable attention recently. This approach evolved from the application of this procedure to patients with recurrent ventricular tachycardia, in whom it has been demonstrated that the ability to induce the clinical arrhythmia in the electrophysiology laboratory, and then to prevent its induction with a specific drug protocol, correlates well with long-term success of therapy.[17,18] Subsequent application of this procedure to survivors of prehospital cardiac arrest carried with it the hope that it would be useful in identifying the specific subgroups of patients at risk, and at the same time would be a useful guide to therapy. The results have been somewhat controversial to date, although the procedure appears useful within certain limits. According to Ruskin,[19] approximately 30 percent of survivors of prehospital cardiac arrest who undergo programmed stimulation studies are inducible into sustained ventricular tachycardia or ventricular fibrillation; an additional 40 percent are inducible into nonsustained forms of ventricular arrhythmias; and 30 percent are noninducible. Most investigators accept the suggestion that inducibility into ventricular fibrillation or sustained ventricular tachycardia is a marker for risk, and that therapy that has been shown to be successful in preventing induction of these arrhythmias indicates protection against spontaneous clinical recurrences.[20,21] The disputes occur in regard to patients who are inducible only into nonsustained forms, particularly with very aggressive pacing protocols, and those who are noninducible. Some data suggest that noninducibility in these patients indicates absence of risk for recurrent events,[20] but this interpretation is not uniformly accepted. At the present time, we believe that the issue has not yet been definitively settled, and that it should be assumed, based on data from our studies,[1] that noninducibility is not helpful in eliminating risk in individual patients. The most heated debates are those that involve patients who have inducibility of nonsustained forms of ventricular arrhythmias. Because of possible nonspecificity of aggressive protocols and uncertainties about the clinical translation of certain forms of nonsustained arrhythmias, the questions of whether or not patients falling into these categories are identified as being at specifically high risk require further evaluating and clarification. Furthermore, additional studies are required to decide the issue of whether or not suppression of inducibility of nonsustained forms is meaningful for predicting successful therapy.

## APPROACHES TO MANAGEMENT

Because survivors of prehospital cardiac arrest have a high risk of recurrence when untreated or inadequately treated,[3,5] and antiarrhythmic therapy may be useful in preventing recurrences,[12,15,20,21] plans for long-term management of such patients are essential. Three approaches are possible at this time: (1) suppression of premature ventricular contractions, with particular emphasis on specific, presumably high-risk complex forms; (2) long-term therapy guided by the results of programmed stimulation with drug intervention; and (3) empiric therapy by monitoring dosages and blood levels of specific antiarrhythmic agents. The empiric approach is limited by the fact that it is statistical and cannot provide identification of specific protection for specific individuals, even though the results in the overall group of survivors of prehospital cardiac arrest are encouraging.[12,22] More individualized therapy is desirable when possible. Quantitative suppression of premature ventricular contractions alone has not proved to be feasible,[13,14] but suppression of complex forms (Class 4-B and 5), as suggested by Graboys and associates,[15] may be an appropriate method of management for patients who demonstrate such forms reproducibly on ambulatory monitor recordings. Unfortunately, not all patients who have recurrent prehospital cardiac arrest have complex forms. Guidance of therapy by programmed stimulation studies has proved useful for identifying risk in certain subgroups as outlined above, but may be limited in its applicability. However, this procedure may prove to be the most individualized and specific of those currently available. The demonstration of loss of inducibility of sustained ventricular tachycardia or fibrillation by a specific dosage and plasma level of an antiarrhythmic agent may provide a combination of approaches that is uniquely useful. Our experience with this combination has been gratifying in recent years; but, as stated above, it may be limited to no more than 30 percent of patients who survive prehospital cardiac arrest. In patients in whom programmed stimulation cannot be used as the guide to therapy, risk of recurrence may be reduced by a combination of the other methods available, such as suppression of specific forms of chronic ventricular arrhythmias,[15] use of newer drugs either empirically or with specific form suppression, or the combination of specific form suppression and maintenance of the plasma levels of standard antiarrhythmic drugs that achieves this goal.[23] In addition, a role for implantable antitachycardia or defibrillating devices is emerging.

## ACKNOWLEDGMENT

We are grateful to Thelma L. Gottlieb for secretarial and administrative support.

## REFERENCES

1. MYERBURG, RJ, CONDE, CA, SUNG, RJ, ET AL: *Clinical, electrophysiologic, and hemodynamic profile of patients resuscitated from prehospital cardiac arrest.* Am J Med 68:568, 1980.

2. NAGEL, EL, LIBERTHSON, RR, HIRSCHMAN, JC, ET AL: *Emergency care.* In PRINEAS, JR AND BLACKBURN, H (EDS): *Sudden Coronary Death Outside Hospital.* Circulation 52(Suppl III):216, 1975.

3. LIBERTHSON RR, NAGEL, EL, HIRSCHMAN, JC, ET AL: *Prehospital ventricular defibrillation: Prognosis and follow-up course.* N Engl J Med 291:317, 1974.

4. BAUM, RS, ALVAREZ, H, AND COBB, LA: *Survival after resuscitation from out-of-hospital ventricular fibrillation.* Circulation 52:1231, 1974.

5. SCHAEFFER, WA AND COBB LA: *Recurrent ventricular fibrillation and modes of death in survivors of out-of-hospital ventricular fibrillation.* N Engl J Med 293:259, 1974.

6. EISENBERG, MS, COPASS, MK, HALLSTROM, AP, ET AL: *Treatment of out-of-hospital cardiac arrests with rapid defibrillation by emergency medical technicians.* N Engl J Med 302:1379, 1980.

7. THOMPSON, RG, HALLSTROM, AP, AND COBB, LA: *Bystander-initiated cardiopulmonary resuscitation in the management of ventricular fibrillation.* Ann Intern Med 90:737, 1979.

8. LIBERTHSON, RR, NAGEL, EL, HIRSCHMAN, JC, ET AL: *Pathophysiologic observations in prehospital ventricular fibrillation in sudden death.* Circulation 49:790, 1974.

9. LIE, KI, LIEM, KL, SCHUILENBURG, RM, ET AL: *Early identification of patients developing late in-hospital ventricular fibrillation after discharge from the CCU.* Am J Cardiol 41:674, 1978.

10. RITCHIE, JL, HAMILTON, GW, TROBAUGH, GB, ET AL: *Myocardial imaging and radionuclide angiography in survivors of sudden cardiac death due to ventricular fibrillation.* Am J Cardiol 39:852, 1977.

11. COBB, LA, BAUM, RS, ALVAREZ, H, ET AL: *Resuscitation from out-of-hospital ventricular fibrillation: 4 year follow-up.* Circulation 52(Suppl III):223, 1975.

12. MYERBURG, RJ, CONDE, CA, SHEPS, DS, ET AL: *Antiarrhythmic drug therapy in survivors of prehospital cardiac arrest: Comparison of effects on chronic ventricular arrhythmias and on recurrent cardiac arrest.* Circulation 59:855, 1979.

13. MYERBURG, RJ, BRIESE, FR, CONDE, CA, ET AL: *Long-term antiarrhythmic therapy in survivors of prehospital cardiac arrest: Initial 18 months' experience.* JAMA 238:2621, 1977.

14. LOWN, B AND GRABOYS, TB: *Management of patients with malignant ventricular arrhythmias.* Am J Cardiol 39:910, 1977.

15. GRABOYS, TB, LOWN, B, PODRID, PJ, ET AL: *Long-term survival of patients with malignant ventricular arrhythmias treated with antiarrhythmic drugs.* Am J Cardiol 50:437, 1982.

16. MYERBURG, RJ, KESSLER, KM, KIEM, I, ET AL: *Relationship between plasma levels of procainamide, suppression of premature ventricular complexes and prevention of recurrent ventricular tachycardia.* Circulation 64:280, 1981.

17. HOROWITZ, LN, JOSEPHSON, ME, FARSHIDI, A, ET AL: *Recurrent sustained ventricular tachycardia: 3. Role of the electrophysiologic study in selection of antiarrhythmic regimens.* Circulation 58:986, 1978.

18. MASON, JW AND WINKLE, RA: *Electrode-catheter arrhythmic induction in the selection and assessment of antiarrhythmic drug therapy for recurrent ventricular tachycardia.* Circulation 58:971, 1978.

19. RUSKIN, JN: Personal communication.

20. RUSKIN, JN, DIMARCO, JP, AND GARAN, H: *Out-of-hospital cardiac arrest: Electrophysiologic observations and selection of long-term antiarrhythmic therapy.* N Engl J Med 303:607, 1980.

21. JOSEPHSON, ME, HOROWITZ, LN, SPIELMAN, SR, ET AL: *Electrophysiologic and hemodynamic studies in patients resuscitated from cardiac arrest.* Am J Cardiol 46:949, 1980.

22. MYERBURG, RJ, KESSLER, KM, ZAMAN, L, ET AL: *Survivors of prehospital cardiac arrest.* JAMA 247:1485, 1982.

23. MYERBURG, RJ, ZAMAN, L, LUCERI, RM, ET AL: *Prehospital cardiac arrest survivors: Classification of risk groups on the basis of electrophysiologic testing.* Ann NY Acad Sci (in press).

# Coronary Artery Spasm: A Mechanism for Sudden Death*

*Joseph Kmonicek, M.D., and Sheldon Goldberg, M.D.*

Coronary artery spasm was proposed as a mechanism for sudden death as early as 1934, when Leary[1] described three patients who died suddenly with a prior history of angina. At postmortem examination, he found insignificant atherosclerotic lesions of the coronary arteries. He postulated that coronary artery spasm with subsequent reduction of flow was the mechanism for angina and sudden death. The concept that dynamic reduction in coronary blood flow caused myocardial ischemia was most elegantly hypothesized by Prinzmetal. In 1959, Prinzmetal and associates[2] described the clinical syndrome of variant angina pectoris with ST segment elevation and ventricular arrhythmias in 32 patients. These episodes, in contrast to classic angina, occurred at rest or spontaneously; and the clinical and electrocardiographic evidence of ischemia reversed with nitroglycerin. In the animal laboratory, the electrocardiographic phenomena were reproduced by intermittently occluding the left anterior descending coronary artery. These investigators concluded that " . . . intermittent occlusion of a diseased vessel by hypertonus is the cause of this syndrome."[2] The arteriographic documentation of coronary spasm was not described until 1973 when Oliva and coworkers fortuitously observed coronary spasm during a spontaneous anginal attack in the cardiac catheterization laboratory.[3]

Coronary spasm is now believed to be a significant factor in the pathogenesis of a number of clinical syndromes in addition to variant angina,[4-6] including unstable angina, myocardial infarction,[7] and postoperative cardiovascular collapse following coronary artery bypass graft surgery.[8] Although there are few series with adequate long-term followup, it appears that sudden death occurs in approximately 4 to 20 percent of patients with coronary artery spasm.[9] Conti and colleagues[10] reported sudden death in 5 of 28 patients with variant angina, whereas Maseri and associates[5] noted a 4 percent incidence in 138 patients. In a series of 114 patients with variant angina, Miller and coworkers[11] reported 6 sudden deaths and 13 patients resuscitated from sudden death. Although sudden death may be relatively common in the syndrome of variant angina, the relative incidence of coronary spasm in the clinical syndrome of sudden death is uncertain. We can perhaps gain a perspective on this interrelationship by examining patients with variant angina whose clinical course is characterized by myocardial infarction or sudden death.

## CLINICAL PROFILE OF CORONARY ARTERY SPASM

Since the original description of variant angina by Prinzmetal, the clinical profile of coronary spasm has broadened to include a wide spectrum of myocardial ischemic states.[5-7]

---

*Supported in part by a grant from W. W. Smith Charitable Trust.

Nonetheless, certain clinical characteristics remain similar. Patients with variant angina develop chest pain at rest, the pain often being more severe than classic exertional angina. A cyclic or circadian pattern of the pain is evident. The pain is classically associated with transient ST segment elevation and with ischemia-related ventricular arrhythmias. These electrocardiographic abnormalities generally subside with resolution of pain. Characteristically, the pain is nitrate responsive. Physical examination during episodes of pain frequently reveals signs of left ventricular dysfunction that return to normal upon relief. It is noteworthy that Prinzmetal suggested ventricular fibrillation as a mechanism for sudden death in variant angina. Since this initial description, there are experimental and clinical data to support additional mechanisms.

## HEMODYNAMIC MECHANISMS OF SUDDEN DEATH

Over the past 25 years, the hemodynamic and arteriographic correlates of variant angina have been well defined.[5–7,12] During episodes of chest pain with ST segment elevation, total or subtotal occlusion of a major coronary artery occurs. This spasm occurs most frequently in association with a pre-existing atherosclerotic narrowing. Less commonly, spasm may occur without underlying coronary artery disease. Selzer and associates[13] suggested that patients with coronary spasm could be categorized into two clinical groups based on the presence or absence of underlying coronary artery disease. Patients with fixed coronary artery lesions frequently had an antecedent history of exertional chest pain and myocardial infarction, and they developed ST segment elevation anterolaterally with associated ventricular arrhythmias. Patients without fixed coronary artery disease did not have exertional angina, usually had no previous infarction, and were more likely to demonstrate ST segment elevation in the inferior leads with associated bradyarrhythmias or atrioventricular block. This dichotomy, however, has not been observed by other investigators.[14]

The hemodynamic consequences of coronary artery spasm have been evaluated extensively. In contrast with patients with classic angina pectoris in whom an increase in myocardial oxygen demand precedes clinical episodes of ischemia, variant angina does not occur in response to an increase in oxygen demand, but is due instead to a decrease in oxygen supply.[5–7,12] Heart rate, blood pressure, and left ventricular end-diastolic pressure are all constant just prior to the pain. Following the onset of pain, left ventricular dysfunction develops, as reflected by a decrease in left ventricular dp/dt, an increase in left ventricular end-diastolic pressure, and systemic hypotension. Maseri and coworkers[5] continuously monitored right and left ventricular, pulmonary artery, and aortic pressures in 22 patients who demonstrated frequent episodes of coronary artery spasm. They observed no increase in heart rate, blood pressure, or dp/dt before the onset of ECG changes. Following the onset of pain, left ventricular dp/dt decreased markedly, with a subsequent increase in left ventricular end-diastolic pressure to levels as high as 40 mm Hg. Using myocardial scintigraphy,[5] it was shown that these hemodynamic changes were associated with a transmural myocardial perfusion defect. The areas of hypoperfusion correlated with the ECG abnormality and returned to normal with resolution of pain. Other investigators demonstrated altered myocardial lactate production during pain,[6] as well as decreased coronary blood flow as measured by the coronary sinus thermodilution technique.[12,15] Ergonovine testing has been demonstrated to be both sensitive and specific as a provocative test for coronary artery spasm.[16] Thus, the hemodynamic consequences of ergonovine-provoked coronary artery spasm accurately reflect the clinical response to spontaneous episodes. The deleterious hemodynamic effect of coronary artery spasm is dramatically illustrated in the following illustrative cases.[21]

### Case 1

A 36-year-old woman developed refractory angina at rest. Coronary arteriography with ergonovine-provocative stimulation was performed. Following two 0.05-mg intravenous doses

120

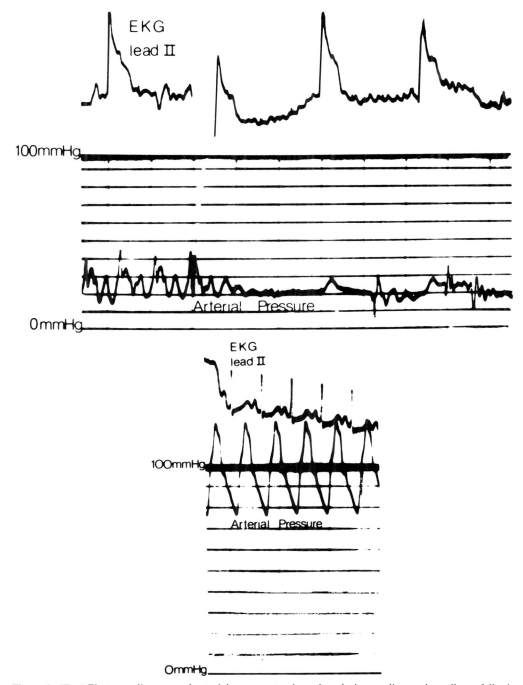

**Figure 1.** *(Top)* Electrocardiogram and arterial pressure tracing taken during cardiovascular collapse following ergonovine administration. *(Bottom)* Electrocardiographic and hemodynamic findings following reversal of coronary vasospasm after intracoronary nitroglycerin. (From BUXTON, A, GOLDBERG, S, HIRSHFELD, JW, ET AL: *Refractory ergonovine induced coronary vasospasm: Importance of intracoronary nitroglycerin.* Am J Cardiol 46:329, 1980, with permission.)

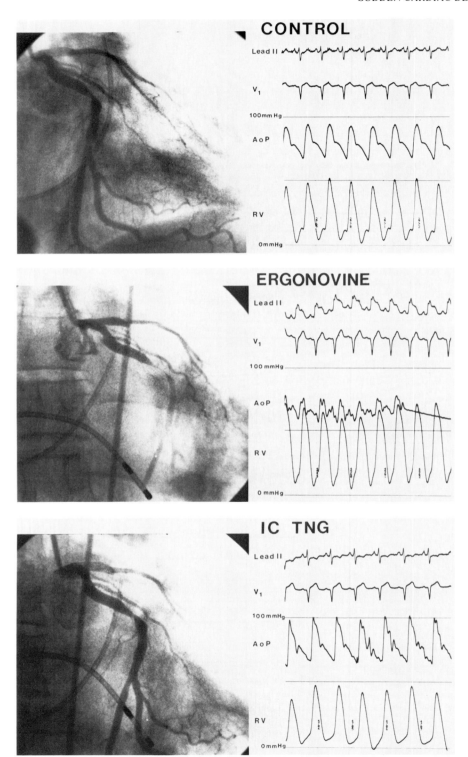

of ergonovine, the patient developed substernal chest discomfort with ST segment elevation in lead $V_1$. Coronary arteriography revealed spasm of the left coronary artery. Despite administration of sublingual nitroglycerin, chest pain persisted and additional ST segment elevation developed in lead $V_1$ accompanied by ST segment elevation in lead II. Intravenous nitroglycerin (300 $\mu$g) failed to alleviate symptoms, and systemic hypotension developed, followed by complete AV block and eventual electromechanical dissociation with cardiopulmonary arrest (Fig. 1, top). Coronary arteriography done at that time revealed severe spasm of the right coronary artery, which responded to intracoronary nitroglycerin (Fig. 1, bottom). Interestingly, the patient developed several episodes of ventricular tachycardia during resolution of the vasospasm. Approximately 1½ hours following cardiac arrest, the patient was hemodynamically stable. The patient remained asymptomatic on medical therapy 12 months after this episode. This patient demonstrates severe cardiovascular collapse caused by refractory coronary vasospasm. In this instance, prompt administration of intracoronary nitroglycerin relieved the vasospasm, and hemodynamic improvement resulted.

## Case 2

A 34-year-old man sustained an acute anterior myocardial infarction. Several days after the acute event, recurrent angina developed in association with ST segment elevation in the inferior leads. Cardiac catheterization revealed total occlusion of the left anterior descending coronary artery. In addition, a high-grade stenosis in the proximal portion of a dominant circumflex coronary artery was present (Fig. 2, top). Following ergonovine stimulation, spastic obliteration of the circumflex coronary artery occurred at the site of stenosis. The vasospasm was associated with chest pain, ST segment elevation in lead II, systemic hypotension, and a rise in right ventricular systolic pressure reflecting left ventricular dysfunction (Fig. 2, center). Immediate administration of intracoronary nitroglycerin resulted in relief of chest pain and resolution of the electrocardiographic and hemodynamic abnormalities (Fig. 2, bottom).

These two cases demonstrate that coronary artery spasm can produce severe myocardial ischemia and attendant left ventricular dysfunction. Depending on the severity and duration of ischemia, myocardial infarction, cardiovascular collapse, or death may follow.

## ELECTROCARDIOGRAPHIC CHANGES AND ARRHYTHMIAS DURING CORONARY ARTERY SPASM

The electrocardiographic findings observed during episodes of coronary artery spasm are a reflection of transmural myocardial ischemia. Classically, there is marked ST segment elevation. With less severe degrees of ischemia, however, ST segment depression may be observed.[17] If myocardial ischemia is of sufficient severity, transient Q waves may occur.[18] Prinzmetal and colleagues[2] noted increased R wave amplitude and width during attacks in those cases with more severe episodes of myocardial ischemia. Subsequently, experimental studies have suggested that increased R-wave amplitude correlates with increased end-diastolic and systolic volumes, reflecting left ventricular dysfunction.[19,20] Kerin and coworkers[14] found a higher incidence of increased R wave amplitude in variant angina patients who dem-

**Figure 2.** *(Top)* Baseline coronary angiogram, electrocardiogram (leads II and $V_1$), and pressure tracings in Case 2. Ao P = aortic pressure; RV = right ventricular pressure. Note total LAD occlusion and circumflex stenosis. *(Center)* Administration of ergonovine maleate results in spastic obliteration of the circumflex coronary artery. Note ST segment elevation in lead II, with systemic hypotension. In addition, right ventricular pressure is elevated, reflecting left ventricular dysfunction. *(Bottom)* Following reversal of spasm with intracoronary nitroglycerin, ST segment elevation resolves and arterial pressure is restored. In addition, right ventricular systolic pressure declines toward the baseline. (From Goldberg, S: *Provocative testing for coronary artery spasm: Specific methodology.* Cardiovasc Clin 14(1):106, 1983, with permission.)

onstrated arrhythmias during their ischemic episodes. R wave amplitude increased by more than 10 percent in 10 of 12 patients with arrhythmias during episodes of variant angina as compared with 6 of 14 patients without arrhythmias during ischemic attacks ($p < 0.05$). These latter investigators suggested that increased R wave amplitude was a marker of severe myocardial ischemia during episodes of chest pain, as reflected by the higher incidence of arrhythmias in this group. There was, however, little correlation between the change in R wave amplitude and the degree of ST segment elevation.

Malignant arrhythmias have been reported to occur during coronary artery spasm. In a series of 127 patients with documented variant angina in whom the clinical efficacy of nifedipine therapy was being assessed, serious arrhythmias occurred in 58 percent (Fig. 3); there was a relatively high incidence of ventricular tachycardia (34 percent) and ventricular fibrillation (13 percent). Similarly, Severi and associates[4] noted serious ventricular arrhythmias in 27 of 138 patients (20 percent). Ten of these 27 patients developed one or more episodes of syncope, and 5 of these 10 patients manifested asymptomatic episodes of ST segment elevation. In 2 of the 10 patients, ventricular tachycardia or fibrillation occurred during the resolution phase of the ischemic episode.

The most frequently documented arrhythmias are ventircular extrasystoles.[11,14] These ventricular ectopic beats occur as often during asymptomatic ischemic attacks as during symptomatic episodes. Although progression to ventricular tachycardia or fibrillation is not uncommon, the frequency of this progression is difficult to determine, and its exact incidence is unknown.

Varying degrees of atrioventricular block, atrial fibrillation, and bradyarrhythmias have been reported to occur with a somewhat greater frequency when spasm involves the right coronary artery.

Continuous electrocardiographic and hemodynamic observations of patients with variant angina have revealed a surprisingly high incidence of asymptomatic ST segment elevation. These episodes may or may not be followed by clinical symptoms.[5] Asymptomatic periods of ST segment elevation appear to be of shorter duration, lasting 30 seconds to 6 minutes. Those episodes followed by or accompanied by symptoms tended to last longer, varying from 2 to 20 minutes in duration.

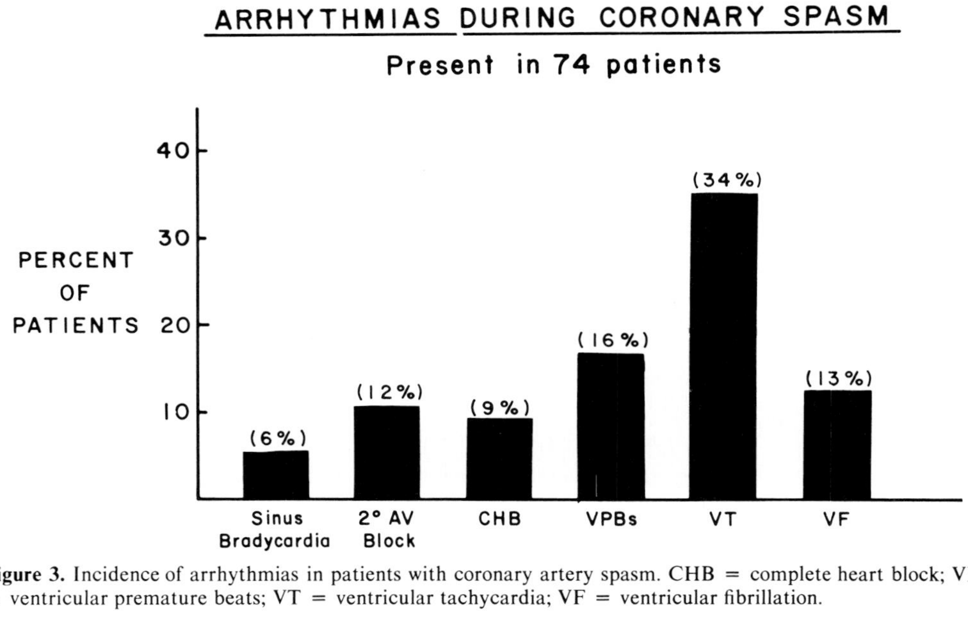

## ARRHYTHMIAS DURING CORONARY SPASM
### Present in 74 patients

Figure 3. Incidence of arrhythmias in patients with coronary artery spasm. CHB = complete heart block; VPBs = ventricular premature beats; VT = ventricular tachycardia; VF = ventricular fibrillation.

Of particular note, Maseri and coworkers[5] observed that episodes of ventricular tachycardia and/or fibrillation may occur during asymptomatic periods of ST segment elevation. Because many patients with sudden death have no antecedent chest pain, it is appealing to hypothesize that episodes of asymptomatic myocardial ischemia, secondary to coronary artery spasm, may lead to arrhythmias of sufficient severity to cause sudden death.

Although there are few data on the incidence of coronary artery spasm in patients with sudden death, several investigators have examined patients with coronary spasm who have progressed to myocardial infarction and/or death. Clinical characteristics of patients with sudden death and variant angina were evaluated by Miller and associates.[11] Of 114 patients with variant angina followed for periods of up to 26 months, there were 6 (5 percent) deaths and 13 (11 percent) patients resuscitated from sudden death. Fifty-six (49 percent) patients had documented serious arrhythmias during their episodes of chest pain. These arrhythmias included ventricular fibrillation (2), ventricular tachycardia (28), grouped ventricular beats (7), second- or third-degree AV block (6), and asystole (3). Interestingly, the maximal degree of ST segment elevation was significantly greater in those patients with more serious arrhythmias. Maximal ST segment elevation in the arrhythmia group was 7.4 $\pm$ 5.7 mm versus 3.3 $\pm$ 2.3 mm in the nonarrhythmia group ($p < 0.01$). Serious arrhythmias were observed in 16 of 19 (84 percent) sudden death patients compared with 36 of 86 (41 percent) survivors ($p < 0.01$). The incidence of sudden death was 42 percent, occurring in 15 of 36 patients with ventricular fibrillation, ventricular tachycardia, high-degree AV block, or asystole during their episodes of chest pain; whereas only 4 of 69 (6 percent) patients without these arrhythmias died suddenly. Thus, it appeared that patients with a greater degree of ST segment elevation were at a greater risk of developing severe arrhythmias and therefore at greater risk of sudden death (Fig. 4). A similar observation had been made earlier by Kerin,[14] who observed serious arrhythmias in 12 of 26 (46 percent) patients with variant angina. All patients with serious arrhythmias had ST segment elevation greater than 4 mm, whereas in those without significant arrhythmias, ST segment elevation ranged from 1.5 to 3 mm. These findings were recently confirmed by Prevetali and coworkers[22] who also noted more severe degrees of ST segment elevation (5.2 $\pm$ 3.7 mm compared with 1.8 $\pm$ 1.0 mm, $p < 0.001$) in those patients with ventricular tachyarrhythmias compared with those without such arrhythmias. In each of these studies, there was little correlation between arrhythmias observed during episodes of pain and pre-existing coronary disease or left ventricular dysfunction. These findings contrast to those reported in patients with classic angina, in whom left ventricular dysfunction and the extent of coronary artery disease seem to correlate with the frequency and complexity of ventricular arrhythmias.[23] Thus, it appears that the presence of coronary artery spasm per se is of paramount importance in the production of myocardial ischemia and resultant arrhythmias.

Several investigators have postulated that ventricular arrhythmias may occur during the reperfusion phase (resolution of coronary artery spasm). The effect of pre-existing stenoses in the development of reperfusion arrhythmias has been evaluated in an experimental dog model. Sheenan and Epstein[24] produced a flow-limiting stenosis upon which complete occlusion was superimposed and subsequent reperfusion allowed to occur. The peak flow during reperfusion was therefore reduced by the flow-limiting stenosis. Interestingly there was a significant inverse correlation between survival during reperfusion and the peak rate at which blood flow returned to the ischemic myocardium. That is, animals with pre-existing stenoses and therefore lower reflow rates had a lower incidence of significant ventricular arrhythmias with a higher survival. Those animals with higher reflow rates in the absence of pre-existing stenoses had a higher incidence of ventricular tachycardia and lower survival. Based upon these observations, one might speculate that patients without underlying coronary artery disease and coronary artery spasm would be at greater risk of sudden death owing to greater peak flows during resolution of spasm. The clinical correlate of this observation has not been evaluated. There has, however, been some clinical evidence supporting the experimental find-

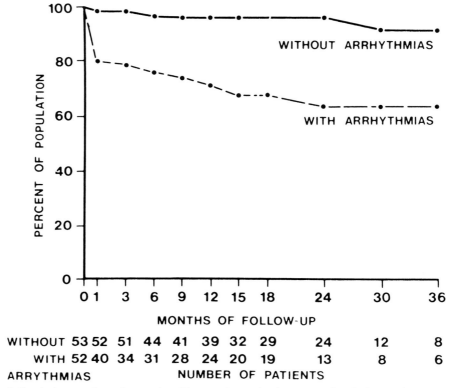

| | | 0 | 1 | 3 | 6 | 9 | 12 | 15 | 18 | 24 | 30 | 36 |
|---|---|---|---|---|---|---|---|---|---|---|---|---|
| WITHOUT | | 53 | 52 | 51 | 44 | 41 | 39 | 32 | 29 | 24 | 12 | 8 |
| WITH | | 52 | 40 | 34 | 31 | 28 | 24 | 20 | 19 | 13 | 8 | 6 |

ARRYTHMIAS                    NUMBER OF PATIENTS

**Figure 4.** Survival curves in variant angina. Those patients who demonstrated arrhythmias during episodes of coronary spasm were at greater risk for sudden death. The difference between the curves is statistically significant (p < 0.001). (From Miller et al,[11] with permission.)

ings of reperfusion arrhythmias. Prevetali and coworkers[22] observed 56 patients with variant angina pectoris. In 29 patients, no ventricular arrhythmias were observed, whereas significant arrhythmias were noted in 27. A more detailed analysis of these patients revealed that in 23 of the 27 patients ventricular arrhythmias developed during periods of maximal ST segment elevation. In 10 of the 27 patients, these arrhythmias were noted during the resolution of the ST segment changes. Those patients with reperfusion arrhythmias had longer periods of ST segment elevation as well as greater degrees of ST segment elevation, reflecting more severe ischemia. However, there was no significant influence of pre-existing coronary artery disease. Thus, there appears to be experimental as well as clinical evidence that significant arrhythmias may occur during resolution of coronary artery spasm. However, the role of concomitant coronary artery disease in patients with coronary artery spasm remains problematic.

A recent evaluation of a continuing series of 169 patients with followup for a period of 3 years demonstrated that the strongest predictor of survival in patients with variant angina pectoris was the presence or absence of coronary artery disease.[25] The highest percentage of complications, including death or myocardial infarction, occurred in patients with three-vessel coronary artery disease. Thirteen deaths occurred in 169 patients. There was only one death among 62 patients with no stenoses. Three deaths occurred in 59 patients who had single-vessel disease. However, nine deaths occurred in the 40 patients (22.5 percent) with multi-vessel disease. Left ventricular function was also predictive of survival; however, multivariate analysis indicated that left ventricular function correlated with coronary artery disease and was not an independent variable. Patients with normal left ventricular function had survival rates of 97 percent, 95 percent, and 91 percent at 1, 2, and 3 years respectively, whereas those patients with left ventricular dysfunction exhibited 88 percent, 84 percent, and 84 percent survival rates of 1, 2, and 3 years respectively. As an index of disease activity, these investigators divided their patients into three groups. One group consisted of patients in whom coronary artery spasm could be demonstrated only after provocative testing. A second group included those patients in whom episodes of coronary artery spasm were accompanied by significant arrhythmias. The third group demonstrated no significant arrhythmias in association with episodes of variant angina. In contrast to previous observations,[11] there was no difference in survival rates between those patients with and without associated arrhythmias. Those patients in whom coronary artery spasm occurred only upon provocative testing did, however, have an improved prognosis. It is noteworthy that those patients in whom coronary artery spasm could only be demonstrated upon provocative testing also had the lowest incidence of multivessel coronary artery disease.

It is difficult to determine the significance of the extent of coronary artery disease in the prediction of sudden death in patients with variant angina. In two large series, the extent of coronary disease was defined differently. In the series of Maseri and colleagues,[4,5] stenoses of 50 percent were considered significant, whereas in the series of Miller and associates,[11] stenoses of 70 percent were considered significant. Maseri and coworkers concluded that overall mortality and myocardial infarction were more common in patients with multivessel disease.

The role of left ventricular dysfunction is equally difficult to assess. Severi and colleagues[4] found the incidence of myocardial infarction and death was significantly greater in 24 patients with diffuse hypokinesis, akinesis, or aneurysm compared with 75 patients with normal left ventricular function or localized hypokinesis. As noted by Waters and associates,[25] the relative role of left ventricular dysfunction may be a reflection of the extent of coronary artery disease and not an independent variable.

In all series with adequate followup reported to date, the incidence of serious complications of coronary spasm—myocardial infarction or death—appears to be greatest within the first 1 to 3 months, with a rapid decline in morbidity and mortality thereafter. Severi and associates[4] reported 28 cases of myocardial infarction and 5 deaths within the first month of symptom onset in his evaluation of 138 patients, whereas there were only 4 deaths within the subsequent 2 years. Waters and coworkers[26] similarly noted 18 cases of myocardial infarction or death within the first month of symptom onset in their series of 132 patients. Thus, it appears that factors that are operative in the production of coronary spasm during the acute phase, which lead to sudden death or myocardial infarction, may not be operative at a later date. Another possibility is that patients with variant angina consist of two subgroups, one of which is characterized by a rapidly progressive course that progresses to myocardial infarction or sudden death.[25]

## THERAPEUTIC IMPLICATIONS

A number of calcium antagonists are presently available for the treatment of coronary artery spasm. These agents effectively decrease the severity and number of ischemic episodes.[27] Whether treatment will affect long-term survival is unclear. Several cases have been reported in which myocardial infarction was the eventual and unheralded outcome[26] despite a decrease in the number of severity of ischemic episodes. Thus, despite control of the ischemic symptoms, ultimate prognosis was not altered. This finding was supported by Water's series in which long-term survival was not affected by therapy.

It is our recommendation that patients with variant angina should be treated in an aggressive fashion with nitrates and calcium antagonists. The role of additional antiarrhythmic therapy has not yet been determined. Those patients with coronary artery spasm and coexistent multivessel coronary disease with left ventricular dysfunction are also at a greater risk of myocardial infarction or sudden death. If recent observations are correct,[25] medical therapy of this subgroup of patients is suboptimal, and consideration should be given to an aggressive surgical approach.

## CONCLUSIONS

Coronary spasm is being recognized as a significant mechanism in a variety of ischemic clinical syndromes. Depression in left ventricular function and malignant arrhythmias are two mechanisms whereby coronary spasm plays a role in the syndrome of sudden death. Sudden death may occur as a result of ventricular arrhythmias that develop either at peak ischemia or during the resolution phase of spasm. Certain electrocardiographic findings such as increased R wave amplitude, marked ST segment elevation, and the complexity of associated arrhythmias may serve as markers in identifying patients at greatest risk for sudden death. Early recognition and appropriate therapy offer the best hope for improvement in prognosis.

## REFERENCES

1. Leary, T: *Coronary spasm as a possible factor in producing sudden death.* Am Heart J 10:338, 1934.

2. Prinzmetal, M, Hennamer, R, Merliss, R, et al: *Angina pectoris: I. A variant form of angina pectoris.* Am J Med 27:375, 1959.

3. Oliva, PB, Potts, DE, and Pluss, RG: *Coronary arterial spasm in Prinzmetal's angina: Documentation by coronary arteriography.* N Engl J Med 288:745, 1973.

4. Severi, S, Davies, G, Maseri, A, et al: *Long term prognosis of "variant" angina with medical treatment.* Am J Cardiol 46:226,1980.

5. Maseri, A, Severi, S, DeNes, M, et al: *"Variant angina": One aspect of a continuous spectrum of vasospastic myocardial ischemia.* Am J Cardiol 42:1019, 1978.

6. Weiner, L, Kasparian, H, Duca, P, et al: *Spectrum of coronary arterial spasm: Clinical, angiographic and myocardial metabolic experience in 29 cases.* Am J Cardiol 38:945, 1976.

7. Oliva, PB and Breckenridge, JC: *Arteriographic evidence of coronary arterial spasm in acute myocardial infarction.* Circulation 56:366, 1977.

8. Buxton, A, Goldberg, S, Harken, A, et al: *Coronary artery spasm after revascularization: Recognition and management.* N Engl J Med 304:1249, 1981.

9. Silverman, ME and Flamm, MD: *Variant angina pectoris: Findings and prognostic implications.* Ann Intern Med 75:339, 1971.

10. Conti, CR, Feldman, RL, and Mehta, J: *Coronary artery spasm.* In Rappaport, E (ed): *Cardiology Update.* Elsevier North Holland, New York, 1981.

11. Miller, D, Waters, D, and Szlachlic, J: *Clinical characteristics associated with sudden death in patients with variant angina.* Circulation 66:588, 1982.

12. Goldberg, S, Lam, W, Mudge, G, et al: *Coronary hemodynamics and myocardial metabolic alterations accompanying coronary spasm.* Am J. Cardiol 43:481, 1979.

13. Selzer, A, Langston, M, Ruggeroli, C, et al: *Clinical syndrome of variant angina with normal coronary arteriogram.* N Engl J Med 295:1343, 1976.

14. Kerin, N, Rubenfire, M, Naini, M, et al: *Arrhythmias in variant angina pectoris: Relationship to ST segment elevation and R wave changes.* Circulation 60:1343, 1979.

15. Ricci, DR, Orlick, AE, Doherty, PW, et al: *Reduction of coronary blood flow during coronary artery spasm occurring spontaneously and after provocation by ergonovine maleate.* Circulation 57:392, 1978.

16. Curry, RC, Jr, Pepine, CJ, Sabom, MB, et al: *Effects of ergonovine in patients with and without coronary disease.* Circulation 56:803, 1977.

17. Yasue, H, Omote, S, Takizawa, A, et al: *Comparison of coronary arteriographic findings during angina pectoris associated with ST elevation or depression.* Am J Cardiol 47:539, 1981.

18. Meller, J, Conde, C, and Donoso, E: *Transient Q waves in Prinzmetal's angina.* Am J Cardiol 35:691, 1975.

19. Nelson, CV, Chatterjee, M, and Angelakos, ET: *Model studies on the effect of the intracardiac blood on the ECG.* Am Heart J 62:83, 1961.

20. Voukydis, PC: *Effect of intracardiac blood on the electrocardiogram.* N Engl J Med 291:612, 1974.

21. Antman, E, Muller, J, Goldberg, S, et al: *Nifedipine therapy for coronary artery spasm: Experience in 127 patients.* N Engl J Med 302:1269, 1980.

22. PREVETALI, M, KLERSY, C, AND SALERNO, J: *Ventricular tachyarrhythmias in Prinzmetal's variant angina: Clinical significance and relation to the degree and time course of ST segment elevation.* Am J Cardiol 52:19, 1983.

23. SCHULZE, RA, HUMPHRIES, JO, GRIFFITH, LS, ET AL: *Left ventricular and coronary angiographic anatomy relationship to ventricular irritability in the late hospital phase of acute myocardial infarction.* Circulation 55:839, 1977.

24. SHEEHAN, F AND EPSTEIN, SE: *Determinants of arrhythmic death due to coronary spasm: Effect of pre-existing coronary artery stenosis on the incidence of reperfusion arrhythmia.* Circulation 65:259, 1982.

25. WATERS, D, MILLER, D, SZLACHLIC, J, ET AL: *Factors influencing the long term prognosis of treated patients with variant angina.* Circulation 68:258, 1983.

26. WATERS, D, SZLACHCIC, J, AND MILLER, D: *Clinical characteristics of patients with variant angina complicated by myocardial infarction or death within one month.* Am J Cardiol 49:658, 1982.

27. KIMURA, E AND KISHIDA, H: *Treatment of variant angina with drugs: A survey of 11 cardiology institutes in Japan.* Circulation 63:84, 1981.

# Identification of Patients at Risk
# for Arrhythmic Death: Role
# of Holter ECG Recording*

## *J. Thomas Bigger, Jr., M.D., and James Coromilas, M.D.*

The widespread development of coronary care units (CCUs) 20 years ago provided an opportunity to observe the rhythm disturbances in acute myocardial infarction. Because the mortality is substantial in the CCU phase of myocardial infarction, the association between ventricular fibrillation (VF) and death was readily established. This association lead to further studies in the CCU phase of myocardial infarction and studies of the prehospital phase of myocardial infarciton. In the past 10 years, several studies have attempted to relate ventricular arrhythmias recorded 10 to 30 days after infarction to long-term outcome. Also, there have been several reports of Holter recordings on persons who have died while a Holter recorder was attached. We will review this information here in order to address the following questions: (1) What is considered normal and abnormal in Holter ECG recordings? (2) When is the best time to evaluate cardiac rhythm with Holter ECG recordings after myocardial infarction? (3) Which ventricular arrhythmias are the best predictors of mortality? (4) Do ventricular arrhythmias predict subsequent mortality independent of left ventricular dysfunction? (5) What are the actual mechanisms of sudden cardiac death?

## VENTRICULAR ARRHYTHMIAS IN NORMAL PERSONS

To recognize what is abnormal, we need a clear definition of normal. Although the definition of normal rhythm in humans is far from complete, a number of studies have been done in apparently normal subjects to determine the prevalence of ventricular arrhythmias and their possible significance. Two studies in normal persons are contrasted to two studies in abnormal groups in Table 1. Brodsky and coworkers[1] studied 50 male medical students, mean age 25 years, with 24-hour continuous ECG recordings. Students were carefully screened and were excluded if they had an abnormality in any of the following: physical examination, chest x-ray, 12-lead ECG, or echocardiogram. These workers found that 25 persons (50 percent) had some ventricular arrhythmias, but only 2 (4 percent) had repetitive ventricular premature depolarizations (VPDs). A study by Kostis and associates[2] provides information on ventricular arrhythmias in normal persons over a much wider range of age, 16 to 68 (average age of 49) years. To avoid including persons with asymptomatic coronary disease, the latter investigators selected 101 persons for analysis from a total of 1500 who had coronary angiography

*Supported in part by NIH Grants HL-22982, HL-12738 and HL-70204 from the National Heart, Lung and Blood Institute, Bethesda, Maryland; by a Grant RR-00645 from the Research Resources Administration, Bethesda, Maryland; by a Grant-in-Aid from the American Heart Association, Dallas, Texas; and by grants from the Winthrop and Chernow Foundations, New York, New York.

**Table 1.** Prevalence of ventricular arrhythmias in normal subjects and those with coronary heart disease

|  | Brodsky | Kostis | Hinkle | Bigger |
|---|---|---|---|---|
| No. of subjects | 50 | 101 | 301 | 616 |
| Median age | 25 | 56 | 55 | 59 |
| Sex | M | 51M, 50F | M | 480M, 136F |
| Status | Normal | Normal | Random sample | Post-infarction |
| *VPD frequency* |  |  |  |  |
| > 1 per hour | 6% | 39% | 30% | 50% |
| > 10 per hour | 0% | 20% | 20% | 25% |
| > 100 per hour | 0% | 4% | 4% | 5% |
| *Complex VPD* |  |  |  |  |
| VT | 2% | 0% | 3% | 11% |
| Pairs | 2% | 0% | 13% | 30% |
| R on T | 6% | 2% | — | 27% |
| Multiform | 12% | 4% | 33% | 54% |

at their center. These 51 men and 50 women had normal hearts as judged by physical examination, 12-lead ECG, exercise test, echocardiogram, coronary angiogram, and left ventriculogram. It can be seen in Table 1 that VPD frequency is much higher in this group than in the young male medical students. The marked difference in VPD frequency between the Brodsky study and the Kostis study could be due either to age or sex differences. Further examination of the Kostis study suggests that age is more likely to be the important variable. There were no significant differences in VPD frequency between the 51 men and 50 women. However, Table 2 shows the strong direct relationship between age and VPD frequency. It should be noted that no repetitive VPDs were found in 24-hour ECG recordings in the Kostis study of normal persons. These two studies in normal persons are compared in Table 1 with studies done in abnormal groups. Hinkle and colleagues[3] studied a random population sample of 301 middle-aged men (mean age 55). Some of these men had obvious heart or lung disease upon examination, but the majority did not have heart disease detectable by history, physical examination, 12-lead ECG, or chest x-ray. The VPD frequency in this group was almost identical to that found in normal persons, but the incidence of repetitive VPDs was increased. The last column of Table 1 provides data on a group of patients studied at the Columbia-Presbyterian Medical Center, all of whom had had myocardial infarction 2 to 4 weeks previously.[4] The median age in this group was similar to that in the studies of Kostis and Hinkle. The VPD frequency found in patients after infarction is remarkably similar to that found in middle-age normal men and women or a random sample of middle-aged men. However, the

**Table 2.** Effect of age on the prevalence of ventricular premature depolarizations in persons with normal hearts (Kostis, 1981)

| Age (years) | No. of patients | VPDs per 24 hours | | |
|---|---|---|---|---|
|  |  | > 0 | > 50 | > 100 |
| 10–29 | 6 | 17% | 0% | 0% |
| 30–39 | 11 | 18% | 0% | 0% |
| 40–49 | 29 | 28% | 4% | 0% |
| 50–59 | 39 | 51% | 13% | 5% |
| 60–69 | 12 | 58% | 25% | 17% |
| Total | 97 | 39% | 9% | 4% |

prevalence of repetitive VPDs is substantially higher in the post-infarction group. Taken together, these studies suggest that although VPD frequency rises as a function of age, this finding is not a strong indicator of heart disease. However, repetitive VPDs appear to be almost always absent in persons with normal hearts and, when present, they suggest the presence of heart disease.

Kennedy and coworkers[5] investigated a similar question using a totally different approach. They wanted to know if patients who have frequent and complex ventricular arrhythmias and normal noninvasive workups are likely to have significant but asymptomatic coronary heart disease. From a group of 62 patients with 100 or more VPDs per hour and repetitive VPDs but normal 12-lead ECG, M-mode echocardiogram, and exercise test, 25 were selected for coronary angiography. The primary indication for angiography was the presence of ventricular arrhythmias in association with coronary risk factors. The average age in the group was 47 years, and the ventricular arrhythmias had been present for an average of 3 years. Coronary angiography showed significant coronary lesions in 25 percent (6 of 25) of the group. This result is ambiguous. It shows that many patients who have frequent and complex VPDs but a normal noninvasive cardiac evaluation do have significant coronary artery lesions. However, this is by no means invariably the case. The increase in the odds of having coronary disease given the finding of repetitive VPDs could not be estimated in Kennedy's study because the study lacked a control group. Additional studies will be needed before we can fully clarify the significance of repetitive VPDs in apparently normal persons.

## TIME COURSE OF VENTRICULAR ARRHYTHMIAS AFTER INFARCTION

The time course of VPD frequency and tachyarrhythmias after myocardial infarction is still poorly defined. Rough estimates for the prevalence as a function of time for VPD frequency, for ventricular tachycardia (VT) and for ventricular fibrillation (VF) are given in Table 3. In the prehospital phase of myocardial infarction, that is, the first 4 to 6 hours, frequent VPDs and VT are not common.[6] Between 6 and 72 hours, the prevalence of frequent VPDs and VT increases markedly. Preliminary data suggest that VPD frequency and VT reach a nadir 3 to 5 days after myocardial infarction. By 10 to 16 days, 20 to 25 percent of the patients have $\geq$ 10 VPDs per hour, and 10 percent have VT. The prevalence of $\geq$ 10 VPDs and VT continues to increase after discharge, reaching a second peak at 6 to 12 weeks after infarction and then remaining relatively constant for at least a year. The prevalence of VF as a function of time after onset of infarction is completely different. About 15 percent of patients with myocardial infarction will experience VF in the first 4 to 6 hours.[6] The incidence falls rapidly to 3 to 4 percent in the 6- to 72-hour period. The incidence of primary VF is about 5 percent between 3 and 16 days after infarction and perhaps 5 to 6 percent between hospital discharge and the 1-year anniversary of infarction.

Interestingly, ventricular arrhythmias recorded in the coronary care unit (CCU) phase of myocardial infarction have much less prognostic significance than those recorded just before hospital discharge. Most patients in the United States are treated in CCUs and have contin-

**Table 3.** Time course of ventricular arrhythmias after myocardial infarction

| Time after infarction | 10 or more VPDs/hour | Nonsustained VT | VF |
|---|---|---|---|
| 0–6 hours | 10% | 4% | 15% |
| 6–72 hours | 70% | 40% | 3% |
| 4–6 days | 10% | 5% | 2% |
| 10–16 days | 20% | 10% | 2% |
| 6–12 weeks | 30% | 15% | — |

**Table 4.** Concordance between VT/VF in the CCU and VT at the time of hospital discharge

| VT/VF in CCU | VT at hospital discharge | | |
| --- | --- | --- | --- |
| | Present | Absent | Total |
| Present | 35 | 188 | 223 |
| Absent | 32 | 295 | 327 |
| Total | 67 | 483 | 550 |

VT at discharge: VT in CCU 16%; no VT in CCU 10%
$X^2 = 3.79$; $p > 0.05$; odds ratio $= 1.7$

uous ECG monitoring for 48 to 72 hours. Although CCU monitoring is not very effective for quantitating VPDs,[8,9] repetitive ventricular arrhythmias, particularly ventricular tachycardia or fibrillation, are often detected. If the presence of VT or VF in the CCU has the same significance as ventricular arrhythmias at the time of hospital discharge, then detection of patients at risk for arrhythmias after discharge would be simple, timely, and inexpensive. Therefore, we examined the concordance between the presence of ventricular tachycardia in the CCU and at the time of hospital discharge (Table 4). The association between ventricular tachycardia in the CCU and ventricular tachycardia at the time of hospital discharge was not statistically significant. Only about half of the patients who had VT or VF 2 weeks after infarction had VT in the CCU. Also, the predictive accuracy of VT detected in the CCU was quite low; only 16 percent of the 223 patients who had ventricular tachyarrhythmias in the CCU had VT detected in their 24-hour ECG recording 2 weeks later.

## VENTRICULAR PREMATURE DEPOLARIZATIONS NEAR THE TIME OF HOSPITAL DISCHARGE

### Frequency of Ventricular Premature Depolarizations

The prevalence and significance of ventricular arrhythmias in coronary heart disease have been studied most after acute myocardial infarction. Most studies were done at about the time of discharge after a myocardial infarction because this is a convenient time for both physician and patient and because the high mortality in the 6 to 12 months after infarction dictates early treatment.[10-13] The prevalence of VPDs 10 to 16 days after myocardial infarction is shown in Figure 1. Between 15 and 20 percent have no VPDs in a 24-hour recording; about 50 percent have an average of less than 1 per hour; 20 to 25 percent have 10 or more per hour; and only 5 percent have 100 or more per hour. As already mentioned, the time between myocardial infarction and the 24-hour ECG recording is an important determinant of VPD prevalence: ventricular arrhythmias are at a minimum at 3 to 5 days after infarction and at a maximum 6 to 12 weeks after infarction. The relationship between VPD frequency and first year post-discharge mortality is shown in Figure 2. Interestingly, the relationship is S-shaped. About half of the VPD-associated mortality increase is achieved at frequencies of 3 per hour, and the mortality plateaus are at about 10 VPDs per hour. The mortality is between 20 and 25 percent for patients with 10 or more VPDs; patients with 100 or more per hour are at no greater risk than those with 10 to 100 per hour. There has been no definitive trial to evaluate whether or not reducing VPD frequency will have a beneficial influence on mortality after infarction.[14] If one assumes that treatment can reduce mortality, the relationship in Figure 2 calls into question the conventional frequency criteria for treatment of ventricular arrhythmias after infarction, usually 60 or 100 per hour or more. One could reasonably conclude that patients with VPD frequencies above 10 per hour should be treated. Recent results from the Multicenter Post-Infarction Program (MPIP) provide a rationale for

134

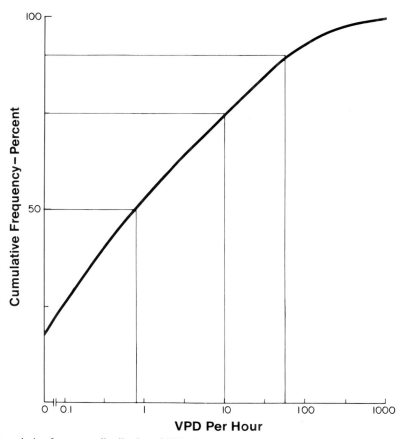

**Figure 1.** Cumulative frequency distribution of VPD frequency expressed as the hourly average over a 24-hour period. The 50th percentile is just below 1 VPD per hour, the 75th percentile is at 10 VPDs per hour, and the 90th percentile is at 60 VPDs per hour. (From Bigger et al,[18] with permission)

using an even lower frequency value as the criterion for treatment, for example, 3 VPDs per hour.[15]

**Repetitive Ventricular Premature Depolarizations**

The complex feature of post-infarction VPDs with the greatest significance is repetitiveness. Multiform VPDs have very little significance and R-on-T complexes have less prognostic significance than repetitive forms.[11,13] About 25 percent of 24-hour predischarge ECG recordings contain repetitive VPDs; about 15 percent contain paired complexes only; and 10 percent contain both paired complexes and one or more episodes of unsustained VPD runs (three or more consecutive ventricular complexes at any rate). Recordings with runs but no pairs are extremely rare, comprising only about 5 percent of the recordings with runs. A study done in 616 post-infarction patients at the Columbia-Presbyterian Medical Center evaluated the mortality risk associated with repetitive VPDs independent of VPD frequency. VPD frequency and repetitiveness were quantitated by a sensitive and specific computer program in 24-hour predischarge ECG recordings.[16] The results are summarized in Table 5. Adjusted for VPD frequency, the overall odds of dying are 2.5 times as great for patients who have repetitive VPDs compared with those who do not. Although there is a significant and moderately strong

135

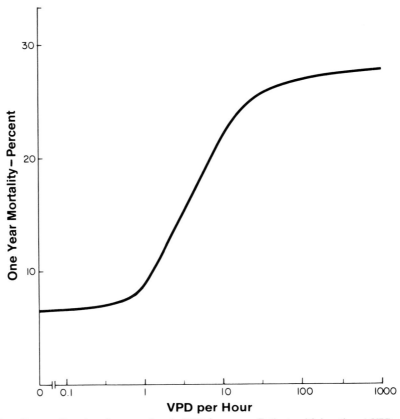

**Figure 2.** Mortality as a function of average hourly VPD frequency. Patients with less than 1 VPD per hour have a low mortality. The mortality rises sharply as a function of VPD frequency and reaches a plateau between 10 and 30 VPDs per hour. (From Bigger et al,[18] with permission)

**Table 5.** The relationship between repetitive VPDs and mortality adjusted for the effects of VPD frequency

| Frequency of VPD (per hr) | Repetitive VPDs | Status | | Total | Mortality | Odds ratio |
|---|---|---|---|---|---|---|
| | | Dead | Alive | | | |
| < 10 | Absent | 31 | 349 | 380 | 8% | |
| | Present | 16 | 68 | 84 | 19% | 2.7 |
| ≥ 10 | Absent | 6 | 36 | 42 | 14% | |
| | Present | 31 | 79 | 110 | 28% | 2.2 |
| | Total | 84 | 532 | 616 | 14% | |

$X^2$−total = 12.11, df = 2; $X^2$−interaction = 0.59, df = 1
$X^2$−association = 11.52, df = 1; summary odds ratio = 2.5

**Table 6.** Studies of nonsustained ventricular tachycardia recorded about 2 weeks after myocardial infarction

|  | Anderson | Bigger | Kleiger | Bigger |
|---|---|---|---|---|
| Number of patients | 915 | 430 | 289 | 819 |
| Age limit | < 66 | <76 | < 71 | < 70 |
| One-year mortality | 4% | 13% | 9% | 9% |
| Duration of ECG recording (hours) | 6 | 24 | 10 | 24 |
| *Definition of VT* |  |  |  |  |
| Consecutive Complexes | ≥ 3 | ≥ 3 | ≥ 3 | ≥ 3 |
| Rate | ≥ 100/min | Any | Any | Any |
| *Prevalence of VT* |  |  |  |  |
| Number | 10 | 50 | 10 | 92 |
| Percent | 1.1% | 11.6% | 3.4% | 11.2% |
| Follow-up time (months) | 48 | 36 | 12 | 24 |
| *Mortality* |  |  |  |  |
| With VT | 25% | 38% | 14% | 25% |
| Without VT | 13% | 19% | 7% | 9% |

association between VPD frequency and repetitive VPDs,[12] there is no interaction between these two factors with respect to mortality, that is, repetitive VPDs add significantly and independently to the risk of dying in the year after myocardial infarction. Also, the mortality for patients with VT is significantly higher than for patients with paired VPDs but no VT. A more recent study of 866 post-infarction patients by MPIP confirmed the finding that repetitive VPDs are associated with 2-year post-infarction mortality independent of any effect of VPD frequency.[15] In the MPIP study also, VT was associated with a higher mortality than paired VPDs, but this difference was not statistically significant.

Nearly every sizable post-infarction study has found that VT (runs of three or more consecutive VPDs) has the strongest association with mortality of all the ventricular arrhythmia variables. Table 6 summarizes four major studies of unsustained VT in patients with recent myocardial infarction.[15,17–19] The prevalence of VT at the time of hospital discharge varies with (1) age and base mortality rate, (2) the recording duration, (3) the sensitivity of the analysis method, and (4) the definition of VT. If predischarge 24-hour recordings are done in a representative cross-sectional sample of the United States post-infarction population with a 10 percent 1-year mortality and are analyzed by sensitive digital computer methods, the prevalence of VT is about 10 percent.[15] Table 6 shows that the mortality influence of VT is large and remarkably constant across these four major studies. In patients with VT, no relationship has been found between the number of episodes of VT or their length and mortality in a year or more of followup.[17,18] However, the studies to date that have addressed this question have been small and, therefore, have had limited power to detect such relationships should they exist. Nearly all episodes of VPD runs (VT) recorded predischarge are brief, infrequent, and asymptomatic.[17–19] Half of the patients have only three VPDs in the longest run, and 30 percent have but a single run of VT in the 24-hour recording. Considering these facts, it is remarkable that patients with unsustained VT have such a high mortality during followup after myocardial infarction.

## RELATIONSHIP BETWEEN VENTRICULAR ARRHYTHMIAS AND LEFT VENTRICULAR DYSFUNCTION

The relationship among left ventricular dysfunction and ventricular arrhythmias and death in patients who have had myocardial infarction is a key to secondary preventive measures for arrhythmic death after infarction. Currently, there are two alternate hypotheses about the relationship between ventricular arrhythmias and left ventricular dysfunction: (1) that ventricular arrhythmias contribute independent mortality force after adjusting for the effects of left ventricular dysfunction, and (2) that ventricular arrhythmias are so stongly associated with left ventricular dysfunction that ventricular arrhythmias do not contribute independently to mortality after adjusting for left ventricular dysfunction. The major studies that address these hypotheses are summarized in Table 7.

Ruberman[13] and Moss[11] and their associates sought a relationship between "complex" ventricular arrhythmias (bigeminy, multiform, pairs, runs, or R-on-T) and mortality after infarction, adjusting for left ventricular dysfunction using the clinical diagnosis of heart failure. Both of these studies were large, 1739 and 940 patients respectively; used fairly brief ECG recordings, 1 hour and 6 hours respectively; and used clinical heart failure to adjust for left ventricular dysfunction. Both analyses yielded a similar result, that is, complex ventricular arrhythmias were significantly associated with followup mortality after adjusting for left ventricular dysfunction.

In a study of 395 coronary heart disease patients referred for cardiac catheterization, Califf and colleagues[20] addressed the same question. Strictly speaking, this was not a post-infarction study; only 53 percent of their patients had a previous myocardial infarction, most of them in the remote past. Angiographic left ventricular ejection fraction (LVEF) was used to adjust for left ventricular dysfunction. A hierarchical scoring system using frequency, multiformity, pairs, and runs was used to grade the ventricular arrhythmias detected using a conventional Holter scanner to analyze 24-hour ECG recordings. R-on-T was not accounted for. As a univariate, the ventricular arrhythmia score had a very strong association with mortality during followup. When Califf and associates used only clinical measures to adjust for left ventricular dysfunction, they obtained a result similar to that of Ruberman and Moss. This adjustment failed to eradicate the relationship between ventricular arrhythmias and mortality. However, after adjusting for left ventricular dysfunction with left ventricular ejection fraction (LVEF), there was no significant independent relationship between ventricular arrhythmias and mortality. Thus, they concluded that the adjustment procedure of Ruberman and Moss failed because they used inadequate variables to represent left ventricular dysfunction. Although the findings of Califf were not obtained in patients with recent myocardial infarction (47 percent had no infarction at all), they, nevertheless, seriously challenge the conclusions of Ruberman and Moss.

**Table 7.** Independence of ventricular arrhythmias and left ventricular dysfunction in coronary heart disease

|  | *Ruberman* | *Moss* | *Califf* | *MILIS* | *MPIP* |
|---|---|---|---|---|---|
| No. of patients | 1739 | 940 | 395 | 388 | 766 |
| Time after infarction (weeks) | 12 | 2–3 | — | 1–2 | 1–2 |
| Measure of LV dysfunction | Clinical | Clinical | Angio EF | RNEF | RNEF |
| Duration of ECG recording (hours) | 1 | 6 | 24 | 24 | 24 |
| Ventricular arrhythmia variable | Complex | Complex | Score | Repetitive | Frequency, Repetitive |
| Duration of followup (years) | 3 | 4 | 3 | 1 | 2 |
| Number of deaths | 208 | 115 | 58 | 25 | 86 |
| Ventricular arrhythmias and LV dysfunction found to be independent | Yes | Yes | No | Yes | Yes |

Angio EF = angiographic ejection fraction; complex ventricular arrhythmias = R-on-T VPDs, $\geq 2$ consecutive VPDs, multiform, bigeminy; repetitive VPDs = $\geq 2$ consecutive VPDs; RNEF = radionuclide ejection fraction; Ventricular arrhythmia score = 0—no VPD; 1—< 30 VPDs/hour; 2—$\geq$ 30 VPDs/hour; 3—multiform VPDs; 4—paired VPDs; 5—$\geq$ 3 consecutive VPDs.

**Table 8.** Mortality 1 year after infarction as a function of left ventricular ejection fraction and repetitive ventricular premature depolarizations

| Ejection fraction | Repetitive VPDs | Number of patients | | Mortality | | Odds ratio | |
|---|---|---|---|---|---|---|---|
| | | *MILIS* | *MPIP* | *MILIS* | *MPIP* | *MILIS* | *MPIP* |
| $\geq 40\%$ | No | 199 | 391 | 2% | 5% | | |
| | Yes | 55 | 119 | 7% | 12% | 4.9 | 2.4 |
| $\geq 40\%$ | No | 87 | 157 | 7% | 17% | 4.4 | 1.7 |
| | Yes | 47 | 99 | 25% | 25% | | |
| | Total | 388 | 766 | 6% | 11% | | |

More recently, two multicenter groups have studied the relationships among left ventricular dysfunction, ventricular arrhythmias, and mortality after myocardial infarction. The Multicenter Investigation of the Limitation of Infarct Size (MILIS) reported their findings in 388 patients[21] and the Multicenter Post-Infarction Program (MPIP) in 766 patients.[22] Both of these studies used sensitive and specific computer methods to analyze the 24-hour ECG recordings and radionuclide methods to measure LVEF. The cross-tabulation of repetitive VPDs, LVEF < 40 percent and 1-year mortality for the MILIS and MPIP studies is shown in Table 8. The MILIS study showed a much stronger unadjusted univariate relationship between repetitive VPDs and mortality than MPIP. The odds ratio for dying during followup for patients with repetitive VPDs versus those without repetitive VPDs was 5.6 for MILIS and only 2.3 for MPIP. The unadjusted univariate relationship between LVEF < 40 percent and mortality was more comparable between the two studies, that is, odds ratio 5.2 for MILIS and 3.4 for MPIP. Within the studies, repetitive VPDs and LVEF < 40 percent contributed almost equally to mortality risk in the MILIS study, whereas LVEF < 40 percent was a much stronger risk factor than repetitive VPDs in the MPIP study. In MILIS, repetitive VPDs were strongly related to mortality after adjusting for left ventricular dysfunction with LVEF < 40 percent. No data on the mortality effect of VPD frequency have been published by MILIS. In MPIP, Bigger and coworkers[15] applied multivariate survivorship techniques and found that VPD frequency, repetitive VPDs, and LVEF each was independently associated with mortality.

## IMPLICATIONS FOR ANTIARRHYTHMIC DRUG TRIALS

The best present evidence favors an independent association between ventricular arrhythmias and death in the early years after myocardial infarction. Because arrhythmic risk is independent of other important post-infarction risk factors, it seems reasonable to believe that reducing ventricular arrhythmias would reduce the risk of arrhythmic death in the years after infarction.[23] However, no study has been done to show that antiarrhythmic drug treatment can reduce mortality after infarction. Inasmuch as we are ignorant of the factors that link spontaneous, asymptomatic ventricular arrhythmias after infarction to arrhythmic death, it is possible that this approach, although reasonable, might fail because of factors that we do not yet understand. Several preliminary or feasibility post-infarction antiarrhythmic trials have been done, but none has selected a group of post-infarction patients with ventricular arrhythmias and treated enough patients in order to detect a moderate but significant reduction in arrhythmic deaths, for example, a 30 to 40 percent decrease.[14] Therefore, a study is strongly needed to test the hypothesis that reducing ventricular arrhythmias after myocardial infarction will increase survival. In our opinion, enrollment into such trials should be restricted to patients who have significant ventricular arrhythmias within 2 months of acute myocardial infarction. The drug treatment protocol should be flexible enough to achieve a marked reduction in VPD frequency and total eradication of repetitive VPDs. The treatment regimen also should markedly decrease the likelihood of VF during transient ischemic episodes. Finally, the drugs used for the trial should not themselves cause serious morbidity or mortality. The Cardiac Arrhythmia Pilot Study (CAPS) sponsored by the National Heart, Lung and Blood Institute is aimed at determining the feasibility of doing such a study. CAPS is trying to determine whether a treatment strategy can be found that will reduce VPD frequency by 70 percent and repetitive VPDs by 90 percent during the entire year following myocardial infarction in at least 80 percent of the patients who have frequent ($\geq$ 10 per hour) or repetitive (10 or more episodes of VT per day) VPDs.

## SUDDEN CARDIAC DEATH DURING HOLTER ECG RECORDING

Ventricular fibrillation is present in about 75 percent of out-of-hospital sudden cardiac death victims when the mobile coronary care unit arrives.[24] The chance occurrence of sudden death while a patient is undergoing ambulatory ECG (Holter) recording has provided us with detailed information both about the arrhythmias present at the time of cardiovascular collapse and about the antecedent electrocardiographic changes and arrhythmias. Thus far, 63 cases have been described in the literature where a patient was undergoing Holter recording at the time of out-of-hospital cardiac arrest or at the time of an in-hospital cardiac arrest.[25-36] An additional 38 cases of sudden cardiac death during ambulatory ECG recording have recently been reported in preliminary form.[37,38] Thirty-two of the case reports come from studies that selected only recordings with VF or torsades de pointes VT and thus provide no information about the prevalence of VF during cardiac arrest.[31,34,35]

The remaining 69 case reports were unselected episodes of sudden cardiac death during ambulatory ECG recording, and these reports confirmed the findings of the mobile coronary care units; VT/VF was the fatal arrhythmia in 80 percent (55 of 69) of the cases, whereas bradyarrhythmias (heart block, marked sinus or junctional bradycardia, or asystole) accounted for only 20 percent (14 of 69) of cases of sudden cardiac death.[24,30,32,33,36-38] In addition, the bradyarrhythmias often occurred in patients without prior bundle branch block or AV block, and patients dying of bradyarrhythmias were indistinguishable from patients who develop VF, in terms of cardiac disease, ventricular arrhythmias, and so on.[24,30,32,33,36-38] Of interest, patients with bifascicular block often died in VF rather than with AV block.[33] Holter results have substantiated the frequent occurrence of VF as the arrhythmia responsible for cardiac arrest, and they also have demonstrated that VF is almost always preceded by at least three complexes of an organized VT.[35-38]

Analysis of the 87 cases of VT, torsades de pointes VT, or VF during ambulatory ECG recording demonstrated that VT/VF is initiated by an R-on-T VPD in 32 percent (28 of 87) of the cases and by a late cycle VPD in the remaining 68 percent (59 of 87) of the cases.[25-38] There is some overlap between early and late cycle VPDs because some authors use a prematurity index (RR'/QT) $\leq$ 1.00 to define R-on-T VPDs, whereas others reserve the term R-on-T for VPDs with a prematurity index $\leq$ 0.85.[26,30,34,35] All the initial case reports of sudden cardiac death during Holter recording showed an R-on-T VPD initiating VT and VF.[25-29] Many of these cases also showed ST segment changes preceding the terminal ventricular arrhythmia, suggesting that these cases were "ischemic" arrhythmias. This finding would be in agreement with the recent studies of Campbell,[39] Adgey,[40] and their colleagues showing the high prevalence of R-on-T VPDs and VF in the first hours following onset of myocardial ischemia or infarction. Many of the other reports of R-on-T VPDs initiating VT/VF therapy occurred in the setting of antiarrhythmic therapy (usually quinidine) and a prolonged Q–T interval.[31,34] In these cases, the VPD initiating VT is often R-on-T despite a relatively long R–V interval (> 440 msec) because the Q–T interval is prolonged. The vast majority of cases of VF recorded during ambulatory ECG recording start with an episode of VT beginning with late cycle rather than an R-on-T VPD.[35-38]

**Table 9.** Relationship between treatment with type 1 antiarrhythmic drugs and torsades de pointes

| Torsades de pointes | Antiarrhythmic treatment | | |
| --- | --- | --- | --- |
| | Present | Absent | Total |
| Present | 14 | 4 | 18 |
| Absent | 9 | 29 | 38 |
| Total | 23 | 33 | 56 |

$X^2 = 12.62$; $p < 0.001$; odds ratio = 10.0

Torsades de pointes VT (polymorphic VT) may be the cause of cardiac arrest in 25 to 33 percent of patients.[34,36] Table 9 examines the relationship between treatment with a Type 1 antiarrhythmic drug and torsades de pointes. Eighty-three percent (15 of 18) of the reported cases of torsades de pointes VT during ambulatory ECG recording have occurred in patients being treated with antiarrhythmic drugs, and 73 percent (11 of 15) of the patients on antiarrhythmic drugs were on quinidine. When the Q–T interval has been prolonged by pharmacologic therapy, mid or late cycle VPDs often initiate torsades de pointes VT. These episodes of torsades de pointes VT degenerated into VF, were terminated by DC cardioversion or ended spontaneously.[31,34-36]

The characteristics of VT/VF (coupling interval of the initial VPD, QRS morphology during VT/VF) may provide a clue to the mechanism of the arrhythmia. Ischemic VF usually is initiated by R-on-T VPDs with a short R–V interval. R-on-T VPD in acute ischemia often initiates ventricular flutter that rapidly degenerates into VF.[25-29] VT/VF initiated by VPDs with a long R–V interval suggests scar-related re-entry as the mechanism of the arrhythmia. The occurrence of a polymorphic VT (torsades de pointes) in the setting of a prolonged Q–Tc interval strongly suggests a proarrhythmic drug effect.[30,31,33-36]

Lewis,[34] Pratt,[35] and their associates performed detailed analyses of the prevalence and frequency of ventricular arrhythmias in the hours preceding ventricular fibrillation or torsades de pointes VT. Both groups found a marked increase in the prevalence of VT and an increase in VPD frequency in the 2 to 3 hours preceding VF or torsades de pointes VT. Increasing prevalence of repetitive ventricular arrhythmia in the hours preceding VF has been noted by several other investigators. Changes in heart rate and ventricular repolarization pattern in the hours preceding sudden death also have been reported, but are not consistent findings. Some groups report a significant increase in heart rate in the hour just before VF,[34,35] whereas other groups find no consistent change.[37] Often the R–R interval preceding the VPD initiating VF is markedly prolonged; and authors have suggested that the prolonged R–R interval increases the dispersion of refractoriness, creating favorable conditions for VF.[30,31] The pre-arrest Q–T behavior has been examined in patients whose arrest arrhythmia is torsades de pointes VT. Although some investigators report sudden prolongation of the Q–Tc in the hour before the episode of torsades de pointes VT,[30,31] the majority of patients show no additional Q–Tc prolongation in the hours preceding sudden death.[34,35] Pre-arrest Q–T prolongation seems to be more common in the congenital long Q–T syndromes than in the drug-induced syndrome.

## REFERENCES

1. BRODSKY, MWD, DENES, P, KANAKIS, C, ET AL: *Arrhythmias documented by 24 hour continuous electrocardiographic monitoring in 50 male medical students without apparent heart disease.* Am J Cardiol 39:390, 1977.

2. KOSTIS, JB, McCRONE, K, MOREYRA, AE, ET AL: *Premature ventricular complexes in the absence of identifiable heart disease.* Circulation 63:1351, 1981

3. HINKLE, LE, CARVER, ST, AND STEVENS, M: *The frequency of asymptomatic disturbance of cardiac rhythm and conduction in middle-aged men.* Am J Cardiol 24:629, 1969.

4. BIGGER, JT, JR, ROLNITZKY, LM, COROMILAS, J, ET AL: *How should ventricular arrhythmias be classified and which patients should be treated?* In MORGANROTH, J AND MOORE, EN (EDS): *Sudden Cardiac Death and Congestive Heart Failure: Diagnosis and Treatment.* Martinus Nijhoff, Boston, pp 46–63.

5. KENNEDY, HL, PESCARMONA, JE, BOUCHARD, RJ, ET AL: *Coronary artery status of apparently healthy subjects with frequent and complex ventricular ectopy.* Ann Intern Med 92:179, 1980.

6. PANTRIDGE, JF, WEBB, SW, AND ADGEY, AAJ: *Arrhythmias in the first hours of acute myocardial infarction.* Prog Cardiovasc Dis 23:265, 1981.

7. BIGGER, JT, JR, WELD, FM, COROMILAS, J, ET AL: *Prevalence and significance of arrhythmias in 24-hour ECG recordings made within one month of acute myocardial infarction.* In KULBERTUS, H AND WELLENS, HJJ (EDS): *The First Year after a Myocardial Infarction.* Martinus Nijhoff, Boston, 1983, p xx.

8. ROMHILT, DW, BLOOMFIELD, SS, CHOU, T, ET AL: *Unreliability of conventional electrocardiographic monitoring for arrhythmia detection in a coronary care unit.* Am J Cardiol 31:457, 1973.

9. VETTER, NJ AND JULIAN DG: *Comparison of arrhythmia computer and conventional monitoring in coronary care unit.* Lancet 1:1151, 1975.

10. KOTLER, MN, TABATZNIK, B, MOWER, MM, ET AL: *Prognostic significance of ventricular ectopic beats with respect to sudden death in the late post-infarction period.* Circulation 47:959, 1973.

11. MOSS, AJ, DAVIS, HT, DECAMILLA, J, ET AL: *Ventricular ectopic beats and their relation to sudden and nonsudden cardiac death after myocardial infarction.* Circulation 60:998, 1978.

12. BIGGER, JT, JR AND WELD, FM: *Analysis of prognostic significance of ventricular arrhythmias after myocardial infarction.* Br Heart J 45:717, 1981.

13. RUBERMAN, W, WEINBLATT, E, GOLDBERG, JD, ET AL: *Ventricular premature beats and mortality after myocardial infarction.* N Engl J Med 297:750, 1977.

14. MAY, GS, EBERLEIN, KA, FURBERG, CD, ET AL: *Secondary prevention after myocardial infarction: A review of long-term trials.* Prog Cardiovasc Dis 24:331, 1982.

15. BIGGER, JT, JR, FLEISS, JL, KLEIGER, R, ET AL: *The relationship between ventricular arrhythmias, left ventricular dysfunction and mortality in the two years after myocardial infarction.* Circulation 69:250, 1984.

16. BIRMAN, KP, ROLNITZKY, LM, AND BIGGER, JT, JR: *A shape oriented system for automated Holter ECG analysis.* Computers in Cardiology, IEEE Computer Society, Long Beach, CA, 1978, p 217.

17. ANDERSON, KP, DECAMILLA, J, AND MOSS, AJ: *Clinical significance of ventricular tachycardia (3 beats or longer) detected during ambulatory monitoring after myocardial infarction.* Circulation 57:890, 1978.

18. BIGGER, JT, JR, WELD, FM AND ROLNITZKY, LM: *Prevalence, characteristics and significance of ventricular tachycardia (three or more complexes) detected with ambulatory electrocardiographic recording in the late hospital phase of acute myocardial infarction.* Am J Cardiol 48:815, 1981.

19. KLEIGER, RC, MILLER, JP, THANAVARO, S, ET AL: *Relationship between clinical features of acute myocardial infarction and ventricular runs two weeks to one year following infarction.* Circulation 63:64, 1981.

20. CALIFF, RM, MCKINNIS, RA, BURKS, J, ET AL: *Prognostic implications of ventricular arrhythmias during 24-hour ambulatory monitoring in patients undergoing cardiac catheterization for coronary artery disease.* Am J Cardiol 50:23, 1982.

21. MUKHARJI, J, RUDE, RE, POOLE, K, ET AL: *Late sudden death following acute myocardial infarction, importance of combined presence of repetitive ventricular ectopy and left ventricular dysfunction.* Clin Res 30:108A, 1982.

22. THE MULTICENTER POSTINFARCTION RESEARCH GROUP: *Risk stratification and survival after myocardial infarction.* N Engl J Med 309:331, 1983.

23. BIGGER, JT, WELD FM, AND ROLNITZKY, LM: *Which postinfarction ventricular arrhythmias should be treated?* Am Heart J 103:660, 1982.

24. LIBERTHSON, RR, NAGEL, EL, HIRSCHMAN, JC, ET AL: *Pathophysiologic observations in prehospital ventricular fibrillation and sudden cardiac death.* Circulation 49:790, 1974

25. BLEIFER, SB, BLEIFER, DJ, HANSMANN, DR, ET AL: *Diagnosis of occult arrhythmias by Holter electrocardiography.* Prog Cardiovasc Dis 16:569, 1974.

26. HINKLE, LE, ARGYROS, DC, HAYES, JC, ET AL: *Pathogenesis of an unexpected sudden death: Role of early cycle ventricular premature contractions.* Am J Cardiol 39:373, 1977.

27. GRADMAN, AH, BELL, PA, AND DeBUSK, RF: *Sudden death during ambulatory monitoring.* Circulation 55:210, 1977.

28. POOL, I, KUNST, K, AND VAN WERMESKERKEN, JL: *Two monitored cases of sudden death outside hospital.* Br Heart J 40:627, 1978.

29. Lahiri, A, Balasubramanian, V, and Raftery, EB: *Sudden death during ambulatory monitoring.* Br Med J 1:1676, 1979.

30. Bissett, JK, Watson, JW, Scovil, JA, et al: *Sudden death in cardiomyopathy: Role of bradycardia-dependent repolarization changes.* Am Heart J 99:625, 1980.

31. Denes, P, Gabster, A, and Huang, SK: *Clinical electrocardiographic and follow-up observations in patients having ventricular fibrillation during Holter monitoring.* Am J Cardiol 48:9, 1981.

32. Salerno, D, Hodges, M, Graham, E, et al: *Fatal cardiac arrest during continuous ambulatory monitoring.* N Engl J Med 305:700, 1981.

33. Nikolic, G, Bishop, RL, and Singh, JB: *Sudden death recorded during Holter monitoring.* Circulation 66:218, 1982.

34. Lewis, BH, Antman, EM, and Grayboys, TB: *Detailed analysis of 24 hour ambulatory electrocardiographic recordings during ventricular fibrillation or torsade de pointes.* J Am Coll Cardiol 2:426, 1983.

35. Pratt, CM, Francis, MJ, Luck, JC, et al: *Analysis of ambulatory electrocardiograms in 15 patients during spontaneous ventricular fibrillation with special reference to preceding arrhythmic events.* J Am Coll Cardiol 2:789, 1983.

36. Panidis, I and Morganroth, J: *Sudden death in hospitalized patients: Cardiac rhythm disturbances by ambulatory electrocardiographic monitoring.* J Am Coll Cardiol 2:798, 1983.

37. Kempf, FC and Josephson, ME: *Sudden cardiac death recorded on ambulatory electrocardiogram.* Circulation 68(II):355, 1983.

38. Milner, PG, Platia, EV, Reid, PR, et al: *Holter monitoring recording at the time of sudden cardiac death.* Circulation 68(II):423, 1983.

39. Campbell, RWF, Murray, A, and Julian, DJ: *Ventricular arrhythmias in the first 12 hours of acute myocardial infarction: Natural history study.* Br Heart J 46:351, 1981.

40. Adgey, AAJ, Devlin, JE, Webb, SW, et al: *Initiation of ventricular fibrillation outside hospital in patients with acute heart disease.* Br Heart J 47:55, 1982.

# Signal Averaging Methods to Select Patients at Risk for Lethal Arrhythmias*

*Michael B. Simson, M.D., Martin S. Kanovsky, M.D.,
Carol A. Dresden, M.S., Rita A. Falcone, M.S., and
Mark E. Josephson, M.D.*

In recent years, several groups have reported that patients and animals prone to ventricular tachycardia or fibrillation have a distinctive electrocardiographic finding: microvolt-level, high-frequency potentials that are continuous with the QRS complex and last a variable time into the ST segment.[1-11] These signals, which require specially processed electrocardiograms to detect, appear to arise from slowly conducting areas of the myocardium.[1,2,12] Many observers have recorded delayed and disorganized activation from directly infarcted myocardium,[14-21] and there is considerable experimental evidence for the concept that slow conduction through damaged tissue is related to re-entrant ventricular arrhythmias.[14,16-18,21] In this chapter, we will review the techniques used in the signal-averaged electrocardiogram and the results in patients with ventricular tachycardia and fibrillation.

## METHODOLOGY

The major problem in recording microvolt-level bioelectric signals from the heart is extraneous noise that masks the waveforms of interest. The noise has three primary origins: (1) skeletal muscle noise, principally from respiratory muscles; (2) interference induced from power lines (50 or 60 Hz and higher-frequency harmonics); and (3) electronic noise from amplifiers and electrodes. Modern amplifier design and good recording techniques can minimize noise from instruments, electrodes, and power line interference, but reduction of artifact from skeletal muscle activity generally requires a signal-averaging technique. The technique averages together multiple samples of a repetitive waveform, such as the electrocardiogram; nonrepeating, random noise cancels and is reduced in amplitude.[22]

How is a waveform that continuously varies over time, such as the QRS complex, averaged together? The process begins by measuring the voltage of a highly amplified electrocardiogram frequently at 1000 times or more per second. A list of numbers, each corresponding to the voltage level at a particular instant of time, is formed inside the computer memory. The computer scans this list and tentatively identifies a QRS complex. It then tests the new beat against a template of previous QRS complexes to ensure that the new beat is not an ectopic one. If it is not, the computer adds together the new beat to the previously processed waveforms by summing the list of numbers point by point. After division by the number of cycles processed, an averaged value of the electrocardiogram for each discrete point in time is

*Supported in part by grants from the National Heart, Lung and Blood Institute (HL24278 and HL22315), the American Heart Association, Southeastern Pennsylvania Chapter, Philadelphia, PA, and Arrhythmia Research Technology, Inc. Dr. Simson is the Samuel Bellet Associate Professor of Medicine in Cardiology.

obtained. The averaged waveform appears smooth and continuous when it is plotted because the time between each point is brief, 1 msec or less, and because of the high resolution of the voltage measurements.

The reduction of noise by the signal-averaging process is proportional to the square root of the number of cycles averaged together.[22] Averaging 100 cycles will decrease the noise level to one tenth of its former value. Noise level in most studies is under 1 $\mu$V or less than 0.01 mm at standard ECG gain. Signals that could not be appreciated on conventional electrocardiographic recordings can be clearly detected. The noise reduction occurs because random disturbances, for example, from skeletal muscle activity, are independent in time from the repeating signal, the electrocardiographic complex. An artifact or noise in one beat does not repeat in synchrony with each cardiac cycle; hence, the contaminating noise tends to cancel and is minimized.

Once the electrocardiogram has been signal averaged, it is usually high-pass filtered to reduce large-amplitude, low-frequency signals that are not of interest. The high-pass filter allows high-frequency signals to pass without attenuation but blocks lower-frequency waveforms. The rationale behind high-pass filtering is that the depolarization of cells generates rapid changes in membrane voltage, fast movements of activation wavefronts, and consequently high frequencies on the body surface. The plateau or repolarization phases of the action potential produce more slowly changing membrane voltages and lower-frequency signals on the body surface. The ST segment, for example, commonly contains either a baseline shift or a slowly changing potential that can be 100 $\mu$V or more. If it were displayed at high-gain, microvolt-level signals, corresponding to the late depolarization of small areas of the myocardium, would be difficult to perceive. The usual high-pass filter frequencies for signal-averaging studies range from 25 to 100 Hz.

A technical problem with high-pass filters of conventional design is that they ring or create other artifacts when large signals abruptly end. This property impedes the detection of low-amplitude waveforms that may occur just after larger signals such as the QRS complex. Digital filtering techniques, which use computer programs for the filtering process, can minimize filter artifact or ringing.[23] We have used a "bi-directional" filter to study ventricular late potentials.[8,9,13] The filter operates in normal time until the middle of the QRS. It then processes the electrocardiogram in reverse time, beginning at the end of the T wave, until the middle of the QRS is reached. Filter artifact or ringing from the QRS complex is eliminated completely because the QRS complex is processed after the late potential.

Bipolar X, Y, and Z leads are used in our investigations. Recordings are made at the patient's bedside in an unshielded room and require about 15 minutes. Approximately 150 beats are averaged; each new beat is tested against a strict template in order to exclude ectopic and grossly noisy beats. The frequency content of each signal-averaged lead is 0.05 to 250 Hz. Each lead is then high-pass filtered with a 25-Hz bi-directional filter and combined into a vector magnitude, a measure that sums the high-frequency information contained in all leads. This measure is termed the "filtered QRS complex" in this chapter. To date, there is no consensus among investigators on recording techniques for signal-averaged electrocardiograms. There are differences in the location and number of leads used, the type of high-pass filter used, and the filter frequency.

## FINDINGS IN PATIENTS WITH VENTRICULAR TACHYCARDIA

Several groups of investigators using the signal-averaging technique have reported evidence of microvolt-level, high-frequency waveforms in patients with ventricular tachycardia (VT).[2-11] The low-amplitude signals, termed "late potentials," are continuous with the QRS complex and last 20 to 60 msec into the ST segment. The late potentials appear to correspond to delayed and asynchronous ventricular activation that has been observed with direct electrogram recordings in patients with VT.[12,18,20,24] The delayed and fragmented electrograms typically occur in only a few areas of the heart, usually on the endocardium, and are less than 1 mV when recorded directly. Conventional electrocardiographic techniques cannot record evidence of these signals on the body surface because of their low amplitude.

Using the signal-averaging technique, we searched for late potentials in 66 patients after myocardial infarction.[8] One group of 39 patients had repeated episodes of sustained ($> 30$ seconds) VT, and the arrhythmia could be reliably induced with programmed ventricular stimulation. A control group of 27 patients had no history of complex ventricular arrhythmias, and a 24-hour Holter recording revealed fewer than 200 premature ventricular contractions (PVCs) daily as well as the absence of multiform PVCs, couplets, or VT. No patient in either group had bundle branch block, and all were studied during normal sinus rhythm when they were not receiving antiarrhythmic medications.

Figure 1 shows examples of records obtained from patients without VT. The unfiltered, signal-averaged leads (top) are shown at high gain. The filtered QRS complex (bottom) is a measure that depicts the high-frequency information ($> 25$ Hz) contained in all three leads. The filtered QRS complex in patients without VT is symmetric, has a peak of high-frequency voltage 40 to 60 msec after QRS onset, and abruptly declines to noise level at the end of the QRS complex. There is no signal above noise level ($< 1$ $\mu$V) in the ST segment. The end-points of the filtered QRS complex (dashed lines) are determined by a statistical algorithm similar to a student's t-test.

In patients with VT (Fig. 2), the initial portion of the QRS complex is similar to that of control patients. At the end of the filtered QRS complex, however, there is a low-amplitude signal that is not present in recordings from patients without VT. The microvolt-level signal, a late potential, is continuous with the QRS complex and corresponds to low-amplitude ripples and notches that can be seen at the end of the QRS complex in the unfiltered leads. The filtering process does not create a new signal. It merely supresses the low-frequency infor-

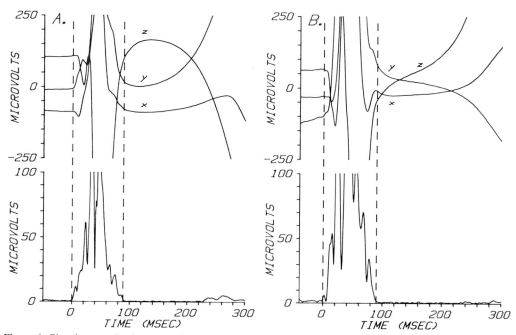

**Figure 1.** Signal processing in two patients who did not have ventricular tachycardia. On the top is the signal-averaged leads shown at high gain. On the bottom is the filtered QRS complex. In both patients, the filtered QRS complex is $< 100$ msec in duration, and there is a large-amplitude signal in the last 40 msec of the filtered QRS complex (41 and 67 $\mu$V, respectively). The patients had an anterior ($A$) and an inferior ($B$) myocardial infarction.

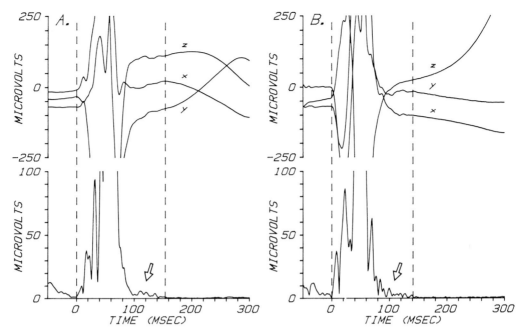

**Figure 2.** Signal processing in two patients with ventricular tachycardia. The filtered QRS complex has a longer duration, and low-amplitude late potentials (arrows) are present, in contrast to the filtered QRS complexes from the control patients (Fig. 1). The voltage in the last 40 msec of the filtered QRS complex measured 3 mV in both cases. The patients had an anterior (*A*) and an inferior (*B*) myocardial infarction.

mation in the ST segment and makes the high-frequency activity relatively more apparent. The amplitude of the late potential varies from 1 to 20 $\mu$V.

The late potential extends the duration of the filtered QRS complex in patients with VT. The filtered QRS duration was longer in patients with VT, 139 $\pm$ 26 versus 95 $\pm$ 10 msec for the control patients (mean $\pm$ S.D., p < 0.001). Seventy-two percent of the patients with ventricular tachycardia, but none of the control patients, had a filtered QRS duration longer than 120 msec.

Patients with VT had low-amplitude signals at the end of the filtered QRS complex. A measurement of the voltage over the last 40 msec of the filtered QRS complex was found to be a distinguishing feature between patients with and without the arrhythmia. Patients with VT had a 15 $\pm$ 14 $\mu$V of high-frequency signal at the end of the QRS complex, whereas in control patients, in contrast, late potential measured 74 $\pm$ 47 $\mu$V (p < 0.001). A threshold of 25 $\mu$V clearly separated the two groups. Ninety-two percent of the patients with, but only 7 percent of the patients without, VT had late potentials less than 25 $\mu$V. In this study, the low-amplitude late potential was present regardless of the location of the infarct or the presence of a ventricular aneurysm.

Late potentials have been recorded by several groups in patients with VT. Fontaine and coworkers[5] demonstrated low-level, polyphasic waveforms early in the ST segment in a patient with arrhythmogenic right ventricular dysplasia. Uther and associates[11] recorded 2-$\mu$V level potentials continuous with the QRS complex in five patients with recurrent ventricular tachycardia; the waveforms lasted up to 170 msec after onset of QRS complex. Hombach, Rozanski and their colleagues[6,7] have detected late potentials in patients with VT. Breithardt and coworkers[3] reported that 45 of 63 patients (71 percent) with documented ventricular tachycardia or fibrillation had late potentials lasting a mean of 51 msec after the end of the surface QRS complex; no late potentials were recorded in 27 control patients. Denes and associates[4] demonstrated that quantitative analysis of the high-frequency components of the terminal portion of the signal-averaged QRS complex could separate patients with ventricular tachycardia from normal subjects, with 58 to 83 percent sensitivity and 90 to 100 percent specificity depending on the discriminant used.

## FINDINGS IN PATIENTS WITH VENTRICULAR FIBRILLATION

The aforementioned studies indicated that patients with sustained and inducible ventricular tachycardia have a high incidence of abnormalities on the signal-averaged electrocardiogram, but the findings in patients with ventricular fibrillation also needed to be defined. Accordingly, we have studied 123 patients with a prior transmural myocardial infarction and a history of ventricular tachycardia or ventricular fibrillation occurring more than 1 week after an acute myocardial infarction.[25] No patient had bundle branch block, and all were studied during sinus rhythm. The patients underwent programmed electrophysiologic stimulation tests and a signal-averaged electrocardiogram while they were off antiarrhythmic medications. One group, 82 patients, had a history of sustained VT. The other group, 41 patients, had an observed episode of ventricular fibrillation; 32 of these patients (78 percent) were known also to have had repeated episodes of sustained VT.

The patients with VT only had a 90 percent incidence of abnormalities on the signal-averaged electrocardiogram, defined as either a filtered QRS complex $> 120$ msec or the presence of a late potential, that is, voltage late in the filtered QRS complex of $< 25 \mu V$. In contrast, those patients with a history of ventricular fibrillation had a lower incidence of abnormalities, 73 percent (p = 0.03). The findings on the signal-averaged electrocardiogram were similar to those during the electrophysiologic stimulation study. When tested with up to three premature ventricular depolarizations, 95 percent of the group with VT had sustained, induced VT; 78 percent of the group with ventricular fibrillation had inducible VT (p = 0.02). Denniss and colleagues[36] found a lower incidence of delayed ventricular activation potentials on an averaged vectorcardiogram in patients with ventricular fibrillation as compared with patients with VT. Several groups have noted that patients with ventricular fibrillation have a lower incidence of inducible ventricular arrhythmias than patients with a history of ventricular tachycardia only. These findings suggest that patients with VT after myocardial infarction may have a more uniform substrate for the arrhythmia than patients with ventricular fibrillation, which may be caused by diverse etiologies such as transient severe myocardial ischemia.

## COMPARISONS OF THE SIGNAL-AVERAGED ELECTROCARDIOGRAM, HOLTER MONITORING, AND CARDIAC CATHETERIZATION

The accurate identification by noninvasive methods of patients after myocardial infarction who are prone to serious ventricular arrhythmias is highly desirable in order to treat rationally the subgroup of patients at very high risk. Holter monitoring, cardiac catheterization, exercise testing, and clinical findings have been used separately and in combination in an attempt to define the characteristics of patients with ventricular tachyarrhythmias after infarction.[25−30] Recently, electrophysiologic stimulation testing has been proposed as a means to identify patients at high risk for lethal arrhythmias.[31−34] However, because of the expense and the invasive nature of the electrophysiology test, it is not an ideal screening test for large numbers of patients.

A signal-averaged electrocardiogram has been shown to be a marker for VT after myocardial infarction. We performed a study to determine whether the signal-averaged electrocardiogram provided information that was independent from that which can be obtained from

Holter monitoring and cardiac catheterization, and to determine the combination of findings from the signal-averaged electrocardiogram, cardiac catheterization, and Holter monitoring that best characterizes patients with ventricular tachycardia after myocardial infarction.[35] A study population with a high incidence of VT was used on the assumption that if a test cannot identify patients with ventricular tachycardia in that group, it would be unlikely to distinguish patients with arrhythmia in a study group with a lower incidence of the arrhythmia.

The study population consisted of 174 patients with a prior transmural myocardial infarction at least 2 weeks old. The VT group (98 patients) was referred for electrophysiologic studies because of repeated episodes of documented, sustained VT. The control group (76 patients) had no clinical history of sustained VT; most patients were referred for cardiac catheterization after myocardial infarction. Patients with left ventricular hypertrophy, valvular heart disease, nonischemic cardiomyopathy, or bundle branch block were excluded. There was no significant difference in age, sex, or infarct location between the control and VT groups. However, the patients with VT did have a higher median age of the infarction (46 weeks) than the control patients (8 weeks).

Ninety-six of the patients with VT were studied in the electrophysiology laboratory and 93 of them were found to have sustained VT inducible by one to three ventricular premature depolarizations. Fourteen of the control patients were also studied, and none of them had inducible, sustained VT. All patients were tested while in sinus rhythm and off antiarrhythmic drugs.

The individual parameters for each test that were significantly different between the control and VT groups by univariate analysis ($2 \times 2$ chi square) are listed in Table 1. An abnormal signal-averaged electrocardiogram was defined as a low-amplitude signal ($< 25 \mu V$) in the last 40 msec of the filtered QRS complex or a filtered QRS complex $> 120$ msec. Abnormal signal-averaged ECGs were found in 90 percent of the VT group and 30 percent of the control group. It should be emphasized that the control group in this study was not preselected for minimal ventricular arrhythmias on Holter monitoring; and, hence, these patients are different from the control group reported earlier in this chapter.

Eight parameters from 24-hour Holter monitoring were examined, and in most there was a higher incidence of abnormalities in the VT group. Patients with VT had a higher incidence

**Table 1.** Comparison of the signal-averaged electrocardiogram, Holter monitoring, and cardiac catheterization in control and ventricular tachycardia groups

|  | Control | VT |
|---|---|---|
| Signal-averaged ECG: | (N = 76) | (N = 98) |
| Abnormal | 23 (30%) | 88 (90%)† |
| Holter monitoring: | (N = 57) | (N = 64) |
| Multifocal | 26 (46%) | 45 (70%)* |
| Couplets | 21 (37%) | 40 (62%)* |
| Complex ventricular ectopy | 32 (56%) | 51 (79%)* |
| Mean PVC/hr > 5 | 20 (35%) | 42 (66%)† |
| Mean PVC/hr > 10 | 13 (23%) | 41 (64%)† |
| Peak PVC/hr > 10 | 23 (40%) | 49 (77%)† |
| Peak PVC/hr > 100 | 8 (14%) | 36 (56%)† |
| Cardiac cathetherization: | (N = 58) | (N = 83) |
| Aneurysm | 15 (26%) | 59 (71%)† |
| Wall motion abnormalities | 42 (72%) | 79 (95%)† |
| Ejection fraction < 40% | 19 (32%) | 59 (71%)† |

*p < .01
†p < .001

of multiform PVCs, couplets, complex ventricular ectopy (defined as multifocal PVCs, couplets, or unsustained VT), and a higher rate of PVCs. However, the control group also had a high incidence of abnormalities on the Holter monitoring. Complex ventricular ectopy, for example, was present in 79 percent of the VT patients but was found also in 56 percent of the control patients. Nonsustained VT on Holter monitoring tended to be more frequently found in the VT group (38 percent) than in the control group (25 percent, p = 0.13).

Univariate analysis of the results from cardiac catheterization showed that the group with VT had a higher incidence of aneurysm, wall motion abnormalities, and an ejection fraction of < 40 percent. There was no signficant difference in coronary artery anatomy between the two groups.

Stepwise, multivariate statistical analysis (logistic regression) was used to determine the significance of the parameters simultaneously. Logistic regression determines which variables are independently significant and then ranks the variables. The process generates an equation that can be used to determine the probability of VT in a given patient.

When the findings from the signal-averaged electrocardiogram, Holter monitoring, and cardiac catheterization were analyzed by multivariate analysis, only three parameters were found to be independently significant. Ranked in order of the power to predict ventricular tachycardia, they were an abnormal signal-averaged electrocardiogram, a peak PVC rate of > 100 per hour, and the presence of an aneurysm (each p < 0.001). No other parameter from the test was found to be significant once those three parameters were included. Patients in whom all three parameters were abnormal had a 99 percent probability of VT, whereas patients with none of the three had a probability of VT of only 4 percent. Patients with only one of the parameters abnormal and the other two normal had a probability of VT of about 30 percent. Patients with any two of the three parameters positive, and the other negative, had an 80 to 90 percent probability of VT. With the logistic regression model, the accuracy of identifying patients with VT was 85 percent (sensitivity 81 percent, specificity 90 percent). When the model was applied to subgroups with different ages of infarctions, the accuracy was similar; this finding suggests that age of infarction was not a significant confounding variable.

The results of the multivariate testing demonstrated that the signal-averaged electrocardiogram is a powerful independent descriptor when compared with the results of Holter monitoring and cardiac catheterization. This study also suggests that the combination of findings from various tests can more accurately describe a subgroup of patients with a high incidence of lethal ventricular arrhythmias. Because the study was retrospective and biased by considering patients referred for electrophysiology testing and cardiac catheterizations, the findings must be applied with caution to different population groups. The results, however, suggest that a signal-averaged electrocardiogram will play an important role as an independent marker for lethal ventricular arrhythmias.

## REFERENCES

1. BERBARI, EJ, SCHERLAG, BJ, HOPE, RR, ET AL: *Recording from the body surface of arrhythmogenic ventricular activity during the ST segment.* Am J Cardiol 41:697, 1978.

2. BREITHARDT, G, BECKER, R, SEIPEL, L, ET AL: *Noninvasive detection of late potentials in man—a new marker for ventricular tachycardia.* Eur Heart J 2:1, 1981.

3. BREITHARDT, G, BORGGREFE, M, KARBENN, U, ET AL: *Prevalence of late potentials in patients with and without ventricular tachycardia: Correlation with angiographic findings.* Am J Cardiol 49:1932, 1982.

4. DENES, P, SANTARELLI, P, HAUSER, RG, ET AL: *Quantitative analysis of the high-frequency components of the terminal portion of the body surface QRS in normal subjects and in patients with ventricular tachycardia.* Circulation 67:1129, 1983.

5. FONTAINE, G, GUIRAUDON, G, FRANK, R, ET AL: *Stimulation studies and epicardial mapping in ventricular tachycardia: Study of mechanisms and selection for surgery.* In KULBERTUS, HE (ED): *Reentrant Arrhythmias.* MTP Press, Lancaster, 1977, p 334.

6. HOMBACH, V, BRAUN, V, HOPP, H-W, ET AL: *The applicability of the signal averaged technique in clinical cardiology.* Clin Cardiol 5:107, 1982.

7. ROZANSKI, JJ, MORTARA, D, MYERBURG, RJ, ET AL: *Body surface detection of delayed depolarization in patients with recurrent ventricular tachycardia and left ventricular aneurysm.* Circulation 63:1172, 1981.

8. SIMSON, MB: *Use of signals in the terminal QRS complex to identify patients with ventricular tachycardia after myocardial infarction.* Circulation 64:235, 1981.

9. SIMSON, MB, SPIELMAN, SR, HOROWITZ, LN, ET AL: *Late potentials in man and cardiac arrhythmias.* In HOMBACH, V AND HILGER, HH (EDS): *Signal Averaging Technique in Clinical Cardiology.* FK Schattauer Verlag, New York, 1981, p 253.

10. SIMSON, MB, SPIELMAN, SR, HOROWITZ, LN, ET AL: *Effects of antiarrhythmic drugs on body surface late potentials in patients with ventricular tachycardia.* Am J Cardiol 49:1030, 1982.

11. UTHER, JB, DENNETT, CJ, AND TAN, A: *The detection of delayed activation signals of low amplitude in the vectorcardiogram of patients with recurrent ventricular tachycardia by signal averaging.* In SANDOR, E, JULIAN, DJ, AND BELL, JW (EDS): *Management of Ventricular Tachycardia—Role of Mexiletine.* Excerpta Medica, Oxford, 1978, p 80.

12. SIMSON, MB, UNTEREKER, WJ, SPIELMAN, SR, ET AL: *The relationship between late potentials on the body surface and directly recorded fragmented electrograms in patients with ventricular tachycardia.* Am J Cardiol 51:105, 1983.

13. SIMSON, MB, EULER, D, MICHELSON, EL, ET AL: *Detection of delayed ventricular activation on the body surface in dogs.* Am J Physiol 241:H363, 1981.

14. BOINEAU, JP AND COX, JL: *Slow ventricular activation in acute myocardial infarction: A source of reentrant premature ventricular contraction.* Circulation 48:702, 1973.

15. EL SHERIF, N, SCHERLAG, BJ, AND LAZZARA, R: *Electrode catheter recordings during malignant ventricular arrhythmias following experimental acute myocardial ischemia.* Circulation 51:1003, 1975.

16. EL-SHERIF, N, SCHERLAG, BJ, LAZZARA, R, ET AL: *Reentrant ventricular arrhythmias in the late myocardial infarction period: I. Conduction characteristics in the infarction zone.* Circulation 55:686, 1977.

17. EL-SHERIF, N, SCHERLAG, BJ, LAZZARA, R, ET AL: *Reentrant ventricular arrhythmias in the late myocardial infarction period: II. Patterns of initiation and termination of reentry.* Circulation 55:702, 1977.

18. JOSEPHSON, ME, HOROWITZ, LN, AND FARSHIDI, A: *Continuous local electrical activity: A mechanism of recurrent ventricular tachycardia.* Circulation 57: 659, 1978.

19. MYERBURG, RJ, GELBAND, H, NILSSON, K, ET AL: *Long-term electrophysiological abnormalities resulting from experimental myocardial infarction in cats.* Circ Res 41:73, 1977.

20. SPIELMAN, SR, UNTEREKER, WJ, HOROWITZ, LN, ET AL: *Fragmented electrical activity-relationship to ventricular tachycardia.* Am J Cardiol 47:448, 1981.

21. WALDO, AL AND KAISER, GA: *A study of ventricular arrhythmias associated with acute myocardial infarction in the canine heart.* Circulation 3:1222, 1973.

22. ROS, HH, KOELEMAN, ASM, AND AKKER, TJ: *The technique of signal averaging and its practical application in the separation of atrial and His Purkinje activity.* In HOMBACH, V AND HILGER, HH (EDS): *Signal Averaging Technique in Clinical Cardiology.* FK Schattauer Verlag, New York, 1981, p 3.

23. OPPENHEIM, AV AND SCHAFFER, RW: *Digital Signal Processing.* Prentice Hall, Englewood Cliffs, NJ, 1975, pp 195–283.

24. JOSEPHSON, ME, SIMSON, MB, HARKEN, AH, ET AL: *The incidence and clinical significance of epicardial late potentials in patients with recurrent sustained ventricular tachycardia and coronary artery disease.* Circulation 66:1199, 1982.

25. SIMSON, MB, FALCONE, R, DRESDEN, C, ET AL: *The signal averaged ECG and electrophysiologic studies in patients with ventricular tachycardia and fibrillation.* Circulation 68(Suppl III):III-173, 1983.

26. HAMMERMEISTER, KE, DEROVEN, TA, AND DODGE, HT: *Variables predictive of survival in patients with coronary disease.* Circulation 59:421, 1979.

27. HARRIS, PJ, HARRELL, FE, LEE, KL, ET AL: *Survival in medically treated coronary artery disease.* Circulation 60:1259, 1979.

28. SCHULZE, RA, HUMPHRIES, JO, GRIFFITH, LSC, ET AL: *Left ventricular and coronary angiographic anatomy: Relationship to ventricular irritability in the late hospital phase of acute myocardial infarction.* Circulation 55:839, 1977.

29. WEAVER, WD, LORCH, GS, ALVAREZ, HA, ET AL: *Angiographic findings and prognostic indicators in patients resuscitated from sudden cardiac death.* Circulation 54:895, 1976.

30. COHEN, M, WIENER, I, PICHARD, A, ET AL: *Determinants of ventricular tachycardia in patients with coronary artery disease and ventricular aneurysm.* Am J Cardiol 51:61, 1983.

31. GREENE, HL, REID, PR, AND SCHAEFFER, AH: *The repetitive ventricular response in man: A predictor of sudden death.* N Engl J Med 299:729, 1978.

32. FARSHIDI, A, MICHELSON, EL, GREENSPAN, AM, ET AL: *Repetitive responses to ventricular extrastimuli: Incidence, mechanism and significance.* Am Heart J 100:59, 1980.

33. RUSKIN, JN, DIMARCO, JP, AND GARAN, H: *Repetitive responses to single ventricular extrastimuli in patients with serious ventricular arrhythmias: Incidence and clinical significance.* Circulation 63:767, 1981.

34. RICHARDS, DA, CODY, DV, DENNISS, AR, ET AL: *Ventricular electrical instability: A predictor of death after myocardial infarction.* Am J Cardiol 51:75. 1983.

35. KANOVSKY, MS, FALCONE, RA, DRESDEN, CA, ET AL: *Identification of patients with ventricular tachycardia after myocardial infarction: Signal averaged ECG, Holter monitoring, and cardiac catheterization.* Circulation (in press).

36. DENNISS, AR, HOLLEY, LK, CODY, DV, ET AL: *Ventricular tachycardia and fibrillation: Differences in ventricular activation times and ventricular function.* J Am Coll Cardiol 1:606, 1983.

# Mechanism of Lethal Arrhythmias: Results of Programmed Electrical Stimulation*

*Alfred E. Buxton, M.D.,† Francis E. Marchlinski, M.D.,†*
*John U. Doherty, M.D.,‡ Harvey L. Waxman, M.D., and*
*Mark E. Josephson, M.D.§*

Sudden death is the most pressing problem in cardiology today. Epidemiologic studies performed initially more than a decade ago and repeated subsequently have demonstrated that greater than 50 percent of deaths in patients with coronary artery disease occur suddenly and unexpectedly. Moreover, most victims of sudden cardiac death when studied by autopsy or (in the case of survivors) by cardiac catheterization have severe, extensive coronary artery disease. Conventional approaches to the prevention of this problem are based on observations made in the 1960s and 1970s when coronary care units came into existence for the treatment of patients with acute myocardial infarction. Because the majority of sudden deaths occurring within the first 24 hours of acute myocardial infarction were demonstrated to be caused by ventricular fibrillation,[1] and because prophylactic antiarrhythmic therapy was shown to be effective against this event,[2,3] it was reasoned that (1) recurrent myocardial ischemia or infarction precipitating ventricular fibrillation was the etiology of out-of-hospital sudden death in most cases, and (2) the use of chronic antiarrhythmic therapy should prove as effective for prevention of out-of-hospital sudden death as it had been in preventing ventricular fibrillation in the coronary care unit. Unfortunately, although it is true that ventricular fibrillation is the initial arrhythmia most frequently observed in victims of out-of-hospital arrest, at present there is no evidence that empiric antiarrhythmic therapy can prevent sudden death following myocardial infarction. The reasons for this seeming discrepancy are not established as yet, but recent studies in the clinical electrophysiology laboratory using programmed electrical stimulation have provided much additional insight into this problem.

Multiple potential reasons exist for the failure of empiric antiarrhythmic therapy to prevent sudden death, including inappropriate or incorrect choice of antiarrhythmic agents or dosages. Antiarrhythmic agents and dosing levels most frequently prescribed are based on trials conducted in patients with documented acute myocardial infarction. However, studies of survivors of out-of-hospital cardiac arrest have documented electrocardiographic and enzymatic evidence of acute myocardial infarction in no greater than 50 percent of patients;[4-6] and most victims who survive such events do not give a history of chest pain immediately preceding cardiac arrest, suggesting that acute myocardial ischemia and infarction are not responsible for initiating many episodes of cardiac arrest. In addition, data from a number of sources

*Supported in part by grants from the American Heart Association, Southeastern Pennsylvania Chapter, Philadelphia, Pennsylvania, and National Heart, Lung, and Blood Institute, Bethseda, Maryland (RO1HL28093).

†Supported by the University of Pennsylvania Department of Medicine Measey Foundation.

‡Recipient of the Southeastern Pennsylvania Heart Association Grant-in-Aid, Philadelphia, Pennsylvania.

§Recipient of Research Career Development Award No. HL00361, National Heart, Lung, and Blood Institute, Bethesda, Maryland.

indicate that ventricular fibrillation is not the only, or perhaps even the most frequent, rhythm disturbance precipitating out-of-hospital cardiac arrest. Ambulatory electrocardiographic monitors have been recorded fortuitously at the time of cardiac arrest in a number of patients.[7-9] Most frequently, the initial dysrhythmia observed was not ventricular fibrillation, but rather rapid ventricular tachycardia that caused cardiac arrest by itself or else degenerated into ventricular fibrillation. Data from our institution and others suggest that the earlier patients are monitored in the course of cardiac arrests, the higher the detection of ventricular tachycardia as the initiating rhythm rather than ventricular fibrillation.[10,11] Although studies of survivors of cardiac arrest may be skewed because patients whose arrest is initiated by ventricular tachycardia appear more likely to survive their event than those whose arrest is initiated by ventricular fibrillation,[6] increasing data support the importance of ventricular tachycardia as the cause of cardiac arrest.

The differentiation between ventricular tachycardia and fibrillation as the initiating arrhythmia has important mechanistic and therapeutic implications. Although ventricular fibrillation may occur as a primary arrhythmia without precipitating factors, it also may result from acute myocardial ischemia or may follow degeneration of an organized ventricular tachycardia. In contrast, ventricular tachycardia occurring in the setting of chronic coronary artery disease most frequently appears to be related to re-entry arising from a fairly stable substrate.[12,13] Such arrhythmias do not require metabolic factors such as acute myocardial ischemia for initiation, as evidenced by the ability to initiate them with timed ventricular extrastimuli in the electrophysiology laboratory and by a lack of angina preceding spontaneous episodes. In addition, such uniform-morphology ventricular tachycardias are rarely observed during acute ischemic events such as coronary artery spasm or within the first hours of acute myocardial infarction. A greatly simplified schema of spontaneous re-entrant ventricular arrhythmias would include two components: (1) a potential re-entrant circuit, and (2) a trigger. In the case of patients with previous myocardial infarctions, the circuit probably consists of a generally stable region of tissue on the periphery of the infarction that has developed arrhythmogenic properties (that is, the potential for slow conduction and unidirectional block). This circuit remains quiescent until the appropriate trigger(s)—usually a ventricular depolarization(s) with a critical degree of prematurity—activates the circuit, initiating ventricular tachycardia.

If such a model of re-entrant ventricular tachyarrhythmias is accurate, one might be able to predict patients at risk of these arrhythmias by identifying those patients in whom either the appropriate triggers are present or the proper substrate exists, or both. Likewise, one might approach the prevention of such arrhythmias by abolishing either the triggers (ventricular premature depolarizations) or the arrhythmogenic substrate. The conventional approach to the identification of patients at high risk for sudden death and the evaluation of antiarrhythmic therapy has been based on evaluation of the triggers. That is, spontaneous ventricular ectopy has been assessed using ambulatory electrocardiographic monitoring. Unfortunately, this technique has serious limitations: the prevalence of spontaneous ventricular arrhythmias in patients with underlying heart disease increases markedly with duration of monitoring, and there is a marked variability in prevalence and characteristics of spontaneous ventricular ectopy over time that may actually mimic the effects of antiarrhythmic therapy.[14,15] Finally, no form of ventricular ectopy has been shown to specifically predict risk of sudden cardiac death versus overall cardiac deaths. Abolition of all spontaneous ventricular ectopy may not be necessary in order to prevent sustained ventricular tachyarrhythmias, and, conversely, suppression of spontaneous ventricular ectopy does not necessarily indicate successful prophylaxis of sustained arrhythmias.[16,17]

The limitations and frustrations of evaluating high-risk patients on the basis of "triggers" using ambulatory monitoring have encouraged the use of other diagnostic and therapeutic approaches based on analysis of the arrhythmogenic substrate, principally using programmed electrical stimulation. Programmed stimulation, by evaluating the inducibility of sustained ventricular arrhythmias, assesses the degree to which the arrhythmogenic substrate is present and able to sustain a continuous re-entrant circuit, while ignoring the spontaneous triggers for this circuit. The proper interpretation of the results of programmed electrical stimulation in patients with ventricular tachyarrhythmias is dependent on three major factors. The first factor is documentation of the electrocardiographic characteristics of the spontaneous arrhythmia with regard to morphology, rate, and duration in order to ensure that the arrhythmia induced in the laboratory is the same as the spontaneous arrhythmia. The second factor is evaluation of potential precipitating factors for the arrhythmia such as acute myocardial ischemia, exercise, or drug toxicity. Third, the use of electrophysiologic studies to guide antiarrhythmic therapy is based on the assumption that the acute response of induced arrhythmias to antiarrhythmic agents assessed in the electrophysiology laboratory correlates with the results of chronic antiarrhythmic therapy for the prevention of the same arrhythmia. The remainder of this chapter will discuss the results of programmed electrical stimulation in a large group of patients with potentially lethal arrhythmias studied in our laboratory over the past 3 years.

## ELECTROPHYSIOLOGIC STUDY PROTOCOL

The initial electrophysiologic study is performed after all antiarrhythmic agents have been discontinued for at least five half-lives of the drugs employed. Multipolar electrode catheters are inserted and placed at one or more right ventricular sites. In our laboratory, stimulation is performed using rectangular impulses 1 msec in duration at twice diastolic threshold. One to three premature ventricular stimuli are introduced during sinus rhythm and during at least two ventricular paced rates. The extrastimuli are initially introduced in late diastole, and repeated with progressively more prematurity. If programmed stimulation fails to induce sustained ventricular tachycardia, rapid pacing without premature stimuli is performed. The protocol is performed at two disparate right ventricular sites, most often the apex and outflow tract, until sustained ventricular tachycardia is induced or ventricular refractoriness is reached. If right ventricular stimulation fails to induce sustained tachycardia, this protocol will be repeated at one or more left ventricular sites. In addition, isoproterenol may be infused in an attempt to provoke tachycardia in selected patients. In all patients, the endpoint of stimulation is induction of sustained arrhythmias. Tachycardias are considered inducible if they can be initiated at least twice by similar modes of programmed stimulation. Nonsustained ventricular tachycardia is one that lasts at least three beats and terminates spontaneously in less than 30 seconds, whereas sustained ventricular tachycardia is one that lasts longer than 30 seconds or requires termination within 30 seconds because of hemodynamic decompensation.

## RESULTS OF PROGRAMMED STIMULATION IN PATIENTS WITH POTENTIALLY LETHAL ARRHYTHMIAS

Two groups of patients have been studied: 172 patients who presented with sustained ventricular tachyarrhythmias (113 of whom had hemodynamically stable sustained ventricular tachycardia and 59 who presented as cardiac arrests with documented ventricular fibrillation or ventricular tachycardia), and 71 patients who presented with only nonsustained ventricular tachycardia. These patients ranged in age from 14 to 82 years, with a median age of 58 years. Coronary artery disease with prior myocardial infarction was the most common underlying cardiac disease in all patient groups, but left ventricular aneurysms were present more frequently in the patients with sustained ventricular arrhythmias than in those with only nonsustained ventricular tachycardia. Cardiomyopathy and absence of structural heart disease were found more frequently in the patients presenting with only nonsustained ventricular tachycardia (Table 1).

**Table 1.** Patient population

| Associated cardiac disease | VT-S | Cardiac arrest | VT-NS |
|---|---|---|---|
| CAD | 94 | 43 | 31 |
| MI | 91 | 38 | 30 |
| LV an | 53 | 20 | 13 |
| CM | 6 | 11 | 17 |
| Other | 7 | 5 | 8 |
| NHD | 6 | 0 | 15 |

VT-S = spontaneous sustained ventricular tachycardia; VT-NS = spontaneous nonsustained ventricular tachycardia; CAD = coronary artery disease; CM = cardiomyopathy; MI = prior myocardial infarction; LV an = left ventricular aneurysm; Other = structural heart disease other than CAD or CM; NHD = no organic heart disease.
Figures represent numbers of patients studied.

The inducibility of ventricular tachyarrhythmias is directly related to the spontaneous arrhythmia. Ventricular tachycardia was induced in 98 percent of those patients who presented with hemodynamically stable, sustained ventricular tachycardia, in comparison with 81 percent of those who presented with cardiac arrest, and with 59 percent of those with nonsustained ventricular tachycardia (Table 2). Similarly, induction of sustained versus nonsustained ventricular tachycardia was related in clinical presentation. Sustained ventricular tachycardia was induced in 96 percent of those who presented with stable sustained ventricular tachycardia, versus 75 percent of those presenting with cardiac arrest and 28 percent of those with nonsustained ventricular tachycardia. Clinical presentation also influenced the mode of stimulation necessary for tachycardia induction. Whereas double ventricular extrastimuli were the most common method for inducing tachycardia in the patients with sustained ventricular tachycardia, triple extrastimuli were required with significantly greater frequency in the patients who presented with cardiac arrest and those patients with nonsustained ventricular tachycardia (see Table 2). Left ventricular stimulation was seldom required in patients with nonsustained ventricular tachycardia and those with hemodynamically stable, sustained ventricular tachycardia, but was needed significantly more frequently in patients presented with cardiac arrest (Table 3).

The characteristics of induced arrhythmias were influenced more by the clinical presentation than the mode of arrhythmia induction. Tachycardias induced in patients who presented as cardiac arrest had significantly shorter cycle lengths than those induced in patients with hemodynamically stable, sustained ventricular tachycardia and nonsustained ventricular tachycardia, although there was a large degree of overlap between each group (Table 4). The tachycardias induced by single extrastimuli in the patients with sustained arrhythmias had significantly longer cycle lengths than those induced by double or triple extrastimuli. The morphology of induced tachycardias (that is, uniform versus polymorphic) was also influenced

**Table 2.** Modes of VT induction

| Patient group | S | D | T | RP | Total (% inducible) |
|---|---|---|---|---|---|
| VT-S | 25 | 59 | 25 | 1 | 110 (98%) |
| Cardiac arrest | 2 | 15 | 30 | 1 | 48 (81%) |
| VT-NS | 3 | 17 | 21 | 1 | 42 (59%) |

VT-S = spontaneous sustained ventricular tachycardia; VT-NS = spontaneous nonsustained ventricular tachycardia; S = induction by single ventricular extrastimulus; D = induction by double ventricular extrastimuli; T = induction by triple ventricular extrastimuli; RP = induction only by rapid ventricular pacing. Figures represent numbers of patients studied.

**Table 3.** Modes of VT induction: Requirement for multiple stimulation sites

| Patient group | RVA | RVOT | LV |
|---|---|---|---|
| VT-S | 95 | 12 | 3 |
| Cardiac arrest | 36 | 3 | 9 |
| VT-NS | 30 | 10 | 2 |

VT-S = spontaneous sustained ventricular tachycardia; VT-NS = spontaneous nonsustained ventricular tachycardia; RVA = VT induced by stimulation at right ventricular apex; RVOT = VT induced only by stimulation at right ventricular outflow tract; LV = induced only by stimulation at left ventricle.

primarily by the clinical presentation rather than the mode of induction. Rapid, polymorphic tachycardias were induced much more often in patients with cardiac arrest than in those with hemodynamically stable, sustained ventricular tachycardia, regardless of the mode of stimulation needed for induction. Polymorphic tachycardias were also induced with similar frequency by double and triple extrastimuli in the patients with nonsustained ventricular tachycardia.

The inducibility of tachycardia was not related to underlying heart disease in the patients who presented with sustained arrhythmias—the vast majority of whom had coronary artery disease. However, inducibility was closely related to type of heart disease in those patients who presented with nonsustained ventricular tachycardia. Whereas 94 percent of patients with nonsustained ventricular tachycardia occurring in the setting of coronary artery disease had inducible arrhythmias, only one third of patients with cardiomyopathy, valvular disease, or no structural heart disease had inducible arrhythmias. The induction of sustained ventricular tachycardias was also closely related to the existence and type of underlying heart disease in the patients with nonsustained ventricular tachycardia. Sustained ventricular tachycardia was not induced in any patient without structural heart disease, but was most often induced in patients with coronary artery disease and left ventricular aneurysms: sustained arrhythmias were induced in 15 out of 83 patients presenting with only nonsustained tachycardia, and 13 of these patients had coronary artery disease with prior myocardial infarctions.

The specificity of our stimulation protocol may be determined by examining the frequency with which apparently nonclinical, rapid, polymorphic tachycardias were induced in patients whose spontaneous arrhythmia had a uniform morphology (Table 5). The frequency of induction of these arrhythmias is similar in each patient group and does not differ significantly with various stimulation modes.

In summary, the use of programmed stimulation in these patient groups results in a high sensitivity of arrhythmia induction in patients who present with sustained arrhythmias, but a lower sensitivity in those with nonsustained tachycardias. Specificity of this stimulation pro-

**Table 4.** Characteristics of induced tachycardias

| Patient group | S | | D | | T | |
|---|---|---|---|---|---|---|
| | CL | % Uniform | CL | % Uniform | CL | % Uniform |
| VT-S | 329 ± 52 | 100 | 287 ± 59 | 96 | 291 ± 60 | 95 |
| Cardiac arrest | 325* | 100 | 213 ± 54 | 60 | 218 ± 38 | 50 |
| VT-NS | 295 ± 88 | 67 | 266 ± 58 | 35 | 270 ± 70 | 62 |

VT-S = spontaneous sustained ventricular tachycardia; VT-NS = spontaneous nonsustained ventricular tachycardia; CL = cycle length of induced tachycardia (mean ± S.D.) in msec; % uniform = percent of induced tachycardias having a uniform morphology; S = characteristics of tachycardias induced by single ventricular extrastimulus; D = characteristics of tachycardias induced by double ventricular extrastimuli; T = characteristics of tachycardias induced by triple ventricular extrastimuli.
*Only two patients with cardiac arrest had arrhythmias induced by single extrastimuli.

**Table 5.** Patients with spontaneous VT having uniform morphology/induced polymorphic VT

| Patient group | Mode of polymorphic VT induction | | | Total |
| | S | D | T | |
|---|---|---|---|---|
| VT-S | 6 | 8 | 1 | 15 (13%) |
| CA | 1 | 8 | 2 | 11 (19%) |
| VT-NS | — | 2 | 6 | 11 (19%) |
| Total | 7 | 18 | 9 | |

VT-S = spontaneous sustained ventricular tachycardia; VT-NS = spontaneous nonsustained ventricular tachycardia; S = polymorphic VT induced by single ventricular extrastimulus; D = polymorphic VT induced by double ventricular extrastimuli; T = polymorphic VT induced by triple ventricular extrastimuli; CA = cardiac arrest.

tocol is quite high in all patient groups. The characteristics of arrhythmias induced (including morphology, cycle length, and duration) depend primarily on the spontaneous clinical arrhythmia rather than the mode of stimulation inducing the tachycardia. Finally, the induction of sustained ventricular tachyarrhythmias is found most frequently in patients with previous myocardial infarctions and coexisting left ventricular aneurysms.

## PERSPECTIVE

The results of various studies including our own have shed much light on the mechanisms responsible for the syndrome of sudden cardiac death. It is now clear that whereas such events result primarily from ventricular tachyarrhythmias, sudden cardiac death may result not only from ventricular fibrillation, but frequently from organized ventricular tachycardias that do not require acute myocardial ischemia or infarction as initiating factors. At present, a number of problems remain with regard to the prevention and therapy of sudden cardiac death. More accurate, specific (and hopefully) noninvasive predictors of patients at risk of this event are needed. The methods for assessing antiarrhythmic therapy require improvement, and we desperately need antiarrhythmic agents with fewer side effects and higher degrees of efficacy. Finally, improvement of mechanical ventricular function by pharmacologic and/or surgical methods may be necessary in addition to primary antiarrhythmic therapy if survival of these patients is to be improved.

## REFERENCES

1. PANTRIDGE, JF AND GEDDES, JS: *A mobile intensive-care unit in the management of myocardial infarction.* Lancet 2:271, 1967.

2. LIE, KI, WELLENS, HJ, VAN CAPELLE, FJ, ET AL: *Lidocaine in the prevention of primary ventricular fibrillation.* N Engl J Med 291:1324, 1974.

3. KOCH-WESER, J, KLEIN, SW, FOO-CANTO, LL, ET AL: *Antiarrhythmic prophylaxis with procainamide in acute myocardial infarction.* N Engl J Med 281:1253, 1969.

4. LIBERTHSON, RR, NAGEL, EL, HIRSCHMAN, JC, ET AL: *Pathophysiologic observations in prehospital ventricular fibrillation and sudden cardiac death.* Circulation 49:790, 1974.

5. BAUM, RS, ALVAREZ, H, AND COBB, LA: *Survival after resuscitation from out-of-hospital ventricular fibrillation.* Circulation 50:1231, 1974.

6. MYERBURG, RJ, CONDE, CA, SUNG, RJ, ET AL: *Clinical, electrophysiologic and hemodynamic profile of patients resuscitated from prehospital cardiac arrest.* Am J Med 68:568, 1980.

7. WINKLE, RA: *Ambulatory electrocardiography and the diagnosis, evaluation, and treatment of chronic ventricular arrhythmias.* Prog Cardiovasc Dis 23:99, 1980.

8. PANIDIS, I AND MORGANROTH, J: *Holter monitoring during sudden cardiac death: Clues to etiology and prevention.* Circulation 66:II-25, 1982.

9. PRATT, CM, FRANCIS, MJ, LUCK, JC, ET AL: *Observations on sudden cardiac death recorded during ambulatory electrocardiographic monitoring.* Circulation 66:II-26, 1982.

10. JOSEPHSON, ME, HOROWITZ, LN, SPIELMAN, SR, ET AL: *Electrophysiologic and hemodynamic studies in patients resuscitated from cardiac arrest.* Am J Cardiol 46:948, 1980.

11. LIBERTHSON, RR, NAGEL, EL, HIRSCHMAN, JC, ET AL: *Prehospital ventricular defibrillation: Prognosis and follow-up course.* N Engl J Med 291:317, 1974.

12. WELLENS, HJJ, DURER, DR, AND LIE, KI: *Observations on mechanisms of ventricular tachycardia in man.* Circulation 54:237, 1976.

13. JOSEPHSON, ME, HOROWITZ, LN, FARSHIDI, A, ET AL: *Recurrent sustained ventricular tachycardia: 1. Mechanisms.* Circulation 57:431, 1978.

14. WINKLE, RA: *Antiarrhythmic drug effect mimicked by spontaneous variability of ventricular ectopy.* Circulation 57:1116, 1978.

15. MORGANROTH, J, MICHELSON, EL, HOROWITZ, LN, ET AL: *Limitations of routine long-term electrocardiographic monitoring to assess ventricular ectopy.* Circulation 57:1116, 1978.

16. MYERBURG, RJ, KESSLER, KM, KIEM, I, ET AL: *Relationship between plasma levels of procainamide, supression of premature ventricular complexes and prevention of recurrent ventricular tachycardia.* Circulation 64:280, 1981.

17. HERLING, IM, HOROWITZ, LN, AND JOSEPHSON, ME: *Ventricular ectopic activity following medical and surgical treatment for recurrent sustained ventricular tachycardia.* Am J Cardiol 45:633, 1980.

# Use of Programmed Electrical Stimulation to Predict Sudden Death After Myocardial Infarction*

*Francis E. Marchlinski, M.D.,† Alfred E. Buxton, M.D.,†*
*John U. Doherty, M.D.,‡ Dennis M. Cassidy, M.D.,§*
*Joseph A. Vassallo, M.D., John M. Miller, M.D.,*
*Michael G. Kienzle, M.D., Wayne Grogan, M.D.,*
*Jesus M. Almendral, M.D., Harvey L. Waxman, M.D., and*
*Mark E. Josephson, M.D.*

The risk of death in survivors of myocardial infarction is approximately 10 percent during the first year and 5 percent in subsequent years.[1-5] Up to 80 percent of these deaths are sudden cardiac deaths. The mechanism for most sudden cardiac death has been documented to be ventricular tachycardia and fibrillation.[6] A method for accurately identifying patients at greatest risk for these life-threatening arrhythmias would allow the opportunity to selectively treat the high-risk patient in an attempt to prevent sudden cardiac death.

## BACKGROUND

Previous work has documented an increased number of total and sudden cardiac deaths in patients with evidence of significant left ventricular dysfunction in association with and following myocardial infarction.[5,7,8] Left ventricular dysfunction associated with large myocardial infarction appears to be a nonspecific marker for electrical instability.[8,9] Most arrhythmias that develop following a recent myocardial infarction both in the experimental canine model and in man appear to have a re-entrant mechanism.[9,10] We have previously shown that programmed ventricular stimulation can be used to initiate ventricular arrhythmias in most patients who develop spontaneous episodes of sustained ventricular tachycardia in the early postinfarction period.[10] The possibility that programmed stimulation could be used to predict which patients are likely to develop ventricular arrhythmias is enticing. The use of premature extrastimuli to initiate a re-entrant tachycardia, thus identifying the patient with the necessary anatomic and electrophysiologic substrate for re-entry, may be the ideal method for identifying patients at increased risk for sudden cardiac death (Fig. 1).

## VALUE OF THE REPETITIVE VENTRICULAR RESPONSE

To date, four studies, including one from our institution, have attempted to determine the value of acute electrophysiologic testing in identifying risk of sudden cardiac death after myocardial infarction.[11-14] Differences in stimulation protocols, patient populations, and end-

*Supported in part by grants from the American Heart Association, Southeastern Pennsylvania Chapter, Philadelphia, Pennsylvania, and grants #HL24278 and #HL00361 from the National Heart, Lung, and Blood Institute, Bethesda, Maryland.

†Supported by the University of Pennsylvania Department of Medicine Measey Foundation.

‡Supported by Grant-in-Aid, American Heart Association, Southeastern Pennsylvania Chapter.

§Supported by a grant from the Canadian Heart Foundation Research Fellowship, Ottawa.

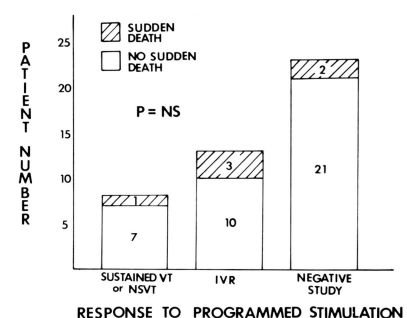

**Figure 1.** Incidence of sudden death (cross-hatched bars) related to response to programmed ventricular stimulation. No response to programmed ventricular stimulation identified patients at increased risk for sudden death. (From Marchlinski et al,[14] with permission.)

points for the response to programmed ventricular stimulation preclude a simple comparison of the results of these studies. Stimulation in all the reported studies was performed within 3 months of infarction. A summary of the protocols used is listed in Table 1.

The first study to be reported was by Greene and colleagues.[11] They studied 48 patients using single ventricular extrastimuli from the right ventricular apex delivered during sinus rhythm or atrial pacing. The endpoint of the stimulation was the development of a repetitive ventricular response. Repetitive ventricular responses were defined as two or more ventricular premature beats in response to a single stimulus. During a followup of 1 year, 15 of the 19 patients who developed a repetitive ventricular response experienced ventricular tachycardia or sudden death, compared with 4 of 29 patients who failed to develop a repetitive ventricular response. These results suggested that the repetitive ventricular response may have predictive value in identifying the risk of life-threatening ventricular tachyarrhythmias.

Initial observations made by Greene and coworkers[11] regarding the frequency of observed repetitive ventricular responses have not been supported by other studies. Hamer and

**Table 1.** Stimulation protocols used in the post-infarction period

| Study | Maximum no. of extrastimuli | Extrastimuli during RV pacing | Current or voltage strength | No. of sites stimulated |
|---|---|---|---|---|
| Greene et al[11] | 1 | No | <4 mA | 1–2 |
| Hamer et al[12] | 1–2 | Yes | 2–10 volts | 1–2 |
| Richards et al[13] | 2 | Yes | 2–20 mA | 2 |
| Marchlinski et al[14] | 2 | Yes | <2 mA | 1 |

RV = right ventricular

associates[12] failed to note intraventricular re-entrant responses in any of the 70 patients receiving single ventricular extrastimuli during sinus rhythm or atrial pacing in the post-infarction period. Our results are consistent with those of Hamer and colleagues[12] in that only 1 of 34 patients studied had intraventricular re-entrant responses with single extrastimuli delivered during normal sinus rhythm. The basis for the discrepancy in results, from those of Greene and coworkers, is not known. Careful exclusion of bundle branch re-entrant repetitive responses (a physiologic response to premature ventricular stimulation) by using additional intracardiac recordings from the His bundle region, may account for some of the difference.[15] Of note, the incidence of repetitive ventricular responses to ventricular extrastimuli delivered during normal sinus rhythm in patients with a history of documented ventricular tachycardia and coronary artery disease but who are not in the peri-infarction period is also relatively low, ranging from 13 to 15 percent.[16,17] Failure to confirm results noted by Greene and colleagues suggests that the repetitive ventricular response still has an unestablished relationship to sudden death in the patient recovering from myocardial infarction. Furthermore, the suppression of the repetitive ventricular response with antiarrhythmic therapy should not be considered an adequate therapeutic endpoint.

## ROLE OF PROGRAMMED VENTRICULAR STIMULATION

The three other studies that assess the value of programmed stimulation in identifying risk of sudden death following myocardial infarction used as endpoints for their stimulation protocols the development of ventricular arrhythmias.[12–14] Hamer and associates[12] studied 70 patients; 37 received only single ventricular extrastimuli during sinus rhythm and right ventricular pacing, and 33 patients received "the complete stimulation protocol," which consisted of single and double ventricular extrastimuli during sinus rhythm and ventricular pacing at a stimulating voltage of 2 to 10 volts. Based on the results of the stimulation, patients were divided into three groups: Group 1 consisted of 12 patients who had at least 5 extra responses (self-limited or nonsustained ventricular tachycardia) to stimulation; Group 2 consisted of 25 patients who had the "complete stimulation protocol" but had fewer than 5 extra responses to programmed ventricular stimulation; and Group 3 consisted of the remaining 33 patients who did not receive the complete protocol and had fewer than 5 extra responses to programmed ventricular stimulation. During a 1-year followup, 4 of the 12 Group 1 patients died suddenly, compared with only 1 of the 25 Group 2 patients ($p < 0.05$). The investigators concluded that a reproducible response of greater than five extra ventricular depolarizations to either single or double extrastimuli might be predictive of an increased risk for subsequent cardiac death. However, inasmuch as the initial design of the study was not to determine the number of the repetitive responses which predicted sudden death, the arbitrary selection of five complexes during data analysis increased the likelihood that differences noted between Groups 1 and 2 occurred by chance alone. Nevertheless, the preliminary findings do suggest a possible role of programmed stimulation in identifying the high-risk patients.

A study by Richards and colleagues[13] reported that a more vigorous stimulation protocol may be important when attempting to identify the patient at risk for sudden death following myocardial infarction. The stimulation protocol used included the introduction of single and double ventricular extrastimuli during ventricular pacing from both the right ventricular apex and outflow tract. Stimuli were initially delivered at twice diastolic threshold using a 2-msec pulse width. If ventricular tachycardia or fibrillation lasting longer than 10 seconds was not initiated, the entire stimulation protocol was repeated using a 20-mA current strength. Based on the response to programmed stimulation, patients were divided into electrically stable (less than 10 seconds of ventricular tachycardia or fibrillation in response to ventricular extrastimuli) and electrically unstable groups. Of the 38 patients who demonstrated electrical instability, 8 died suddenly and 4 developed spontaneous ventricular tachycardia during a mean followup of 8 months. This compared with no sudden deaths and only 2 patients developing ventricular tachycardia in the 127 patients who demonstrated electrical stability. The cumulative 1-year survival was 91 percent for the electrically stable patients and 65 percent for the electrically unstable patients (p < 0.001). It is noteworthy that the sensitivity and specificity of a stimulation protocol using increased current strength have not been established for any clinical situation. In comparison, the introduction of single and double right ventricular extrastimuli at twice diastolic threshold has been demonstrated to result in the induction of sustained ventricular tachycardia in approximately 80 percent of patients with chronic sustained ventricular tachycardia and in over 50 percent of patients with sustained ventricular tachycardia associated with a recent myocardial infarction.[10,18,19] More importantly, the same stimulation protocol also produced a few false-positive results; of the 156 patients in the reported series who had no previously documented arrhythmias, no patient had sustained ventricular tachycardia initiated and only 37 percent of these patients had nonsustained ventricular tachycardia initiated.[18,19] Nevertheless, the study by Richards and colleagues, like that of Hamer and associates,[12] suggests that programmed stimulation may have a role in identifying patients at risk for life-threatening ventricular arrhythmias.

## THE RESPONSE TO PROGRAMMED VENTRICULAR STIMULATION VERSUS EVIDENCE OF LEFT VENTRICULAR DYSFUNCTION IN IDENTIFYING PATIENTS AT RISK OF SUDDEN DEATH

We have also attempted to determine the predictive value of programmed stimulation in identifying patients at risk of sudden death following myocardial infarction.[15] In addition, we wanted to compare the ability of programmed stimulation to identify patients at risk for sudden death versus the ability of indices of left ventricular dysfunction and the degree of spontaneous ectopy to identify risk. Forty-six patients underwent programmed ventricular stimulation at a mean of 22 days after myocardial infarction. The stimulation protocol involved single and double ventricular extrastimuli from the right ventricular apex during ventricular pacing in all patients and normal sinus rhythm in 33 of the 46 patients. All stimulation was performed using a pacing current that was twice diastolic threshold and less than or equal to 2 mA. In 44 of the 46 patients, left ventricular ejection fraction and the presence of a left ventricular aneurysm were determined. None of the patients studied had ventricular tachycardia or fibrillation after the initial 24 hours of hospitalization.

Based on the response to programmed ventricular stimulation, patients were divided into three groups. Group 1 consisted of 10 patients who developed either nonsustained (5 patients) or sustained (5 patients) ventricular tachycardia. Nonsustained ventricular tachycardia was defined as four or more complexes but terminating in less than 30 seconds. Group 2 consisted of 13 patients in whom one to two intraventricular re-entrant repetitive responses were observed. Group 3 consisted of 23 patients in whom bundle branch re-entrant or no repetitive responses were observed. All patients have been followed for at least 6 months with a mean followup of 18 months. During the followup period, there were six sudden cardiac deaths. Two patients, one with nonsustained and one with sustained ventricular tachycardia, were excluded from data analysis because therapy at the request of the referring physician was directed by programmed ventricular stimulation. Both patients are doing well. It is noteworthy that no response to programmed ventricular stimulation using the described protocol indentified the patients at increased risk of sudden death (see Fig. 1). Similarly, the presence of complex ventricular ectopy did not appear to identify the high-risk patient, in that the incidence of sudden death in the patients with Lown grade 0 to 2 ventricular arrhythmias (3 of 23 patients) did not differ from those patients with Lown grades 3 or 4 ventricular arrhythmias (3 of 19 patients). Importantly, however, the presence of an ejection fraction of less than 40 percent or a left ventricular aneurysm appeared useful in identifying patients at highest risk for dying suddenly (Fig. 2).

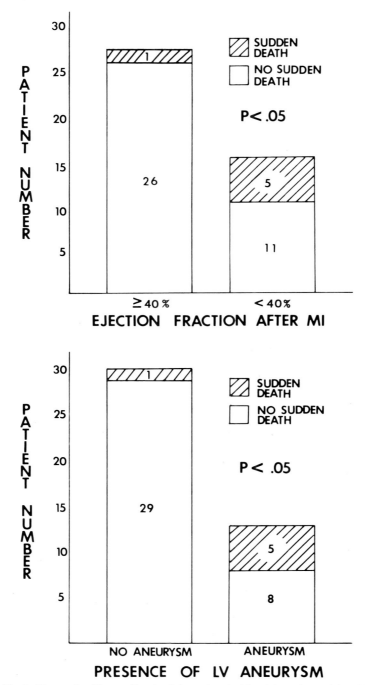

**Figure 2.** *(Top)* The incidence of sudden cardiac death (cross-hatched bars) in patients with an EF of less than 40 percent following MI is significantly greater than in the patients with an EF greater than or equal to 40 percent. *(Bottom)* Similarly, the incidence of subsequent sudden cardiac death is significantly greater in patients who have a LV aneurysm after MI. (From Marchlinski et al,[14] with permission.)

### Characteristics of Induced Ventricular Tachycardia

The sustained ventricular tachycardia induced in five patients had a uniform morphology. The tachycardia cycle length tended to be rapid, ranging in cycle length from 220 to 280 msec with a mean of 235 msec. The induced nonsustained ventricular tachycardia had a uniform morphology in two patients and was polymorphic in three patients. The cycle length of the induced nonsustained ventricular tachycardia also tended to be rapid and ranged between 210 and 250 msec. Double ventricular extrastimuli were required to initiate all episodes of ventricular tachycardia. The short cycle length of the ventricular tachycardia suggests an anatomically or physiologically small re-entrant circuit. This circuit may be less responsive to spontaneous triggers of arrhythmias and thus may account for the unexpected low incidence of spontaneous arrhythmias despite evidence suggesting the presence of the necessary substrate for ventricular arrhythmias.

## COMPARISON OF STUDIES

The basis for the difference in the results of our investigation compared with those reported by others may be related to the stimulation protocol used.[12–14] Both studies suggesting that the response to programmed ventricular stimulation may identify the high-risk patient differed from ours in two major ways: (1) two right ventricular sites were stimulated in all the patients studied by Richards and colleagues and approximately two thirds of the patients studied by Hamer and coinvestigators, and (2) ventricular stimulation was also performed at markedly increased current or voltage strength. Hamer and associates[12] noted that stimulation from a second right ventricular site (outflow tract) did not significantly contribute to the results of programmed stimulation. The frequency of ventricular tachycardia or fibrillation induced from only the second right ventricular site was not discussed by Richards and coworkers;[13] therefore, its importance cannot be determined. When examining the importance of increased current strength, Hamer and associates[12] noted that 4 of the 12 patients who had greater than 5 extra responses to programmed stimulation required increased stimulation voltage to elicit this response. It is not stated, however, whether any of the four patients died suddenly during followup. Similarly, it is not stated by Richards and coworkers[13] how many patients required increased current strength to demonstrate electrical instability, although they did note that four of their patients who did not die suddenly or develop ventricular tachycardia required the increased current strength to demonstrate greater than 10 seconds of ventricular tachycardia or fibrillation in response to programmed ventricular stimulation.

## SUMMARY

The use of programmed ventricular stimulation to identify patients at risk for sudden cardiac death following myocardial infarction has not yet been firmly established. The repetitive ventricular response following extrastimuli does not appear to be useful in identifying patients at risk and should not be used to guide antiarrhythmic therapy. Similarly, the response to single and/or double ventricular extrastimuli delivered at twice diastolic threshold from a single right ventricular site during normal sinus rhythm and ventricular pacing also does not appear to be helpful in identifying patients at risk for life-threatening ventricular arrhythmias. A more vigorous stimulation protocol that involves more than one right ventricular site and increased current strength may be necessary to elicit a predictive electrophysiologic response. The need for a more vigorous stimulation is suggested by two preliminary studies. Confirmation of initial reports is necessary. The predictive value of the response to programmed ventricular stimulation must be compared with other noninvasive and invasive measurements of left ventricular dysfunction and the degree of spontaneous ventricular ectopy to determine its superiority or to ascertain multiple variables that can be used together to identify those patients most likely to die suddenly after myocardial infarction. Stimulation protocols used during programmed stimulation must have sufficient sensitivity without sacrificing specificity. A concerted effort using uniform stimulation protocols in large numbers of patients is essential to resolve this important clinical problem.

# REFERENCES

1. GAZES, PC, KITCHELL, JR, MELTZER, LE, ET AL: *Death rate among 795 patients in first year after myocardial infarction.* JAMA 197:184, 1966.

2. MOSS, AJ, DECAMILLA, J, AND DAVIS, H: *Cardiac death in the first 6 months after myocardial infarction: Potential for mortality reduction in the early post-hospital period.* Am J Cardiol 39:816, 1977.

3. HELMERS, C AND LUNDMAN, T: *Early and sudden death after myocardial infarction.* Acta Med Scand 205:3, 1979.

4. KANNEL, W, STOLLIE, P, AND MCNAMANA, P: *Prognosis after initial myocardial infarction: The Framingham Study.* Am J Cardiol 44:53, 1979.

5. SANZ, G, COSTANER, A, BETRIU, A, ET AL: *Determinants of prognosis in survivors of myocardial infarction.* N Engl J Med 306:1065, 1982.

6. PANIDIS, I AND MORGANROTH, J: *Sudden death in hospitalized patients: Cardiac rhythm disturbances detected by ambulatory electrocardiographic monitoring.* J Am Coll Cardiol 2: 798, 1983.

7. SCHULZE, RA, ROULEAU, J, RIGO, P, ET AL: *Ventricular arrhythmias in the late hospital phase of acute myocardial infarction: Relation to left ventricular function detected by gated cardiac blood pool scanning.* Circulation 52:1006, 1975.

8. LIE, KI, LIEM, KL, SCHUILENBURG, RM, ET AL: *Early identification of patients developing late in-hospital ventricular fibrillation after discharge from the coronary care unit.* Am J Cardiol 41:574, 1978.

9. GANG, ES, BIGGER, JT, AND LIVELLI, FD: *A model of chronic ischemic arrhythmias: The relation between electrically inducible ventricular tachycardia, ventricular fibrillation threshold and myocardial infarct size.* Am J Cardiol 50:469, 1982.

10. MARCHLINSKI, FE, WAXMAN, HL, BUXTON, AB, ET AL: *Sustained ventricular tachyarrhythmias during the early postinfarction period: Electrophysiologic findings and prognosis for survival.* J Am Coll Cardiol 2:240, 1983.

11. GREENE, HL, REID, PR, AND SCHAEFFER, AH: *The repetitive ventricular response in man: A predictor of sudden death.* N Engl J Med 299:729, 1978.

12. HAMER, A, VOHRA, J, HUND, D, ET AL: *Prediction of sudden death by electrophysiologic studies in high risk patients surviving acute myocardial infarction.* Am J Cardiol 50:223, 1982.

13. RICHARDS, DA, CODY, DV, DENNISS, AR, ET AL: *Ventricular electrical instability: A predictor of death after myocardial infarction.* Am J Cardiol 51:75, 1983.

14. MARCHLINSKI, FE, BUXTON, AB, WAXMAN, HL, ET AL: *Identifying patients at risk of sudden death after myocardial infarction: Value of the response to programmed stimulation, degree of ventricular ectopic activity and severity of left ventricular dysfunction.* Am J Cardiol 52:1190, 1983.

15. AKTAR, M, DAMATO, AN, BATISFORD, WP, ET AL: *Demonstration of reentry within the His Purkinje system in man.* Circulation 50:1150, 1974.

16. MASON, J: *Repetitive beating after single ventricular extrastimuli: Incidence and prognostic significance in patients with recurrent ventricular tachycardia.* Am J Cardiol 45:1126, 1980.

17. RUSKIN, JW, MARCO, JP, AND GARAN, H: *Repetitive responses to single ventricular extrastimuli in patients with serious ventricular arrhythmias: Incidence and clinical significance.* Circulation 63:767, 1981.

18. VANDEPOL, CJ, FARSHIDA, A, SPIELMAN, JR, ET AL: *Incidence and clinical significance of induced ventricular tachycardia.* Am J Cardiol 45:725, 1980.

19. LIVELLI, FD, BIGGER, JT, REIFFEL, JA, ET AL: *Response to programmed ventricular stimulation: Sensitivity, specificity and relation to heart disease.* Am J Cardiol 50:452, 1982.

20. LOWN, B AND WOLF, M: *Approaches to sudden death from coronary heart disease.* Circulation 44:130, 1971.

# Electrophysiologic Testing of Survivors
# of Cardiac Arrest*

*Denis Roy, M.D., Francis E. Marchlinski, M.D.,†*
*John U. Doherty, M.D.,‡ Alfred E. Buxton, M.D.,†*
*Harvey L. Waxman, M.D., and Mark E. Josephson, M.D.*

Electrophysiologic testing is increasingly used as a method for identifying and managing patients who are at risk of sudden death. This technique has been performed in at least three groups of patients who are known to be at risk of sudden death: patients with recurrent sustained ventricular tachycardia (VT), survivors of a recent myocardial infarction, and survivors of a cardiac arrest. Electrophysiologic testing has proven helpful in evaluating patients with recurrent sustained VT,[1-6] and recent studies have suggested that electrophysiologic testing may identify survivors of a recent myocardial infarction who are at risk of dying suddenly.[7,8] Previous clinical trials have demonstrated that survivors of a cardiac arrest not related to an acute myocardial infarction who are discharged on empiric antiarrhythmic therapy have a high risk of recurrent sudden death.[9-11] This observation has prompted investigators during the past few years to use electrophysiologic testing to evaluate this small but high-risk group.[12-15] In this chapter, we will describe the technique of electrophysiologic testing and will examine the results of this technique when applied to survivors of a cardiac arrest.

## ELECTROPHYSIOLOGIC TESTING PROTOCOL

Antiarrhythmic drugs are discontinued for at least four half-lives before electrophysiologic testing. Studies are performed in the unsedated postabsorptive state. Two or more electrode catheters are inserted percutaneously or by venous cutdown and positioned in the heart under fluoroscopic guidance. Routinely, quadripolar catheters are placed at the high right atrium, coronary sinus, and right ventricular apex; and a tripolar catheter is used for His bundle recording at the atrioventricular junction.

Electrical stimulation is performed with a programmable stimulator and isolated constant current source. The stimuli are rectangular pulses, 1 msec in duration, delivered at twice diastolic threshold. Intracardiac recordings are filtered at 30 to 500 Hz and simultaneously recorded with three or more electrocardiographic leads (I, AVF, and $V_1$).

Sinus node function, atrioventricular conduction, and response to ventricular stimulation are tested. Atrial stimulation should be performed in particular in patients with the Wolff-

---

*Supported in part by grants from The American Heart Association, Southeastern Pennsylvania Chapter, Philadelphia, Pennsylvania, and grants #HL00361 and #HL24278 from the National Heart, Lung, and Blood Institute, Bethesda, Maryland, and The Fannie E. Ripple Foundation, Morristown, New Jersey.

†Supported by the University of Pennsylvania Measey Foundation.

‡Supported by a Grant-in-Aid from the American Heart Association, Southeastern Pennsylvania Chapter, Philadelphia, Pennsylvania.

Parkinson-White syndrome to rule out rapid supraventricular tachycardia as a cause of cardiac arrest.[16-19]

The stimulation techniques for initiating ventricular arrhythmias[4] consist of the delivery of one, two, or three ventricular extrastimuli during sinus rhythm or paced ventricular rhythm from the right ventricular apex and outflow tract. At least two paced ventricular rhythms are used (usually 600 and 400 msec), and the coupling intervals of the stimuli are decreased by 10-msec steps until they reach ventricular refractoriness. Rapid ventricular pacing at cycle lengths of 400 to 250 msec is also performed for 10 to 30 seconds. The stimulation protocol is repeated during isoproterenol infusion (increasing sinus rate to 100 to 150 beats per min) if VT is not induced in the control state and if the patient does not have significant ischemic heart disease. If VT is not induced with right ventricular stimulation, left ventricular stimulation is then performed.

## RESULTS OF ELECTROPHYSIOLOGIC TESTING

### Atrioventricular Conduction

Atrioventricular nodal refractory periods and paced cycle length to atrioventricular Wenckebach conduction were normal in all 50 survivors of cardiac arrest studied by Josephson and coworkers.[14] Sinus nodal function was normal in all but 1 of 46 patients they tested. Patients with inducible ventricular arrhythmias had longer mean A–H (91 msec versus 77 msec) and H–V (63 msec versus 50 msec) intervals than those without inducible ventricular arrhythmias. Furthermore, intraventricular conduction defects were common in both groups but more frequent in patients (18 of 32) with than in those (7 of 19) without inducible arrhythmias.

### Ventricular Stimulation

Myerburg and associates[12] observed inducible ventricular arrhythmias in 5 of 17 patients (29 percent) resuscitated from cardiac arrest. However, their stimulation protocol was limited to a single ventricular extrastimulus from the right ventricle. Ruskin and colleagues[13] reported inducible ventricular arrhythmias in 25 of 31 survivors (81 percent) of a cardiac arrest, with 13 patients (42 percent) having inducible sustained ventricular tachyarrhythmias. The stimulation protocol used by Ruskin and colleagues[13] consisted of right ventricular stimulation with single and double extrastimuli and brief bursts of rapid ventricular pacing. Using a more rigorous stimulation protocol, which included right and left ventricular stimulations with three extrastimuli and isoproterenol, Morady and coworkers[15] recently reported inducible sustained VT in 26 of 45 patients (58 percent) who survived a cardiac arrest. Nonsustained VT was induced in 8 of their patients.

Using the stimulation protocol described previously, we were able to initiate sustained VT or ventricular fibrillation (VF) in 72 of 119 survivors (61 percent) of a cardiac arrest.[20] Nonsustained VT was induced in 11 patients, and a maximum of three repetitive ventricular responses were observed in 36 patients (Table 1). As in the report of Morady and coworkers,[15] VT was considered sustained if it lasted longer than 30 seconds and/or required termination by direct-current cardioversion or programmed ventricular stimulation. In our study,[20] the arrhythmia responsible for the cardiac arrest was considered non-inducible if the complete stimulation protocol failed to produce a sustained ventricular tachyarrhythmia. We believe that the induction of short-lasting and spontaneously terminating ventricular tachyarrhythmias cannot necessarily be considered a reproduction of the patient's lethal arrhythmia.

The induced arrhythmia was sustained VT in 63 patients (uniform morphology in 45, multiple morphologies or polymorphic in 18 patients), and VF in 9 of our patients. Spontaneous degeneration into VF occurred in 8 of the 63 patients with inducible VT. The mean tachy-

**Table 1.** Electrophysiologic results

| | | |
|---|---|---|
| Inducible sustained ventricular arrhythmia | 72 pts | (61%) |
| ventricular tachycardia | 63 | |
| (degeneration to ventricular fibrillation) | 8 | |
| ventricular fibrillation | 9 | |
| Non-inducible sustained ventricular arrhythmia | 47 pts | (39%) |
| $\leqq 3$ repetitive ventricular response | 36 | |
| nonsustained ventricular tachycardia | 11 | |

cardia cycle length was 277 msec, which is similar to the findings of Ruskin,[13] Morady,[15] and their coworkers, who reported mean VT cycle lengths of 275 msec and 273 msec, respectively.

Sustained ventricular arrhythmias were initiated by right ventricular stimulation in 63 patients (87 percent) and required 1 premature stimulus in 10 patients, 2 premature stimuli in 38 patients (during isoproterenol infusion in 1), 3 premature stimuli in 14 patients, and rapid ventricular pacing in 1 patient. Left ventricular stimulation was required in 9 patients, with 2 premature stimuli in 2 patients, 3 premature stimuli in 4 patients (during isoproterenol infusion in 1), and rapid ventricular pacing in 3 patients (Table 2). Direct-current cardioversion was required to terminate the arrhythmia in 42 patients (58 percent). VT was terminated by programmed ventricular stimulation in 25 patients and by 1 thump version in 1 patient, and spontaneous termination occurred in 4 patients. These findings are similar to those reported by Morady and coworkers.[15] In their series, VT could be induced by right ventricular stimulation in 23 of 26 patients (88 percent), and the arrhythmia required termination by direct-current cardioversion in 15 patients (58 percent).

Thus, electrophysiologic testing in survivors of a cardiac arrest has shown that the frequency of inducing ventricular arrhythmias is related to the aggressiveness of the stimulation protocol. Using a rigorous protocol, a sustained and often lethal ventricular tachyarrhythmia can be produced in approximately 60 percent of survivors of a cardiac arrest.

## RELATIONSHIP BETWEEN CLINICAL AND INDUCED VENTRICULAR ARRHYTHMIAS

Ruskin[13] and Morady[15] and their associates reported that the earliest arrhythmia recorded at the time of cardiac arrest was VF in 23 (74 percent) and 30 (67 percent) of their patients, respectively. In our study,[20] the earliest arrhythmia recorded at the time of cardiac arrest was VF in 70 patients (59 percent) and VT in 34 patients (28 percent); the arrhythmia was not documented before cardioversion in 15 patients.

**Table 2.** Ventricular stimulation protocol in patients with inducible sustained ventricular arrhythmias

| | Inducible (72 patients) |
|---|---|
| Right ventricular stimulation | 63 |
| 1, 2 VES RVP | 49 |
| 3 VES | 14 |
| Left ventricular stimulation | 9 |
| 1, 2 VES RVP | 5 |
| 3 VES | 4 |

RVP = rapid ventricular pacing; VES = ventricular extrastimuli.

**Table 3.** Relation between clinical and induced ventricular arrhythmia

| Earliest rhythm at cardiac arrest | Cases (N) | Induced rhythm | Cases (N) |
|---|---|---|---|
| VF | 70 | VF | 7 |
| | | Sustained VT (degeneration to VF = 5) | 29 |
| | | Nonsustained VT | 8 |
| | | ≦ 3 beats | 26 |
| VT | 34 | VF | 2 |
| | | Sustained VT (degeneration to VF = 1) | 24 |
| | | Nonsustained VT | 2 |
| | | ≦ 3 beats | 6 |
| Not recorded | 15 | Sustained VT (degeneration to VF = 2) | 10 |
| | | Nonsustained VT | 1 |
| | | ≦ 3 beats | 4 |

VT = ventricular tachycardia; VF = ventricular fibrillation

The relation between clinical and induced arrhythmia is shown in Table 3. We were able to induce a sustained VT (29 patients) or VF (7 patients) in 36 patients (51 percent) whose earliest arrhythmia at the time of cardiac arrest was VF. Sustained VT (24 patients) or VF (2 patients) was induced in 26 patients (76 percent) in whom VT was documented during resuscitation. Sustained VT was initiated in 10 of 15 patients (67 percent) whose arrhythmia was not documented at the time of cardiac arrest. Morady and associates[15] found inducible VT in 23 of 30 patients (77 percent) who had VF at the time of resuscitation, and VT was induced in 10 of 12 patients (83 percent) who had VT at cardiac arrest.

Thus, the frequency of induction of sustained VT is highest among patients with VT at cardiac arrest. Although VF is the most frequently recorded arrhythmia at the time of resuscitation, the initiating arrhythmia is rarely recorded. Josephson and colleagues[14] were able to monitor the onset of cardiac arrest in the hospital in 24 patients and found VT to be the initiating mechanism in 17 patients (Fig. 1). This observation and the finding that VT can be initiated in many patients with VF at the time of resuscitation suggest that VT often precipitates sudden death.

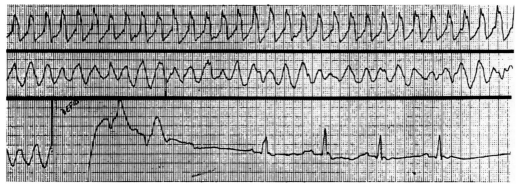

**Figure 1.** Cardiac arrest related to ventricular tachycardia degenerating into ventricular fibrillation. A modified lead 1 was recorded in the coronary care unit. Cardiac arrest is initiated by an episode of sustained ventricular tachycardia at a rate of 170 beats per min *(top)*, that degenerates to ventricular fibrillation *(middle)*. Electrical defibrillation results in sinus rhythm *(bottom)*. Note the presence of an intraventricular conduction defect during sinus rhythm. (From Josephson et al,[14] with permission.)

## ANATOMIC AND ELECTROPHYSIOLOGIC CORRELATES

The great majority of survivors of cardiac arrest have ischemic heart disease, most often with two- and three-vessel involvement.[12,14,21,22] However, we and others have found that patients with inducible arrhythmias have a higher incidence of prior myocardial infarction and greater angiographic ventricular dysfunction than patients with non-inducible arrhythmias.[12,20] These findings suggest that the induction of the arrhythmia by electrophysiologic testing is related to a fixed anatomic substrate, as is the case for most patients with recurrent sustained VT.

## PATIENTS WITH NO INDUCIBLE TACHYARRHYTHMIAS

Kehoe and coworkers[23] reported that 16 of 44 survivors of cardiac arrest (36 percent) with no inducible VT or VF were discharged without antiarrhythmic therapy and have not had recurrent sudden death at 14-month followup. These investigators[24] subsequently reported that acute myocardial ischemia probably precipitated the cardiac arrest in their patients, all of whom were thereafter treated with anti-ischemic drugs or underwent surgery. Ruskin and associates[25] reported that 14 of 60 survivors of cardiac arrest (23 percent) with no inducible VT or VF were not treated with antiarrhythmic drugs and had no recurrence of cardiac arrest over a mean followup of 15 months. However, it is not mentioned in their preliminary report whether these patients were treated with anti-ischemic drugs or had surgery. Morady and coworkers[19] described 11 of 45 survivors of cardiac arrest (24 percent) who had no inducible VT and remained free of recurrent sudden death at a mean followup of 19 months. Three of these patients were discharged on antiarrhythmic therapy, and eight received treatment aimed at the underlying heart disease. Of our 47 patients without inducible sustained ventricular arrhythmias, 15 (32 percent) have died suddenly over a mean followup of 20 months.[20] This high incidence of recurrent sudden death was not changed by treatment in our noninducible patients and was observed in both treated (10 of 29) and untreated (5 of 18) patients (Fig. 2). Treatment consisted of empiric antiarrhythmic drug therapy in 22 patients, whereas 7 patients underwent antiarrhythmic and/or anti-ischemic surgical therapy. Of the 18 patients discharged on no antiarrhythmic therapy, 12 patients with ischemic heart disease received beta-blocking agents. Antiarrhythmic drugs were discontinued in six patients in whom the cardiac arrest was believed to be drug induced. Furthermore, the incidence of recurrent sudden death was not significantly higher in patients with nonsustained VT (5 of 11 patients) as compared with those patients without inducible ventricular arrhythmias (10 of 36 patients).

Thus, recent series concerning survivors of cardiac arrest have shown that 24 to 39 percent have no ventricular arrhythmias inducible in the laboratory. In some of these patients a reversible factor such as myocardial ischemia or drug-induced VT/VF can be identified and, if treated, will prevent recurrent sudden death. In others with no inducible VT or VF, the initiating mechanism of the cardiac arrest remains unclear. Our findings indicate that these patients may die suddenly despite empiric antiarrhythmic therapy or treatment directed at their underlying heart disease. We believe that the inability to initiate ventricular arrhythmias and to test the effect of therapy contributes to the high incidence of recurrent sudden death in these patients.

## SUMMARY AND THERAPEUTIC IMPLICATIONS

Electrophysiologic testing has demonstrated that a poorly tolerated VT or VF can be initiated with an aggressive stimulation protocol in the majority of survivors of a cardiac arrest.[15,20,23,25] The likelihood of inducing a ventricular arrhythmia is greater in patients who

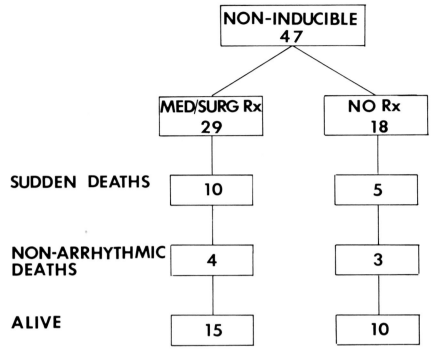

**Figure 2.** Outcome in 47 patients with no inducible sustained ventricular arrhythmias during the control study. MED/SURG Rx = medically and/or surgically treated patients; No Rx = patients discharged on no antiarrhythmic therapy. See text.

have VT at the time of cardiac arrest and in those who have left ventricular dysfunction or intraventricular conduction defects. Observations made during electrophysiologic testing also suggest that VT rather than VF is the primary arrhythmia precipitating sudden death in many of these patients.[13,15,20] The ability to initiate ventricular tachyarrhythmias in most survivors of a cardiac arrest has led investigators to use electrophysiologic testing as a method for evaluating treatment to prevent recurrent sudden death. Therapy guided by electrophysiologic testing will be discussed in the next chapter.

Electrophysiologic testing also may identify a subset of patients without inducible arrhythmias in whom the cardiac arrest was caused by a corrigible abnormality.[15,24] Patients without inducible arrhythmias and in whom a triggering factor for the cardiac arrest cannot be identified are likely to experience recurrent sudden death. However, our results indicate that empiric and conventional antiarrhythmic therapy is ineffective in preventing sudden death in these patients.[20] Although further trials are needed, amiodarone might be useful in lowering the risk of recurrent sudden death in this subgroup of survivors of a cardiac arrest.

## REFERENCES

1. FISHER, JD, COHEN, HL, MEHRA, R, ET AL: *Cardiac pacing and pacemakers II. Serial electrophysiologic-pharmacologic testing for control of recurrent tachyarrhythmias.* Am Heart J 93:658, 1977.

2. HARTZLER, GD AND MALONEY, JD: *Programmed ventricular stimulation in management of recurrent ventricular tachycardia.* Mayo Clin Proc 52:731, 1977.

3. MASON, JW AND WINKLE, RA: *Electrode catheter induction in the selection and assessment of antiarrhythmic drug therapy for recurrent ventricular tachycardia.* Circulation 58:971, 1978.

4. HOROWITZ, LN, JOSEPHSON, ME, FARSHIDI, A, ET AL: *Recurrent sustained ventricular tachycardia: 3. Role of the electrophysiologic study in selection of antiarrhythmic regimens.* Circulation 58:986, 1978.

5. JOSEPHSON, ME AND HOROWITZ, LN: *Electrophysiologic approach to therapy of recurrent sustained ventricular tachycardia.* Am J Cardiol 43:631, 1979.

6. NACCARELLI, GV, PRYSTOWSKY, EN, JACKMAN, WM, ET AL: *Role of electrophysiologic testing in managing patients who have ventricular tachycardia unrelated to coronary artery disease.* Am J Cardiol 50:165, 1982.

7. HAMER, A, VOHRA, J, HUNT, D, ET AL: *Prediction of sudden death by electrophysiologic studies in high risk patients surviving acute myocardial infarction.* Am J Cardiol 50:223, 1982.

8. RICHARDS, DA, CODY, DV, DENNISS, AR, ET AL: *Ventricular electrical instability: A predictor of death after myocardial infarction.* Am J Cardiol 51:75, 1983.

9. LIBERTHSON, RR, NAGEL, EL, HIRSCHMAN, JC, ET AL: *Prehospital ventricular defibrillation: Prognosis and follow-up course.* N Engl J Med 291:317, 1974.

10. COBB, LA, BAUM, RS, ALVAREZ, H, III, ET AL: *Resuscitation from out-of-hospital ventricular fibrillation: 4 year follow-up.* Circulation 51–52(Suppl III):223, 1975.

11. SCHAFFER, WA AND COBB, LA: *Recurrent ventricular fibrillation and modes of death in survivors of out-of-hospital ventricular fibrillation.* N Engl J Med 293:259, 1975.

12. MYERBURG, RJ, CONDE, CA, SUNG, RJ, ET AL: *Clinical, electrophysiologic and hemodynamic profile of patients resuscitated from prehospital cardiac arrest.* Am J Med 68:568, 1980.

13. RUSKIN, JN, DIMARCO, JP, AND GARAN, H: *Out-of-hospital cardiac arrest: Electrophysiologic observations and selection of long-term antiarrhythmic therapy.* N Engl J Med 303:607, 1980.

14. JOSEPHSON, ME, HOROWITZ, LN, SPIELMAN, SR, ET AL: *Electrophysiologic and hemodynamic studies in patients resuscitated from cardiac arrest.* Am J Cardiol 46:948, 1980.

15. MORADY, F, SCHEINMAN, MM, HESS, DS, ET AL: *Electrophysiologic testing in the management of survivors of out-of-hospital cardiac arrest.* Am J Cardiol 51:85, 1983.

16. DREIFUS, LS, HAIAT, R, WATANABE, Y, ET AL: *Ventricular fibrillation: A possible mechanism of sudden death in patients with Wolff-Parkinson-White syndrome.* Circulation 43:520, 1971.

17. WELLENS, HJ AND DURRER, D: *Wolff-Parkinson-White syndrome and atrial fibrillation: Relation between refractory period of accessory pathway and ventricular rate during atrial fibrillation.* Am J Cardiol 34:777, 1974.

18. KLEIN, GJ, BASHORE, TM, SELLERS, TD, ET AL: *Ventricular fibrillation in the Wolff-Parkinson-White syndrome.* N Engl J Med 301:1080, 1979.

19. MORADY, F, SLEDGE, C, SHEN, E, ET AL: *Electrophysiologic testing in the management of patients with the Wolff-Parkinson-White syndrome and atrial fibrillation.* Am J Cardiol 51:1623, 1983.

20. ROY, D, WAXMAN, HL, KIENZLE, MG, ET AL: *Clinical characteristics and long term follow-up in 119 survivors of cardiac arrest: Relation to inducibility at electrophysiologic testing.* Am J Cardiol 52:969, 1983.

21. WEAVER, WD, LORCH, GS, ALVAREZ, HA, ET AL: *Angiographic findings and prognostic indicators in patients resuscitated from sudden cardiac deaths.* Circulation 52(Suppl III):214, 1975.

22. RISSANEN, V, ROMO, M, AND SILTANEN, P: *Prehospital sudden death from ischaemic heart disease: A post-mortem study.* Br Heart J 40:1025, 1978.

23. KEHOE, RF, MORAN, JM, ZHEUTLIN, T, ET AL: *Electrophysiologic study to direct therapy in survivors of prehospital ventricular fibrillation.* Am J Cardiol 49:928, 1982.

24. TOMMASO, C, KEHOE, R, AND ZHEUTLIN, T: *Survivors of ischemic mediated sudden death—clinical angiographic and electrophysiologic features and response to therapy.* Circulation 66(Suppl II):25, 1982.

25. RUSKIN, JN, GARAN, H, DIMARCO, JP, ET AL: *Electrophysiologic testing in survivors of prehospital cardiac arrest: Therapy and long term follow-up.* Am J Cardiol 49:958, 1982.

# Pharmacologic Therapy for Survivors of Sudden Death Based on Programmed Stimulation*

*Denis Roy, M.D., Francis E. Marchlinski, M.D.,†*
*John U. Doherty, M.D.,‡ Alfred E. Buxton, M.D.,† and*
*Mark E. Josephson, M.D.*

Electrophysiologic testing is used to guide therapy[1-9] and has proven effective in the long-term management of patients with recurrent sustained ventricular tachycardia (VT). In the previous chapter, we have shown that VT or ventricular fibrillation (VF) can be reproduced in the electrophysiology laboratory in most survivors of sudden death. This observation has led investigators[10-15] to develop drug therapy based on the results of electrophysiologic testing, as it is done for patients with recurrent sustained VT. This chapter will describe the technique and results of electrophysiologic-pharmacologic testing, pointing out its advantages and current limitations when performed to prevent recurrent sudden death.

## TECHNIQUE OF ELECTROPHARMACOLOGIC TESTING

Survivors of a cardiac arrest undergo acute and/or chronic drug studies to identify an antiarrhythmic regimen that will suppress the induction of sustained ventricular tachyarrhythmias. The stimulation protocol during control and subsequent studies is described in detail in the previous chapter. Therapy is considered effective if the ventricular arrhythmia observed at the time of baseline study can no longer be induced by programmed ventricular stimulation.

Conventional or experimental drugs to be tested are chosen according to each patient's previous clinical response and are administered in the following manner:

*Intravenous administration*
Lidocaine 300 mg intravenously at 20 to 30 mg/min
Procainamide 1 to 2 g intravenously at 50 mg/min
Quinidine gluconate 400 to 600 mg intravenously at 20 mg/min
Propranolol 0.1 to 0.2 mg/kg at 1 mg/min
Phenytoin 1 g intravenously at 20 mg/min.

---

*Supported in part by grants from the American Heart Association, Southeastern Pennsylvania Chapter, Philadelphia, Pennsylvania, and grants #HL00361 and #HL24278 from the National Heart, Lung, and Blood Institute, Bethesda, Maryland, and the Fannie E. Ripple Foundation, Morristown, New Jersey.

†Supported by the University of Pennsylvania Measey Foundation.

‡Supported by a Grant-in-Aid from the American Heart Association, Southeastern Pennsylvania Chapter, Philadelphia, Pennsylvania.

*Oral administration*
Procainamide 2.4 to 8 g/day
Quinidine 1.2 to 2.4 g/day
Disopyramide 400 to 600 mg/day
Propranolol 160 to 480 mg/day
Mexiletine 600 to 1200 mg/day
Tocainide 800 to 1200 mg/day

Drugs administered intravenously should be given until the maximum dose is achieved or until side effects occur. Electrophysiologic testing is performed at the termination of infusion, and plasma concentrations if available are measured after testing or at the time of induction of VT if it occurred.

When an oral agent is selected, electrophysiologic testing is performed after the drug has been administered for five half-lives to assure steady-state levels.

Conventional type 1 antiarrhythmic drugs are usually tested first. If a single agent is found ineffective, combination regimens are sometimes tested. However, it has been reported that patients who do not respond to procainamide will rarely respond to other conventional drugs.[16] Furthermore, combination of type 1 drugs is usually ineffective if large doses of procainamide did not prevent the induction of ventricular arrhythmias. Thus, electrophysiologic testing of one type 1 antiarrhythmic agent will usually suffice in identifying those patients who will respond to conventional drugs and those who might benefit from experimental drugs or surgical treatment.

Of the aforementioned experimental drugs, amiodarone deserves special consideration. It has been found that there is a poor correlation between electrophysiologic testing and clinical outcome in patients treated with this drug.[17-19] For this reason, electrophysiologic testing is probably not required to further guide therapy in patients who have failed other drugs and who are begun on amiodarone treatment.

## ELECTROPHARMACOLOGIC RESULTS

Ruskin and coworkers[10] reported complete suppression of inducible ventricular arrhythmias with conventional and/or experimental drugs in 17 of 23 survivors of cardiac arrest (74 percent) who had inducible VT or VF at baseline study. None of their 17 patients had recurrent VT or VF at 15-month followup. Of six patients in whom inducible arrhythmias could not be suppressed, three died suddenly within 6 months. These authors[12] later reported on a larger series of 47 patients with inducible ventricular arrhythmias. Antiarrhythmic drugs were effective in preventing the induction of VT or VF in 36 (77 percent) of their patients. Two (5 percent) of these patients died suddenly at a followup of 18 months. Of 11 patients in whom they could not find an antiarrhythmic regimen that prevented the induction of VT or VF, 4 (36 percent) died suddenly at a followup of 15 months. In the report by Kehoe and associates,[11] 28 patients had inducible sustained VT at control electrophysiologic testing. VT induction was eventually prevented by antiarrhythmic drugs in 5 patients (18 percent) and by endocardial resection after failure of antiarrhythmic drugs in 11 patients, whereas 9 patients had persistence of inducible VT despite serial evaluations with conventional and/or experimental drugs. Three patients died perioperatively after endocardial resection. All 16 patients discharged on an antiarrhythmic regimen that prevented the induction of VT remained free of recurrent VT or VF at 14-month followup. Of the nine patients with persistence of inducible VT, seven (78 percent) had recurrent sudden death during a followup of 9 months.

Morady and colleagues[14] found that conventional antiarrhythmic drugs suppressed the induction of VT in 9 of 34 survivors of a cardiac arrest (26 percent). Three of these nine patients had recurrent VT or sudden death over a followup of 20 months. Of their 25 patients with persistence of inducible VT despite conventional antiarrhythmic drugs, 23 were dis-

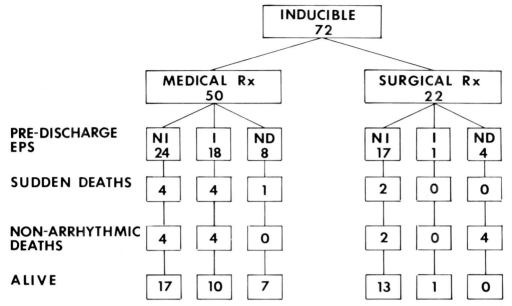

**Figure 1.** Outcome in 72 patients with inducible sustained ventricular arrhythmias at control electrophysiologic study. EPS = electrophysiologic study; I = inducible; NI = noninducible; ND = not done. See text.

charged on amiodarone and 2 underwent surgery. Three of these 25 patients (12 percent) have died suddenly over an 18-month followup.

We[15] have found that antiarrhythmic drugs prevented the induction of VT or VF in 24 of 72 survivors of cardiac arrest (33 percent) (Fig. 1). Recurrent sudden deaths occurred in 4 (17 percent) of these 24 patients at a mean followup of 18 months. Eighteen patients remained with inducible sustained VT or VF despite serial drug evaluations and were discharged on amiodarone therapy (9 patients) or on a drug regimen that slowed the tachycardia or rendered its induction more difficult. There have been four (one patient on amiodarone) sudden deaths (22 percent) among these 18 patients. A predischarge electrophysiologic study was not performed in the remaining eight medically treated patients. There has been one sudden death (at 3-month followup) among these eight patients, three of whom were treated with amiodarone. Twenty-two patients in whom medical therapy had failed to prevent the induction of sustained VT or VF were treated surgically. There have been two sudden deaths (12 percent) among the 17 surgically treated patients in whom sustained VT or VF was not induced postoperatively. One patient with persistence of inducible VT at postoperative electrophysiologic testing is alive without recurrent sudden death at 17-month followup. Four patients died of nonarrhythmic causes 1 to 4 weeks after surgery.

Overall, in our study, 6 of 41 patients (15 percent) discharged on antiarrhythmic drug and/ or surgical therapy that prevented the induction of sustained VT died suddenly at a followup of 18 months. By comparison, 5 of 27 patients (19 percent) discharged on an unsuccessful antiarrhythmic regimen or without a predischarge study died suddenly at a followup of 16 months. However, 12 of these 27 patients were treated with amiodarone, only 1 of whom died suddenly. Therefore, if we exclude the amiodarone-treated patients, 4 of 15 patients (27 percent) discharged with persistence of inducible ventricular arrhythmias (3 of 9) or without electrophysiologic re-evaluation (1 of 6) had recurrence of sudden death.

Thus, electrophysiologic testing in survivors of cardiac arrest has shown that the induction of VT or VF can be prevented by antiarrhythmic drugs in 18 percent to 77 percent of patients.[10,11,12,14,15] Discrepancies in stimulation protocol and in the use of conventional versus

**Table 1.** Cumulative results from four series of survivors of cardiac arrest treated with an antiarrhythmic drug that suppressed the induction of VT/VF

| Investigators | No. pts with inducible ventricular arrhythmias at baseline testing | No. pts with suppression of inducible VT/VF with antiarrhythmic drugs | No. pts with recurrent VT/VF | Followup |
|---|---|---|---|---|
| Ruskin et al[12] | 47 | 36 (77%) | 2 (5%) | 18 months |
| Kehoe et al[11] | 28 | 5 (18%) | 0 | 14 months |
| Morady et al[14] | 34 | 9 (26%) | 3 (33%) | 20 months |
| Roy et al[15] | 72 | 24 (33%) | 4 (17%) | 18 months |
| Total | 181 | 74 (41%) | 9 (12%) | 17.5 months |

experimental drugs (amiodarone) during serial drug testing explain differences in results among series. Furthermore, some investigators[10,14] have included in the serial drug testing studies patients with repetitive ventricular responses or nonsustained VT at control testing, whereas others[11,15] have not done so. The risk of recurrent sudden death among patients in whom suppression of inducible VT or VF was achieved with antiarrhythmic drugs has varied from 0 to 33 percent, with followups ranging from 14 to 20 months (Table 1). Overall, 74 patients from 4 series were discharged on an antiarrhythmic drug that prevented the induction of VT or VF and were followed for a mean of 17.5 months. There have been 9 (12 percent) reported sudden deaths among these patients. These results suggest that electropharmacologic testing can identify those patients with inducible VT or VF who will respond to antiarrhythmic drugs and who appear to have a low risk of recurrent sudden death.

In contrast, patients discharged with persistence of inducible VT or VF despite serial drug evaluations have 12 to 78 percent incidence of recurrent sudden death during followups of 9 to 18 months.[10-12,14,15] Excluding patients from these trials that were reported to be treated with amiodarone, we find that patients with persistence of inducible VT/VF despite antiarrhythmic drug treatment have a 48 percent incidence of recurrent sudden death over 13-month followup (Table 2). This high incidence of recurrent sudden death is similar to the 30 to 40 percent incidence reported in previous studies of survivors of cardiac arrest who were treated empirically with conventional drugs.[20-22]

In the series of Morady and coworkers,[14] 23 patients in whom conventional drugs had failed to prevent the induction of VT or VF were discharged without further electropharmacologic

**Table 2.** Cumulative results from three series of survivors of cardiac arrest treated with an antiarrhythmic drug* that failed to prevent the induction of VT/VF

| Investigators | No. pts discharged on antiarrhythmic drugs that failed to prevent the induction of VT/VF | No. pts with recurrent VT/VF | Followup |
|---|---|---|---|
| Ruskin et al[12] | 11 | 4 (36%) | 15 months |
| Kehoe et al[11] | 9 | 7 (78%) | 9 months |
| Roy et al[15] | 9 | 3 (33%) | 16 months |
| Total | 29 | 14 (48%) | 13 months |

Pts = patients; VT = ventricular tachycardia; VF = ventricular fibrillation.
*Excluding amiodarone.

testing on amiodarone. Only two of these patients had recurrent sudden death over an 18-month followup. In our study,[15] 14 patients who had failed conventional antiarrhythmic drug therapy were treated with amiodarone. Electrophysiologic testing was performed in 11 of these patients and revealed suppression of inducible VT in two patients. Twelve of the 14 patients (86 percent) on amiodarone did not have recurrent sudden death over a 15-month followup. One patient without inducible VT died at 4 months and one patient with inducible VT died at 13 months. These results suggest that amiodarone can be effective in preventing recurrent sudden death in those patients in whom suppression of inducible VT or VF cannot be achieved with other antiarrhythmic drugs. Electropharmacologic testing is not required when patients are treated with amiodarone, inasmuch as the clinical response to this drug cannot be accurately predicted from the laboratory response.[17-19]

## LIMITATIONS

Electrophysiologic studies are expensive, time consuming, and associated with some morbidity and potential mortality. They require sophisticated equipment and highly trained personnel. These studies should be performed in specialized centers so as to minimize the risk and assure an accurate evaluation of the patient's arrhythmia.[23-26] Although much data have been accumulated in recent years regarding electropharmacologic testing in survivors of cardiac arrest, this approach has several limitations and certain areas require further research, to wit, (1) this technique cannot be applied to a significant number of patients who do not have inducible VT or VF; (2) it is unclear whether survivors of cardiac arrest with nonsustained VT should be evaluated by electropharmacologic testing; (3) the results of electropharmacologic testing may not predict accurately the clinical response to some drugs (amiodarone). It must also be recognized that observations made in this chapter are limited by the fact that data were derived from different laboratories. Patients among these studies had heterogeneous clinical characteristics and underwent testing with different stimulation protocols. Furthermore, they received different therapies, and criteria for drug efficacy varied among investigators.

## CONCLUSIONS AND RECOMMENDATIONS FOR THERAPY

The fundamental question raised in this chapter and the previous one is whether electrophysiologic testing is useful in the management of patients resuscitated from a cardiac arrest. The available data suggest that electrophysiologic studies can be useful in identifying those patients who have inducible VT or VF and who will respond to conventional drugs. These patients have a low risk of recurrent sudden death and need not be exposed to potentially toxic experimental drugs. If conventional drug therapy fails to prevent the induction of VT, the patient should receive alternate treatment: amiodarone, cardiac electrosurgery, or an implantable automatic defibrillator. Although amiodarone is a potentially toxic drug, its use in patients with persistence of inducible VT or VF seems justified because of the excellent response to amiodarone therapy in this high-risk subgroup. Surgical therapy and implantable devices to treat lethal arrhythmia will be discussed in other chapters.

Electrophysiologic testing also will identify survivors of cardiac arrest without inducible VT or VF. In some of these patients, a triggering event (such as myocardial ischemia) will be found responsible for the cardiac arrest. If treatment is directed at preventing the transient abnormality, these patients also have a low risk of recurrent sudden death. However, patients without inducible arrhythmias and in whom a triggering factor for the cardiac arrest cannot be identified are likely to experience recurrent sudden death. Empiric trials with amiodarone are needed to determine whether this drug can be useful in this subgroup of survivors of cardiac arrest. Figure 2 summarizes our view of the role of electrophysiologic testing in the management of survivors of a cardiac arrest.

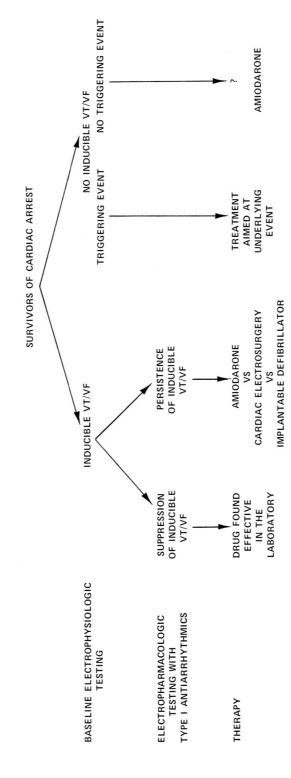

**Figure 2.** A flow diagram for the evaluation and management by electrophysiologic testing of survivors of cardiac arrest. VT = ventricular tachycardia; VF = ventricular fibrillation.

184

# REFERENCES

1. FISHER, JD, COHEN, HL, MEHRA, R, ET AL: *Cardiac pacing and pacemakers II. Serial electrophysiologic-pharmacologic testing for control of recurrent tachyarrhythmias.* Am Heart J 93:658, 1977.

2. HARTZLER, GD and MALONEY, JD: *Programmed ventricular stimulation in management of recurrent ventricular tachycardia.* Mayo Clin Proc 52:731, 1977

3. MASON, JW and WINKLE, RA: *Electrode catheter induction in the selection and assessment of antiarrhythmic drug therapy for recurrent ventricular tachycardia.* Circulation 58:971, 1978.

4. HOROWITZ, LN, JOSEPHSON, ME, FARSHIDI, A, ET AL: *Recurrent sustained ventricular tachycardia: 3. Role of the electrophysiologic study in selection of antiarrhythmic regimens.* Circulation 58:986, 1978.

5. JOSEPHSON, ME and HOROWITZ, LN: *Electrophysiologic approach to therapy of recurrent sustained ventricular tachycardia.* Am J Cardiol 43:631, 1979.

6. HOROWITZ LN, JOSEPHSON, ME, and KASTOR, JA: *Intracardiac electrophysiologic studies as a method for the optimization of drug therapy in chronic ventricular arrhythmia.* Prog Cardiovasc Dis 23:81, 1980.

7. MASON, JM and WINKLE, RA: *Accuracy of the ventricular tachycardia induction study for predicting long-term efficacy and inefficacy of antiarrhythmic drugs.* N Engl J Med 303:1073, 1980.

8. NACCARELLI, GV, PRYSTOWSKY, EN, JACKMAN, WM, ET AL: *Role of electrophysiologic testing in managing patients who have ventricular tachycardia unrelated to coronary artery disease.* Am J Cardiol 50:165, 1982.

9. SWERDLOW, CD, WINKLE, RA, and MASON, JW: *Prognostic significance of the number of induced ventricular complexes during assessment of therapy for ventricular tachyarrhythmias.* Circulation 68:400, 1983.

10. RUSKIN, JN, DIMARCO, JP, and GARAN, H: *Out-of-hospital cardiac arrest: Electrophysiologic observations and selection of long-term antiarrhythmic therapy.* N Engl J Med 303:607, 1980

11. KEHOE, RF, MORAN, JM, ZHEUTLIN, T, ET AL: *Electrophysiologic study to direct therapy in survivors of pre-hospital ventricular fibrillation.* Am J Cardiol 49:928, 1982.

12. RUSKIN, JN, GARAN, H, DIMARCO, JP, ET AL: *Electrophysiologic testing in survivors of prehospital cardiac arrest: Therapy and long term follow-up.* Am J Cardiol 49:958, 1982.

13. TOMMASO, C, KEHOE, R, and ZHEUTLIN, T: *Survivors of ischemic mediated sudden death—clinical angiographic and electrophysiologic features and response to therapy.* Circulation 66(Suppl II):25, 1982.

14. MORADY, F, SCHEINMAN, MM, HESS, DS, ET AL *Electrophysiologic testing in the management of survivors of out-of-hospital cardiac arrest.* Am J Cardiol 51:85, 1983.

15. ROY, D, WAXMAN, HL, KIENZLE, MG, ET AL: *Clinical characteristics and long term follow-up in 119 survivors of cardiac arrest: Relation to inducibility at electrophysiologic testing.* Am J Cardiol 52:969, 1983.

16. WAXMAN, HL, BUXTON, AE, SADOWSKI, LM, ET AL: *The response to procainamide during electrophysiologic study for sustained ventricular tachyarrhythmias predicts the response to other medications.* Circulation 67:30, 1983.

17. HEGER, JJ, PRYSTOWSKY, EN, JACKMAN, WM, ET AL: *Amiodarone: Clinical efficacy and electrophysiology during long term therapy for recurrent ventricular tachycardia or ventricular fibrillation.* N Engl J Med 305:539, 1981.

18. HAMER, AW, FINERMAN, WB, PETER, T, ET AL: *Disparity between the clinical and electrophysiologic effects of amiodarone in the treatment of recurrent ventricular tachyarrhythmias.* Am Heart J 102:992, 1981.

19. WAXMAN, HL, GROH, WC, MARCHLINSKI, FE, ET AL: *Amiodarone for control of sustained ventricular tachyarrhythmia: Clinical and electrophysiologic effects in 51 patients.* Am J Cardiol 50:1066, 1982.

20. LIBERTHSON RR, NAGEL, EL, HIRSCHMAN, JC, ET AL: *Prehospital ventricular defibrillation: Prognosis and follow-up course.* N Engl J Med 291:317, 1974.

21. COBB, LA, BAUM, RS, ALVAREZ, H, III, ET AL: *Resuscitation from out-of-hospital ventricular fibrillation: 4 year follow-up.* Circulation 51–52(Suppl III): 223, 1975.

22. SCHAFFER, WA AND COBB, LA: *Recurrent ventricular fibrillation and modes of death in survivors of out-of-hospital ventricular fibrillation.* N Engl J Med 292:259, 1975.

23. ROSS, DL, FARRÉ, J, BÄR, FWHM, ET AL: *Comprehensive clinical electrophysiologic studies in the investigation of documented or suspected tachycardias.* Circulation 61:1010, 1980.

24. SURAWICZ, B: *Intracardiac extrastimulation studies: How to? Where? By Whom?* Circulation 65:428, 1982.

25. HOROWITZ, LN and MORGANROTH, J: *Can we prevent sudden cardiac death?* Am J Cardiol 50:535, 1982.

26. SCHEINMAN, MM and MORADY, F: *Invasive cardiac electrophysiologic testing: The current state of the art.* Circulation 67:1169, 1983.

# The Selection of Antiarrhythmic Regimens by Electrophysiologic Studies: Techniques and Results

*Leonard N. Horowitz, M.D., Scott R. Spielman, M.D.,*
*Allan M. Greenspan, M.D., and Charles R. Webb, M.D.*

Ventricular tachyarrhythmias present a monumental health care problem in the western world. Nearly half of all deaths in the United States are related to cardiac disorders, and half of these are due to sudden cardiac death and presumably a ventricular tachyarrhythmia.[1] Although admirable, community-based emergency medical systems salvage only a small proportion of victims of these life-threatening arrhythmias, and prevention is clearly preferable. Recurrent ventricular tachyarrhythmias are frequently life-threatening and difficult to treat by empiric drug selection. The development of intracardiac electrophysiologic studies using programmed electrical stimulation has provided a more precise method for selecting effective therapy in certain groups of patients with recurrent ventricular tachyarrhythmias. Thus, the advent of electrophysiologic studies for selection of prophylactic therapy has gained considerable attention. In this chapter, we will review the techniques and results of electrophysiologic testing for selection of treatment for patients with recurrent ventricular tachycardia and fibrillation and survivors of out-of-hospital cardiac arrest. We will discuss those areas of this topic in which consensus has been achieved and highlight those areas in which controversy still exists.

## ELECTROPHYSIOLOGIC TECHNIQUES

The advent of electrophysiologic testing for ventricular tachyarrhythmias occurred in the early 1970s.[2-4] These studies were performed primarily to define the arrhythmogenic mechanisms producing these arrhythmias and to identify patient groups in which electrophysiologic testing might be of clinical value. The therapeutic application of the information derived from these early studies was minimal. Because electrophysiologic testing did not evolve from a unitary source but from several contemporaneous laboratories, certain differences in approach occurred and persist. Therefore, results may not be completely comparable from one laboratory to another.

The electrophysiologic methods described in the following section are based primarily on those used by the authors in the Clinical Cardiac Electrophysiology Laboratory of the Likoff Cardiovascular Institute. They are, however, basically similar to those used in many other institutions and by and large can be considered typical of a modern electrophysiology laboratory. It is, however, important to emphasize again that the results obtained with electrophysiologic testing are dependent on the protocols employed.

Patients undergo electrophysiologic study either unsedated or under mild sedation (usually diazepam) in the postabsorptive state. It is important that all potential proarrhythmic conditions and drugs be eliminated before the study. These cautions include the correction of any electrolyte abnormalities, the removal of proarrhythmic drugs, and the control of myocardial ischemia and congestive heart failure. In addition, baseline studies should be performed in the absence of any antiarrhythmic agents because the baseline observation of the patient's ventricular tachyarrhythmia is critical to assessing the therapeutic response once drug interventions are employed. The presence of any proarrhythmic factors or antiarrhythmic agents during these baseline observations can significantly confound analysis of antiarrhythmic interventions that are subsequently employed.

Electrode catheters are inserted percutaneously or by cutdown and positioned in the heart under fluoroscopic guidance. The number and precise positioning of these electrode catheters are dependent on the data to be obtained. The number varies from one to five catheters, with two to four being the usual number. For serial drug studies, some investigators have advocated the use of an electrode catheter that has been inserted through a jugular, subclavian, or antecubital vein and can be left for a prolonged period of time for sequential studies. We do not currently favor such an approach because the incidence of infection and thrombophlebitis is increased and the ability to move the catheter within the right ventricle to obtain studies at multiple sites is restricted. This latter point is particularly significant and will be discussed below.

**Stimulation Protocols**

Programmed ventricular stimulation consists of the introduction of electrical stimuli during a patient's spontaneous cardiac rhythm or ventricular pacing. The pattern and rate of the stimuli vary widely. The stimuli are generally rectangular pulses of short duration (1 to 2 msec) and two to five times diastolic threshold in amplitude. Our current stimulation protocol during baseline and all subsequent drug evaluation studies includes the introduction of single, double, and triple ventricular extrastimuli delivered during the patient's spontaneous rhythm and ventricular paced rhythms at cycle lengths of 600 and 450 msec. The multiple extrastimuli are scanned in a sequential pattern. In addition, bursts of rapid ventricular pacing at cycle lengths of 600 to 300 msec for brief intervals not exceeding 15 to 30 seconds are used.[4] At other centers, the routine use of more than three premature stimuli, very short ventricular pacing cycle lengths, and alternating current has been advocated;[5,6] the clinical utility of these techniques has yet to be established.

In many patients with recurrent ventricular tachyarrhythmias, stimulation at the right ventricular apex will initiate the arrhythmia.[4,7,8] In certain patients, the tachyarrhythmia may not be inducible by stimulation at the right ventricular apex or might be more easily initiated by stimulation at the right ventricular outflow tract. However, in almost 90 percent of patients with recurrent ventricular tachycardia, the arrhythmia can be initiated by right ventricular stimulation. In some of the remaining patients, ventricular tachycardia can be initiated by left ventricular stimulation, but in a small percentage (5 percent) of patients it cannot be initiated at all. When a recurrent ventricular tachyarrhythmia cannot be initiated by programmed stimulation, a diligent search should be made for intercurrent conditions such as myocardial ischemia, worsening of congestive heart failure, or proarrhythmic drugs.

In some patients, the infusion of isoproterenol to increase sinus rate facilitates the induction of ventricular tachycardia by programmed stimulation.[9] The mechanism by which isoproterenol facilitates the induction of ventricular tachycardia is probably related to its electrophysiologic effects (shortening conduction time and refractoriness), its ability to induce ischemia, or facilitation of an arrhythmogenic mechanism that is dependent upon catecholamine stimulation. The number of patients in whom catecholamine stimulation is necessary is small, and thus it is infrequently employed.

**Results of Programmed Stimulation in Patients With Ventricular Tachyarrhythmias**

The sensitivity and specificity of programmed electrical stimulation protocols vary considerably and are primarily dependent upon the number of extrastimuli employed. The use of fewer than two extrastimuli results in an extremely low rate of ventricular tachycardia induction.[10,11] The use of progressively more extrastimuli produces a commensurate increase in the induction rate. The use of three or more extrastimuli is most likely to produce the maximum percentage of inducible patients.[11-14] When protocols with three or fewer extrastimuli are used, ventricular tachycardia is inducible in 80 to 95 percent of patients with clinically documented sustained ventricular tachycardia. As will be discussed subsequently, the decision made about the therapeutic effects of antiarrhythmic drugs depends on the reproducibility of initiation of the ventricular tachyarrhythmia over the course of the study. Thus, it must be ascertained during the baseline study that programmed stimulation can, indeed, reproducibly initiate the tachyarrhythmia under investigation.

Although some controversy exists regarding the number of stimuli and stimulation sites, the divergent opinions may not be as different as they appear. There is a general consensus that the use of two or fewer extrastimuli produces a highly specific response in ventricular tachycardia induction and that the use of four or more extrastimuli produces a significant reduction in specificity. Controversy centers primarily on the use of triple extrastimuli. However, it is agreed that the use of three extrastimuli increases sensitivity while reducing specificity. This controversy is inconsequential when applied to the baseline electrophysiology study in a patient with a clinically documented sustained ventricular tachycardia, because the response to the stimulation can be validated by comparison with the clinically documented arrhythmia. The controversy assumes more significance when the baseline study is used for the evaluation of patients at high risk for a ventricular tachyarrhythmia but who have not yet had a spontaneous episode. In addition, the use of three extrastimuli during drug testing has produced some controversy because the use of such an aggressive protocol, particularly in patients in whom the arrhythmia was induced with fewer than three extrastimuli during a baseline study, reduces the efficacy of the tested antiarrhythmic drugs. Those laboratories that use triple extrastimuli routinely, as ours does, must do so with the knowledge that their use produces some reduction in specificity of programmed stimulation and also establishes a more stringent requirement for antiarrhythmic drug effect during drug studies. However, this approach results in a more sensitive baseline study and possibly a more effective therapeutic regimen.

Stimulation of more than one right ventricular site increases the sensitivity of electrophysiologic testing without a significant decrease in specificity.[7] Stimulation of the left ventricle also increases sensitivity; however, the effect on specificity has not been widely studied.[15] The risks and difficulty of left ventricular electrophysiologic study, particularly when repeated for drug evaluation, make left ventricular electrophysiologic study for drug evaluation undesirable, and the use of multiple right ventricular sites seems preferable and sufficient for clinical purposes.

The majority of electrophysiologic studies evaluating ventricular tachyarrhythmias and drug evaluations have employed a current amplitude and duration that range from two to four times late diastolic threshold and 1 to 2 msec respectively. It is generally agreed that the use of these stimulus parameters is not associated with frequent induction of nonclinical arrhythmias. Although several notable studies have employed high current amplitudes and greater pulse widths,[16,17] the clinical relevance of these studies remains to be confirmed; and, at present, it would seem appropriate to restrict stimulation studies to the stimulus characteristics in common usage.

## Relationship of Laboratory-Induced Arrhythmia to Clinical Arrhythmia

The use of an electrophysiologic protocol for the selection of drug therapy is based on the hypothesis that the arrhythmia initiated by the stimulation protocol is substantially the same as the clinical arrhythmia. In most patient groups, this assumption appears to be well founded. In early studies[8] and more recent corroborative studies,[7,12] the duration and type of induced arrhythmia closely paralleled those of the previously documented clinical arrhythmia. In certain patients, however, additional dissimilar arrhythmias, particularly polymorphic ventricular tachycardia or ventricular fibrillation, have been initiated by programmed electrical stimulation. The reported incidence of this phenomenon varies from 5 to 25 percent.[8,11,12,14] Inasmuch as polymorphic ventricular tachycardia or ventricular fibrillation may, in fact, be a clinically irrelevant laboratory phenomenon in patients with clinically documented uniform morphology ventricular tachycardia, their occurrence should be considered nonclinical. On the other hand, if the clinical arrhythmia cannot be documented (such as occurs frequently in patients resuscitated from out-of-hospital cardiac arrest) or if it is known to be polymorphic ventricular tachycardia or ventricular fibrillation, then these arrhythmias have been used as a basis for drug testing.

The concept of serial drug testing using electrophysiologic studies is based on the hypothesis that the prevention of initiation of a sustained ventricular tachyarrhythmia by an antiarrhythmic agent in a patient in whom such an arrhythmia was inducible during the baseline study predicts successful antiarrhythmic treatment. This hypothesis appears to be well proven.[2-4,18-21] It is believed that the prevention of initiation of a previously inducible arrhythmia indicates a pharmacologic alteration of the electrophysiologic properties of the myocardium that produces the arrhythmia such that the arrhythmia can no longer be initiated or maintained. Electrophysiologic testing provides an objective basis on which to judge pharmacologic therapy.

## PHARMACOLOGIC PROTOCOLS

Following baseline studies, serial electrophysiologic evaluations are performed during administration of a variety of antiarrhythmic agents. Although we previously advocated intravenous administration of drugs whenever possible, our position has changed over the past few years. The exigency of time notwithstanding, oral administration is preferable for several reasons: (1) many drugs are extensively metabolized and their efficacy is dependent on the extent of metabolism; (2) the relationship between intravenous and oral forms of the same medication is not completely known in many cases; and (3) the oral form of the drug is the one that will be employed chronically.

Studies must be scheduled so as to ensure that the steady-state condition is reached on the drug being tested and that previously administered drugs have been eliminated. We currently evaluate patients on at least one representative drug from classes IA, IB, IC, and III and on appropriate combinations of these agents until a successful antiarrhythmic regimen that prevents induction of the arrhythmia is found. Table 1 lists the dosages and range of blood levels obtained with drugs used during this type of testing.

Programmed electrical stimulation should be performed at a time when the plasma concentration of the agent under evaluation has reached steady-state conditions and preferably at a time when the nadir concentration would be present (typically at the time of a scheduled dose). Plasma concentrations of the tested agents should be measured at the time of the electrophysiologic study. An individual agent or combination of agents suitable for chronic oral administration can therefore be identified. It is imperative that the drug regimen selected be used prior to hospital discharge.

### Measures of Drug Efficacy

There are many potential indices of drug efficacy. There is a general consensus that prevention of initiation of a previously inducible sustained arrhythmia is the best index of drug efficacy. In fact, such prevention of initiation is associated with an excellent subsequent prognosis.[3,4,18,19,20,21] Some controversy has arisen over the definition of noninducibility. Many laboratories have used the criteria of five or fewer induced complexes as being synonymous with noninducibility. Recent evidence suggests that possibly less stringent criteria, that is, 15 or fewer complexes, may be equally effective.[21]

190

**Table 1.** Drugs used during electrophysiologic testing of ventricular tachyarrhythmias

| Drug | Usual oral dose range (mg/day) | Usual plasma concentration range (mcg/ml) |
|---|---|---|
| Type IA | | |
| Procainamide | 3000–8000 | 7.0 –15.0* |
| Quinidine | 800–1600 | 2.0 – 3.5 |
| Disopyramide | 400–1200 | 1.5 – 4.0 |
| Type IB | | |
| Tocainide | 1200–2400 | 3.0 –15.0 |
| Mexiletine | 600–1200 | 1.0 – 2.0 |
| Type IC | | |
| Encainide | 100–400 | 0.05– 0.4 |
| Flecainide | 200–400 | 0.6 – 1.2 |
| Indecainide | 100–400 | 0.5 – 1.0 |
| Type III | | |
| Amiodarone | 800–2000 | 1.0 – 2.5 |
| Sotalol | 320– 640 | |

*Excluding NAPA concentration.

Other criteria for drug efficacy have been suggested. These include changes in the width of the tachycardia zone, alterations in the complexity of the stimulation protocol required to induce ventricular tachycardia, and changes in tachycardia characteristics such as rate and symptoms produced by the arrhythmia. Changes in tachycardia characteristics have proven to be unreliable in estimating drug efficacy. Most antiarrhythmic drugs increase tachycardia cycle lengths and ameliorate the symptoms produced by them; however, recurrence rates remain high in patients in whom the arrhythmia remains inducible despite beneficial alterations in the arrhythmia characteristics.[3,23] Similarly, it has been suggested that an increase in the complexity of the stimulation required to induce ventricular tachycardia can be used to predict drug efficacy. In this regard, drug efficacy would be inferred from a study in which tachycardia could be induced only with triple extrastimuli during drug treatment when, during baseline studies, double extrastimuli were able to initiate the tachycardia.[5,24] This concept will require further confirmation before being accepted. Some investigators have stressed that the reproducibility of the precise stimulation technique used to initiate ventricular tachycardia between studies is low and therefore should not be used as an index of drug efficacy.[25,26] Thus, at this time, the only reliable index of drug efficacy is the prevention of induction of an arrhythmia. The precise definition of what is not inducible is a matter of discussion but does not appear to be a major issue.

Two areas of controversy exist regarding the topic of indices of drug efficacy. One such area of controversy involves the use of more aggressive stimulation protocols during drug evaluation studies than were originally required during the baseline study to initiate the clinical arrhythmia. On the one hand, it has been argued that such a practice is not clinically relevant and reduces the apparent efficacy of antiarrhythmic regimens. Certainly, this type of protocol does reduce the number of successful tests obtained during electrophysiologic testing. In our experience over the past 2 years, 40 percent of drug studies were considered unsuccessful because a clinical tachycardia was induced by a protocol that was more aggressive than that required to induce the tachycardia during baseline conditions. Our use of more aggressive protocols is based on the known variability of induction of clinical arrhythmias by an individual protocol, and thus we have considered induction of arrhythmia as the endpoint and have placed less stress on the type of stimulation required to induce it. Using this protocol, we have had recurrence rates of less than 10 percent in patients treated with a regimen that successfully suppressed induction of the clinical arrhythmia during electrophysiologic testing. Whether similar long-term results can be obtained using other strategies, particularly by limiting the stimulation protocol during followup studies to that which induced the clinical arrhythmia during the baseline study, remains conjectural; however, some evidence to this effect has been presented.[27] Similarly in terms of controversy, it has been suggested that the efficacy of drugs can be overestimated if left ventricular stimulation is not performed during drug studies, even if left ventricular stimulation was not required during the baseline study.[28] Morady and coworkers[28] have shown that in a group of patients who did not undergo left ventricular stimulation during apparently successful drug evaluations, the recurrence rate was 27 percent compared with 0 percent in a group of patients in whom left ventricular stimulation failed to induce ventricular tachycardia that had previously been inducible during right ventricular stimulation.[28] These workers suggest that as many as 50 percent of drug trials may be incorrectly judged as successful if such aggressive stimulation is not performed. Presumably, such questions will be resolved in the future by more careful study design.

The effects of individual agents or drug combinations are unpredictable in individual patients. Certain clinical, hemodynamic, and electrophysiologic data can be used to stratify patients into groups that are likely to respond to drugs during electrophysiologic study.[21,22] However, the precise drug that will be effective in an individual patient cannot be determined by such algorithms.

During electrophysiologic testing, recurrent sustained ventricular tachycardia has appeared to respond most frequently to group IA or membrane-depressant antiarrhythmic drugs. The success of these drugs in preventing initiation of ventricular tachycardia has ranged from 20 to 50 percent.[4] Procainamide, particularly when used in high doses that produce relatively high blood levels (10 to 20 mcg/ml), has produced suppression of inducibility in approximately one third of patients.[30,31] The efficacy of quinidine for recurrent sustained ventricular tachycardia has been shown to be similar to that of procainamide.[32] The plasma concentration of quinidine required to control ventricular tachycardia is approximately 3 mcg/ml. Long-term therapy with either procainamide or quinidine has produced good clinical results. The recurrence rate of ventricular tachycardia has been low (less than 15 percent), and the incidence of drug discontinuation because of side effects has also been low. Disopyramide, another type IA agent, has been shown similarly to prevent induction of ventricular tachycardia in approximately one third of patients.[33] However, the long-term followup in patients treated with disopyramide has shown a greater incidence of side effects, and only slightly over half of the patients can continue on therapy with this agent. Furthermore, a majority of patients with life-threatening ventricular arrhythmias have markedly reduced left ventricular function and cannot tolerate disopyramide because of its negative inotropic effects, so that in many patients it cannot even be evaluated.

When type IA agents fail to prevent initiation of ventricular tachyarrhythmias, they frequently increase the cycle length and reduce the hemodynamic and clinical consequences of the arrhythmia. Therefore, they can be used as adjunctive regimens or in combination with other drugs or devices to treat patients with recurrent ventricular tachyarrhythmias. As with most other antiarrhythmic drug classes, the group IA drugs exhibit a proarrhythmic effect in a small number of patients. Although not widely studied, the incidence of proarrhythmic effect during electrophysiologic studies with this group of drugs is relatively low, occurring in approximately 5 to 10 percent of patients.[34]

The drugs classified as group IB are generally less effective in preventing initiation of ventricular tachycardia. Success with this group of agents ranges from 5 to 20 percent. However, they have been found to be useful in combination with other agents. Tocainide and lidocaine have been used interchangeably during electrophysiologic testing. The efficacy of either of these drugs alone in patients with recurrent sustained ventricular tachycardia has been less than 10 percent.[2-5] Mexiletine has also been evaluated for its ability to prevent induction of sustained ventricular tachycardia, and its efficacy has been similarly low.[35,36] When ventricular tachycardia is not prevented by the type IB agents, the cycle length of the tachycardia may be increased nonetheless; however, it is not increased to the extent noted with type IA drugs nor is the increase in cycle length uniformly observed. Furthermore, occasionally the tachycardia cycle length is shortened and symptoms worsened by the type IB drugs. The incidence of arrhythmia potentiation by these agents is low. Thus, the major proarrhythmic effect that is noted is the increase in tachycardia rate and consequent worsening of symptoms.

The drugs that have been classified as IC agents—encainide, flecainide, indecainide, and others—are a group of agents that are still largely investigational. They are particularly effective in suppressing spontaneous ventricular premature complexes and nonsustained ventricular tachycardia. Encainide, flecainide, and more recently, indecainide have been studied during electrophysiologic testing and have been found to prevent inducible ventricular tachycardia in 10 to 20 percent of patients.[37–40] When ventricular tachycardia remains inducible on these agents, however, a profound increase in tachycardia cycle length and consequent reduction in the hemodynamic impact of these arrhythmias have been noted. The reduction in tachycardia rate is more impressive than that noted with type IA agents. The proarrhythmic effects of the type IC agents has been most noticeable during electrophysiologic testing. The incidence ranges as high as 20 percent or more in certain studies. The proarrhythmic effects of these agents have been noted primarily following their intravenous administration. During chronic oral treatment with these drugs, the incidence of proarrhythmic effect during electrophysiologic testing has been considerably lower.[41,42]

The class III antiarrhythmic agents—the repolarization-prolonging agents—are represented by amiodarone and sotalol at present. Both agents have shown promise in treating sustained ventricular tachyarrhythmias. Some controversy exists regarding the application of electrophysiologic testing to amiodarone. Prevention of arrhythmia initiation following amiodarone treatment has been reported to occur in as few as 8 percent to as many as 60 percent.[43] This disparity can be explained by a number of factors including differences in patient population, route and dose of drug administration, electrophysiologic protocols and criteria used to judge efficacy, and duration of drug administration prior to electrophysiologic testing. Following intravenous administration, amiodarone can prevent induction of ventricular tachycardia in 30 to 50 percent of patients;[43] however, during oral loading, the prevention of arrhythmia induction is considerably less frequent, that is, approximately 15 to 20 percent. Furthermore, some investigators have presented data indicating that electrophysiologic testing is not useful in predicting the clinical efficacy of amiodarone, whereas others have suggested that the opposite is true.[43–45] Nonetheless, most agree that the inability to induce a previously inducible ventricular tachyarrhythmia following amiodarone therapy predicts long-term suppression of this arrhythmia. Recurrence rates in patients in whom ventricular tachyarrhythmias remain inducible are lower than those in patients who are treated with other drugs and in whom the arrhythmia remains inducible. The reasons for this lower incidence of subsequent spontaneous arrhythmia recurrence is not known. We continue to believe that electrophysiologic testing is helpful in the management of patients receiving amiodarone therapy because the severity of an arrhythmia recurrence can be assessed by electrophysiologic study with amiodarone, and the study is helpful in selecting patients who continue to be vulnerable to life-threatening arrhythmia so that more aggressive therapy may be prescribed. Initial reports of the efficacy of sotalol in preventing induction of ventricular tachycardia have also shown prevention of induction of ventricular tachycardia in over 50 percent of patients.[46] Confirmation of these excellent results are required before its place in clinical therapy can be assessed. Like the type IA agents, when the class III agents fail to prevent induction of ventricular tachycardia, the arrhythmia is frequently slower and its hemodynamic consequences less than in the baseline state.

The class II and class IV antiarrhythmic agents—the beta-adrenergic blocking and calcium-channel blocking agents—have shown little if any efficacy in preventing induction of sustained ventricular tachycardia.[23,47] Moreover, because of their negative inotropic effect, they have the potential for producing worsening of hemodynamic status during ventricular tachycardia.

Combination regimens have been frequently used for the treatment of ventricular tachyarrhythmias, but studies of such combinations during electrophysiologic testing have been few. The combination of type IA agents has little to offer except the increased risk of adverse reactions. There are virtually no studies of the combination of IB type agents or IC agents with each other. Combinations of type IA agents with either beta-blocking agents or type IB agents have been shown to be the most useful. Ross and coworkers[48] have reported that the combination of propranolol with quinidine or procainamide was effective in 15 to 20 percent of trials in which all agents administered alone have been ineffective. Similarly, the combination of quinidine or procainamide with mexiletine has been shown to be effective in as many as one third of patients when neither agent was effective alone.[49] In patients in whom the ventricular tachyarrhythmia remained inducible on this latter combination, the rate of the tachycardia was substantially slowed and the hemodynamic consequences and symptoms markedly reduced. Antiarrhythmic drug combinations require further study, but is is noteworthy that the combination of a group IA or IB agent shows early promise.

## EFFECTIVENESS OF ANTIARRHYTHMIC THERAPY DIRECTED BY ELECTROPHYSIOLOGIC TESTING

Using the aforementioned techniques, successful antiarrhythmic regimens can be developed for 50 to 75 percent of patients with recurrent sustained ventricular tachycardia, many of whom had been previously believed to be refractory to pharmacologic therapy. In this group of patients, recurrences of ventricular tachycardia are uncommon (10 to 20 percent) and are frequently due to alterations in drug regimens.[18,19] Moreover, the treatment of patients with regimens that failed to prevent induction of ventricular tachycardia correlate well with arrhythmia recurrences (greater than 80 percent). In addition to defining successful and unsuccessful chronic regimens, serial drug studies using electrophysiologic techniques provide other useful information. Potentially detrimental and proarrhythmic drug effects can be delineated.[34] Also, adjunctive antiarrhythmic effects that can be combined with antiarrhythmic devices or antiarrhythmic surgery can be detected. In other cases, such studies provide the rationale for proceeding to more aggressive treatment modalities such as surgery or implantation of antitachycardia devices.

The role of electrophysiologic studies in selecting therapy for survivors of out-of-hospital cardiac arrest is also clear. The high occurrence rate of life-threatening ventricular tachyarrhythmias in patients who have survived out-of-hospital cardiac arrest requires the institution of effective prophylactic therapy after the first clinical event if a significant salvage rate is to be obtained. The results of electrophysiologic testing for selecting antiarrhythmic regimens has shown suppression of inducible ventricular arrhythmias in approximately 60 to 70 percent of such patients.[50,51] Therapy that prevents induction of ventricular tachycardia or ventricular fibrillation in this group of patients results in recurrence rates of less than 15 percent. Recurrence rates of ventricular tachycardia and cardiac arrest among patients with persistently inducible ventricular arrhythmias despite antiarrhythmic regimens has been 40 to 60 percent. Thus, serial electrophysiologic studies have been shown to be of great benefit in patients who have survived an out-of-hospital cardiac arrest.

## BENEFITS AND LIMITATIONS

Electrophysiologic studies cannot be undertaken lightly. Despite the fact that this technique for selecting antiarrhythmic therapy has been shown to be effective, it is not applicable to all patients. Patients must have inducible ventricular tachyarrhythmia for drug evaluations to be made. Most but not all patients with recurrent ventricular tachyarrhythmias fit into this category. Moreover, provocative tests such as these are not without risk of morbidity or mortality. Complications have been low when performed by experienced and well-trained physicians; however, serious complications may still occur. These untoward effects range from local bleeding, hematoma formation, and phlebitis to serious ones such as cardiac perforation, life-threatening ventricular arrhythmia, and death. Electrophysiologic testing requires the use of sophisticated equipment and many specialized personnel. It requires a major time commitment, as well as substantial financial commitment by the institution in which the studies are being performed.

Despite the obvious limitations of this technique, the risk-benefit ratio favors provocative electrophysiologic testing, both from an economic viewpoint[42] and, even more importantly, from a human viewpoint. The correct selection of antiarrhythmic therapy for lethal ventricular tachyarrhythmias improves survival and reduces the mortality from this common cause of death among cardiac patients.

## REFERENCES

1. MAY, GS, EBERLEIN, KA, FURBERG, CD, ET AL: *Secondary prevention after myocardial infarction: A review of long-term trials.* Prog Cardiovasc Dis 24:331, 1982.

2. MASON JW and WINKLE, RA: *Electrode catheter arrhythmia induction in the selection and assessment of antiarrhythmic drug therapy for recurrent ventricular tachycardia.* Circulation 58:971, 1978.

3. HOROWITZ, LN, JOSEPHSON, ME, FARSHIDI, A, ET AL: *Recurrent sustained ventricular tachycardia: 3. Role of the electrophysiologic study in selection of antiarrhythmic regimens.* Circulation 58:986, 1978.

4. HOROWITZ, LN, JOSEPHSON, ME, and KASTOR, JA: *Intracardiac electrophysiologic studies as a method for the optimization of drug therapy in chronic ventricular arrhythmia.* Prog Cardiovasc Dis 23:81, 1980.

5. FISHER, JD: *Role of electrophysiologic testing in the diagnosis and treatment of patients with known and suspected bradycardias and tachycardias.* Prog Cardiovasc Dis 24:25, 1981.

6. MOWER, MM, REID, PR, WATKINS, L, ET AL *Use of alternating current during diagnostic electrophysiologic studies.* Circulation 67:69, 1983.

7. DOHERTY, JU, KIENZLE, MG, WAXMAN, HL, ET AL: *Programmed ventricular stimulation at a second right ventricular site: An analysis of 100 patients with a special reference to sensitivity, specificity and characteristics of patients with induced ventricular tachycardia.* Am J Cardiol 52:1185, 1983.

8. VANDEPOL, CG, FARSHIDI, A, SPIELMAN, SR, ET AL: *The incidence and clinical significance of induced ventricular tachycardia.* Am J Cardiol 45:725, 1980.

9. REEDY, CP and GETTES, LS: *Use of isoproterenol as an aid to electric induction of chronic recurrent ventricular tachycardia.* Am J Cardiol 44:705, 1979.

10. DENES, P, WU, D, DHINGRA, RC, ET AL: *Electrophysiologic studies in patients with chronic recurrent ventricular tachycardia.* Circulation 54:229, 1976.

11. LIVELLI, FD, BIGGER, JT, REIFFEL, JA, ET AL: *Response to programmed ventricular stimulation: Sensitivity, specificity and relation to heart disease.* Am J Cardiol 50:452, 1982.

12. BRUGADA, P, ABDOLLAH, H, HEDDLE, B, ET AL: *Results of ventricular stimulation protocol using a maximum of 4 premature stimuli in patients without documented or suspected ventricular arrhythmias.* Am J Cardiol 52:1214, 1983

13. MANN, DE, LUCK, JC, GRIFFIN, JC, ET AL: *Induction of clinical ventricular tachycardia using programmed stimulation: Value of third and fourth extrastimuli.* Am J Cardiol 52:501, 1983.

14. BRUGADA, P, GREEN, M, ABDOLLAH, H, ET AL: *Significance of ventricular arrhythmias initiated by programmed ventricular stimulation: The importance of the type of ventricular arrhythmia induced and the number of premature stimuli required.* Circulation 69:87, 1984.

15. MICHELSON, EL, SPIELMAN, SR, GREENSPAN, AM, ET AL: *Electrophysiologic study of the left ventricle: Indications and safety.* Chest 75:592, 1979.

16. HAMER, A, VOHRA, J, HUNT, D, ET AL: *Prediction of sudden death by electrophysiologic studies in high risk patients surviving acute myocardial infarction.* Am J Cardiol 50:223, 1982.

17. RICHARDS, DA, CODY, DV, DENNISS, AR, ET AL: *Ventricular electrical instability: A predictor of death after myocardial infarction.* Am J Cardiol 51:75, 1983.

18. HOROWITZ, LN, SPIELMAN, SR, GREENSPAN, AM, ET AL: *Role of programmed stimulation in assessing vulnerability to ventricular arrhythmias.* Am Heart J 103:604, 1982.

19. MASON, JW and WINKLE, RA: *Accuracy of the ventricular tachycardia-induction study for predicting long-term efficacy and inefficacy of antiarrhythmic drugs.* N Engl J Med 303:1073, 1980.

20. RUSKIN, JN, DIMARCO, JP, and GARAN, H: *Out-of-hospital cardiac arrest: Electrophysiologic observations and selection of long-term antiarrhythmic therapy.* N Engl J Med 303:607, 1980.

21. SPIELMAN, SR, SCHWARTZ, JS, MCCARTHY, DM, ET AL: *Predictors of the success or failure of medical therapy in patients with chronic recurrent sustained ventricular tachycardia: A discriminant analysis.* J Am Coll Cardiol 1:401, 1983.

22. SWERDLOW, CD, GONG, G, ECHT, DS, ET AL: *Clinical factors predicting successful electrophysiologic-pharmacologic study in patients with ventricular tachycardia.* J Am Coll Cardiol 1:409, 1983.

23. WELLENS, HJJ, BAR, FWHM, LIE, KJ, ET AL: *Effect of procainamide, propranolol, and verapamil on mechanism of tachycardia in patients with chronic ventricular tachycardia.* Am J Cardiol 40:579, 1977.

24. DIMARCO, J, GARAN, H, and RUSKIN, JN: *Partial suppression of induced arrhythmias during electrophysiologic testing.* Circulation 62:III-261, 1890.

25. LIVELLI, FD, GANG, ES, REIFFEL, JA, ET AL: *Reproducibility of inducible ventricular tachycardia.* Circulation 66:II-146, 1982.

26. SCHOENFELD, MH, GARAN, H, McGOVERN, B, ET AL: *Long-term reproducibility of programmed cardiac stimulation in patients with recurrent ventricular tachyarrhythmias.* Circulation 66:II-146, 1982.

27. SWERDLOW, CD, BLUM, J, WINKLE, RA, ET AL: *Decreased incidence of antiarrhythmic drug efficacy at electrophysiologic study associated with the use of a third extrastimulus.* Am Heart J 104:1004, 1982.

28. MORADY, F, HESS, D, and SCHEINMAN, MM: *Electrophysiologic drug testing in patients with malignant ventricular arrhythmias: Importance of stimulation at more than one ventricular site.* Am J Cardiol 50:1055, 1982.

29. WAXMAN, HL, BUXTON, AE, SADOWSKI, LM, ET AL: *The response to procainamide during electrophysiologic study for sustained ventricular tachyarrhythmias predicts the response to other medications.* Circulation 67:30, 1983.

30. GREENSPAN, AM, HOROWITZ, LN, SPIELMAN, SR, ET AL: *Large dose procainamide therapy for ventricular tachyarrhythmia.* Am J Cardiol 46:453, 1980.

31. MYERBURG, RJ, KESSLER, KM, KIEM, I, ET AL: *Relationship between plasma levels of procainamide, suppression of premature ventricular complexes and prevention of recurrent ventricular tachycardia.* Circulation 64:280, 1981.

32. DIMARCO, JP, GARAN, H, and RUSKIN, JN: *Quinidine for ventricular arrhythmias: Value of electrophysiologic testing.* Am J Cardiol 51:90, 1983.

33. LERMAN, BB, WAXMAN, HL, BUXTON, AE, ET AL: *Disopyramide: Evaluation of electrophysiologic effects and clinical efficacy in patients with sustained ventricular tachycardia or ventricular fibrillation.* Am J Cardiol 51:759, 1983.

34. POSER, R, LOMBARDI, F, PODRID, P, ET AL: *Aggravation of induced arrhythmias with antiarrhythmic drugs during electrophysiological test.* J Am Coll Cardiol 1:709, 1983.

35. WASPE, LE, WAXMAN, HL, BUXTON, AE, ET AL: *Mexiletine for control of drug-resistant ventricular tachycardia: Clinical and electrophysiologic results in 44 patients.* Am J Cardiol 51:1175, 1983.

36. PALILEO, EV, WELCH, W, HOFF, J, ET AL: *Lack of effectiveness of oral mexiletine in patients with drug-refractory paraoxysmal sustained ventricular tachycardia.* Am J Cardiol 50:1075, 1982.

37. HOROWITZ, LN, SPIELMAN, SR, GREENSPAN, AM, ET AL: Unpublished data, 1984.

38. HOROWITZ, LN, SPIELMAN, SR, GREENSPAN, AM, ET AL: Unpublished data, 1984.

39. ANDERSON, JL: *Experience with electrophysiologically guided therapy of ventricular tachycardia with flecainide: Summary of long-term follow-up.* Am J Cardiol 53:79B, 1984.

40. DIBIANCO, R, FLETCHER, RD, COHEN, AI, ET AL: *Treatment of frequent ventricular arrhythmia with encainide: Assessment using serial ambulatory electrocardiograms, intracardiac electrophysiologic studies, treadmill exercise tests and radionuclide cineangiographic studies.* Circulation 65:1134, 1982.

41. MORGANROTH, J and HOROWITZ, LN: *Flecainide: Its proarrhythmic effect and expected changes on the surface electrocardiogram.* Am J Cardiol 53:89B, 1984.

42. WINKLE, RA, MASON, JW, and GRIFFIN, JC: *Malignant ventricular tachyarrhythmias associated with the use of encainide.* Am Heart J 102:857, 1981.

43. HOROWITZ, LN, SPIELMAN, SR, GREENSPAN, AM, ET AL: *Amiodarone—ventricular arrhythmia: Use of electrophysiologic studies.* Am Heart J 106:881, 1983.

44. WAXMAN, HL: *The efficacy of amiodarone for ventricular arrhythmias cannot be predicted with electrophysiologic studies.* Int J Cardiol 3:76, 1983.

45. McGOVERN, B and RUSKIN, JN: *The efficacy of amiodarone for ventricular arrhythmias can be predicted with clinical electrophysiologic studies.* Int J Cardiol 3:71, 1983.

46. SENGES, J, LENGFELDER, W, JAUERNIG, R, ET AL: *Electrophysiologic testing in assessment of therapy with sotalol for sustained ventricular tachycardia.* Circulation 69:577, 1984.

47. MASON, JW, SWERDLOW, CD, and MITCHELL, LB: *Efficacy of verapamil in chronic, recurrent ventricular tachycardia.* Am J Cardiol 51:1614, 1983.

48. ROSS, DL, SZE, DY, KEEFE, DL, ET AL: *Antiarrhythmic drug combinations in the treatment of ventricular tachycardia.* Circulation 66:1205, 1982.

49. Greenspan, AM, Spielman, SR, Webb, CR, et al: *Efficacy of combination therapy with mexiletine and a type IA agent for sustained ventricular tachyarrhythmias.* J Am Coll Cardiol 3:557, 1984.

50. Ruskin, JN, DiMarco, JP, and Garan, H: *Out-of-hospital cardiac arrest: Electrophysiologic observations and selection of therapy.* N Engl J Med 303:607, 1980.

51. Morady, F, Scheinman, MM, Hess, DS, et al: *Electrophysiologic testing in the management of survivors of out-of-hospital cardiac arrest.* Am J Cardiol 51:85, 1983.

52. Ferguson, D, Saksena, S, Greenberg, E, et al: *Management of recurrent ventricular tachycardia: Economic impact of therapeutic alternatives.* Am J Cardiol 53:531, 1984.

# Clinical Pharmacology of Old and New Antiarrhythmic Drugs*

*Lyle A. Siddoway, M.D., Dan M. Roden, M.D., and Raymond L. Woosley, M.D., Ph.D.*

Treatment of cardiac arrhythmias has led to improvements in quality of life and longevity for many patients with symptomatic arrhythmias, but for others treatment has been limited by ineffectiveness, drug toxicity, or both. Also, the recognition of a relationship between late arrhythmias and mortality from sudden cardiac death in the months following myocardial infarction has led to the hope that arrhythmia suppression can reduce the risk of sudden death. However, attempts to test this still unproven hypothesis have been thwarted by the narrow margin between therapeutic and toxic effects of currently available drugs. In view of this narrow therapeutic index, physicians treating patients with arrhythmias must have a working understanding of the pharmacologic properties of these drugs to provide optimum arrhythmia suppression with minimum side effects. In this chapter, we will review the clinical pharmacology of antiarrhythmic drugs currently available commercially in the United States, several promising investigational drugs, and two drugs already commercially available but not primarily used for arrhythmias.

## BRIEF PHARMACOLOGY REVIEW

Variations in processes involved in the uptake, distribution, effect, and elimination of drugs have potential implications for safety and efficacy of a given treatment regimen.

RELEASE OF DRUG INTO THE GASTROINTESTINAL TRACT. Changes in pharmaceutical preparations can alter the extent and time course of drug release. This recognition several years ago in the case of digoxin[1] led to improved standards for determining the ability of pharmaceutical preparations to release medication.[2] Potential problems nowadays can arise from drugs intentionally designed to release drug slowly. With the recent emphasis on infrequent dosing to improve patient compliance, sustained-release preparations of several cardiovascular drugs have been developed. Although formulations vary, a common feature of these preparations is that the drug is in a form that allows only very slow release into the gut lumen. Because drug is released more slowly, it is carried farther in the gastrointestinal tract before complete absorption has occurred. In conditions leading to decreased bowel transit time, such preparations may be carried past the absorptive sites of the bowel before the drug can be completely absorbed, or before complete tablet dissolution can occur. There are also interindividual differences in completeness of absorption of drug from sustained-release formulations. These variables can lead to a decrease in drug release and absorption, and consequently

*Supported by grants from the United States Public Health Service (GM 07569 and GM31304). Dr. Roden is a recipient of the Clinician Scientist Award of the American Heart Association.

a fall in plasma drug concentration and loss of therapeutic effect. An early sustained-release preparation of procainamide exemplifies this problem: drug from one preparation is sometimes incompletely released during bowel transit in patients with colostomies.[3] (Passing intact tablets in stool does not always imply incomplete absorption. Some patients will pass intact "skeleton" wax matrix tablets in the stool—these are the remnants of tablets that have released all the drug contained in them without being broken down themselves.[3])

ABSORPTION, PRESYSTEMIC CLEARANCE. There is wide variability in the degree to which different drugs (or in some cases the same drug in different patients) reach the systemic circulation. This variability arises from differences in the extent of metabolism of drug in the gut wall, absorption into the portal circulation, and metabolism on passage through the liver via the portal circulation before entering the systemic circulation (so-called presystemic or "first-pass" clearance). The combined efficiency of absorption and presystemic clearance is reflected in the "bioavailability," or systemic availability, of the drug, defined as the ratio of oral and intravenous areas under the concentration–time curve and reflecting the fraction of total drug reaching plasma. Factors influencing bioavailability are listed in Table 1.

CLEARANCE. Drugs can be cleared from plasma at several sites, with liver and kidneys being most important for most drugs. Clearance of drugs extensively metabolized in the liver

**Table 1.** Factors influencing oral bioavailability

| A. Factors affecting absorption | Example |
|---|---|
| 1. Physicochemical properties of the drug (e.g., polarity at physiologic pH) | Bretylium, a quaternary amine, is highly polar and poorly absorbed[4] |
| 2. Decreased absorptive surface area | Decreased Vitamin $B_{12}$ absorption in patients with regional and ileal resection[5] |
| 3. Decreased bowel transit time | Decreased absorption of griseofulvin in patients with diarrhea[6] |
| 4. Formation of poorly absorbed complexes with other gut contents | Decreased tetracycline absorption when given with milk[7] |
| 5. Intraluminal degradation of drug by gut flora | Increased digoxin dosage has been needed in some patients to maintain therapeutic concentrations because of bacterial degradation of digoxin in the bowel; some of these patients have been reported to become digoxin toxic and have decreased fecal digoxin degradation products after receiving broad-spectrum antibiotics[8] |
| 6. Malabsorption syndrome | Decreased Vitamin K absorption in patients with fat malabsorption[9] |
| 7. Medication formulation | Quinidine sulfate is more rapidly absorbed than is quinidine gluconate[10] |
| **B. Factors affecting drug clearance** | |
| 1. Rate of delivery of drug to the liver (ie., rate of absorption) | Clearance of propafenone is lower with large than with small doses, indicating saturation of available metabolizing enzyme[11] |
| 2. Avidity of hepatic enzymes for the drug ("extraction ratio") | Procainamide is metabolized much less on first pass than is propafenone[11,12] |
| 3. Inherited interindividual differences in drug metabolism | Encainide is metabolized to a more active metabolite by an enzyme system deficient in 5–10% of the population[13–15] |
| 4. Treatment with drugs that enhance ("induce") hepatic oxidative metabolism | Decreased systemic availability of quinidine after treatment with rifampin, phenytoin, or phenobarbital, which are hepatic enzyme inducers[16–18] |

can be altered by many factors. As mentioned for presystemic clearance in Table 1, rate of drug delivery to the liver (in this case, liver blood flow), hepatic extraction ratio of the drug, inherited differences in metabolic pathways, plasma protein binding, and administration of enzyme inducers can all play a role.

Liver blood flow can be altered by several factors, including low cardiac output and treatment with beta-adrenergic blockers[18,19] or cimetidine.[20-23] Hepatic extraction ratio defines the fraction of drug metabolized on a single pass through the liver. This ratio varies for different drugs, depending on the enzyme system involved, the rapidity of uptake of the drug in the liver, and the avidity of the enzyme for the drug. Inherited differences in drug metabolism have been demonstrated for some hepatic enzymes. Interindividual differences in acetylation of procainamide, dapsone, hydralazine, and isoniazid have been linked to quantitative differences in N-acetyltransferase. These differences are inherited in a bimodal pattern as the "fast" or "slow" acetylator phenotype, with rapid acetylators having approximately twice as much enzyme as slow acetylators.[24] Oxidative metabolism via some of the P-450 enzymes also is bimodally inherited. The best studied of these is the enzyme metabolizing debrisoquin. Debrisoquin is a guanethidine-like antihypertensive drug that was noted to produce excessive and prolonged hypotension in a small subset of patients.[25] It was subsequently found that 6 to 9 percent of populations are poor metabolizers of debrisoquin.[26] Several other drugs, including encainide and propranolol, were subsequently found to have polymorphic metabolism paralleling that of debrisoquin, suggesting the same enzyme is involved in their metabolism.[14,27-32] These phenotypic differences can have important implications for the duration of a drug's effects and its metabolite profile. Hepatic enzymes can be "activated" (induced) or inhibited by several drugs. These drugs are listed in Table 2.

Renal failure can affect drug clearance in several ways: reduction of clearance of parent drug (e.g., digoxin),[34] reduction of clearance of active metabolities (e.g., N-acetylprocainamide),[35] or altered protein binding (e.g., phenytoin).[36] Other routes of drug clearance, such as lung or plasma metabolism, can be important, particularly for some short-acting compounds.[37,38]

HALF-LIFE, "STEADY STATE." Half-life is the time required for a 50 percent change in any first-order process. Since distribution and elimination of most drugs follow first-order kinetics, half-life can be a useful descriptor for these processes. Distribution half-life reflects the time for distribution of drug from plasma to other organs (most important after an intravenous bolus), and is usually only a few minutes. Elimination half-life is the time required for elimination of half of the drug from the body, or the time taken for plasma concentration to fall by 50 percent. After administration of a drug is discontinued, a time equal to four elimination half-lives is required to reduce drug concentration to less than 7 percent of its original level. This may be helpful in some cases in predicting the duration of a drug's effect. "Steady state"

**Table 2.** Some drugs with known or proposed enzyme induction or inhibition effects in man

| Hepatic enzyme inducers | Hepatic enzyme inhibitors |
| --- | --- |
| Phenytoin | Cimetidine |
| Phenobarbital | Allopurinol |
| Rifampin | Disulfiram |
| Ethanol | Anabolic steroids |
| Carbamazepine | Chloramphenicol |
| Ethchlorvynol | Metronidazole |
| Glutethimide | Quinacrine |
| Griseofulvin | Isoniazid |
| | Estrogens/oral contraceptives |
| | Amiodarone |

defines the time at which drug intake and elimination are equal, resulting in reproducible drug concentrations after each dose. Its time course is dependent on the elimination rate, again with four or five elimination half-lives between the time of initiation of treatment or change in dosage and achievement of a new steady state. If dosage changes are made before steady state is reached, the clinician must be vigilant to the possibility of excessive drug accumulation or unexpected loss of effect later. Although the time course of reaching steady state is dependent on elimination half-life, the magnitude of steady state (i.e., steady-state concentration) is dependent only on clearance and dose. In some cases, the half-life of a drug is discordant with the time course of its effects. For example, in most patients, encainide has an elimination half-life of 2.5 hours but a half-life of effect of 6 to 8 hours, suggesting the presence of an active metabolite with a half-life longer than that of the parent drug.[39] Also, beta-adrenergic blockers can produce antihypertensive effects that persist much longer than would be predicted by elimination half-life, suggesting the presence of an active metabolite or of an effect that, once initiated, continues in the absence of the drug.[40-43]

DISTRIBUTION. Analysis of a drug's pharmacokinetic properties is complicated somewhat by an apparent variability in the rate and extent of uptake of drug by different tissues. Kinetically, these tissues are described as residing in different mass-action "compartments." These compartments do not necessarily define a given group of organs or tissues. These compartments are shown schematically in Figure 1. The organs to which drug is rapidly distributed after reaching the systemic circulation comprise the pharmacokinetic "central compartment." This compartment is believed to generally include highly perfused organs (e.g., kidney, heart, brain, liver, vascular system). For most drugs, a slower distribution can be demonstrated to occur from the central compartment to a second "peripheral" compartment, which usually accumulates larger quantities of drug. A third "deep" compartment can be demonstrated for some drugs, such as guanethidine and amiodarone. A theoretical compartment defined by the time course of a drug's effects (rather than by the time–concentration curve) makes up the "effect" compartment, which may or may not correspond to one of the previously mentioned mass-action compartments.[44] The clinical significance of these compartments is evident in the relationship between drug plasma concentration and effect, and in the way drug must be administered to achieve a rapid effect. Guanethidine exemplifies a drug whose kinetics fit a three-compartment model, with the effect compartment paralleling the deep compartment. If no loading regimen is used, the antihypertensive effect may not be apparent until 4 or 5 days after initiation of treatment, corresponding to the slow accumulation of guanethidine in the

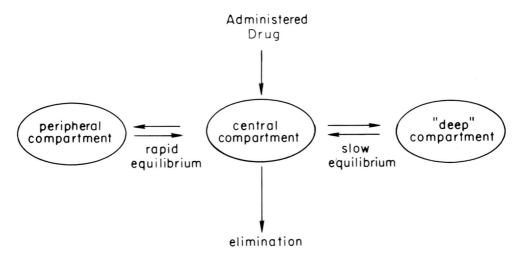

**Figure 1.** Schematic illustration of three-compartment model of drug distribution and elimination.

deep compartment.[45] The size of the central compartment and the rate of drug distribution are important in determining the appropriate dose of an intravenous drug for which a rapid effect is essential. For example, the concentration achieved immediately after a bolus of lidocaine depends primarily on the volume of the central compartment.[46] For lidocaine and several other drugs, this central volume is decreased in such disease states as congestive heart failure, necessitating a decrease in the amount of drug given in a bolus in order to avoid toxic concentrations. The steady-state volume of distribution, defined as the dose divided by steady-state plasma concentration, assumes importance in some specific situations. For example, as an indicator of a large degree of protein binding or tissue accumulation, a large steady-state volume of distribution would indicate that toxic drug concentrations would be unlikely to be rapidly reduced by dialysis.

DRUG ADMINISTRATION. With a knowledge of a drug's means of clearance and patterns of distribution and elimination, a dosing regimen can be developed. The simplest dosage regimen is one in which the patient is simply given a maintenance dosage regimen without any loading doses. This method is preferred in situations in which the drug effect is not urgently needed, or where doses larger than the maintenance dose could be harmful. In more urgent circumstances, it is frequently necessary to give large loading doses at the onset of therapy in order to quickly achieve a therapeutic effect. Lidocaine, procainamide, and amiodarone are among the drugs for which loading regimens are frequently needed. An ideal loading regimen would instantaneously achieve a therapeutic plasma concentration, and subsequently maintain that concentration without fluctuation. This can be done by initially giving a dose sufficient to "fill" the central compartment (i.e., achieve a therapeutic plasma concentration), followed by doses sufficient to replace drug that is distributed to peripheral compartments or eliminated. Because drug distribution is a first-order process, the amount of drug in the peripheral compartment will increase exponentially and, conversely, the amount of drug needed to fill the peripheral compartment will fall exponentially. The amount of administered drug required to replace drug eliminated is constant for a given steady-state plasma concentration and comprises the "maintenance dose." Using lidocaine as an example, in practice the exponential dosing needed early in treatment is frequently approximated by administering one or more bolus doses at the beginning of treatment or increasing the initial infusion rate, followed later by reduction to a maintenance dosage. More sophisticated approximations, with less fluctuation of plasma concentration, may be possible with use of two-bottle dilution administration devices or computer-controlled pumps.[47,48] Figure 2 illustrates idealized lidocaine concentration–time curves with different loading regimens. As has been mentioned previously, the size of the loading and maintenance dosages must be based on the volume of the central and peripheral compartments, clearance, and the presence or absence of concurrent illnesses, and the dosages should be reassessed when a situation arises that could potentially alter one of these factors.

PROTEIN BINDING. Upon entering the circulation, many drugs are partially bound to plasma proteins, primarily albumin for acidic drugs and alpha-1-acid glycoprotein for basic drugs, and an equilibrium is established between bound and unbound drug. It is unbound (or "free") drug, that when distributed to the drug's site of action, leads to a pharmacologic effect. Factors causing changes in protein binding can cause an alteration in the pharmacologic effect encountered with a given drug dosage. Some factors affecting drug protein binding are pH, competition with other drugs for binding sites, drug concentration, concentration of albumin or alpha-1-acid glycoprotein, and the presence of renal or hepatic failure. One example of a clinically significant protein binding alteration is the decrease in plasma protein binding of phenytoin in patients with uremia.[49] A converse example is the increase in protein binding of lidocaine related to elevation of plasma alpha-1-acid glycoprotein in the setting of acute myocardial infarction.[50] These changes lead to an alteration in clearance and in the relationship of total drug to unbound drug concentrations, with a consequent change in the relationship between total drug concentration and therapeutic (or toxic) effect.

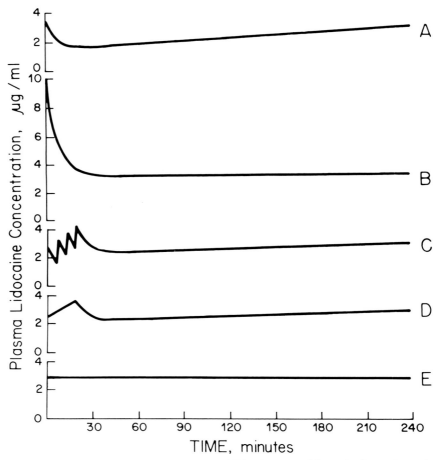

**Figure 2.** Computer modeled time-concentration profiles of lidocaine using different loading regimens for a 70-kg normal individual. (*A*) 100-mg bolus followed by 2 mg/min maintenance infusion. (*B*) 300-mg bolus followed by 2 mg/min maintenance infusion. (*C*) 75-mg loading dose followed by 50-mg boluses at 7, 13, and 19 minutes, followed by 2 mg/min maintenance infusion. (*D*) Loading bolus of 75 mg followed by infusion of 8.3 mg/min for 18 minutes, followed by 2 mg/min maintenance infusion. (*E*) 92-mg bolus followed by 8.33 mg/min exponentially decreasing to 2 mg/min maintenance. (From Riddell et al,[48] with permission.)

"THERAPEUTIC RANGE." The most commonly used means of describing desirable plasma concentrations for a given drug is the therapeutic range. The lower end of this range is the average minimum effective concentration of the drug, whereas the upper end is the concentration providing maximum benefit or, more commonly, the concentration at which frequent side effects begin to be noted. Thus, the therapeutic range is a statistical figure and as such provides rough guidelines but no absolute information for treatment of an individual patient. This must be kept in mind, for there can be marked interindividual differences in tolerance to a drug and responsiveness to its therapeutic effects. Usually these differences are not predictable, and therefore treatment should be started with low dosages and carefully titrated upward as needed for each individual. In some cases, such as antiarrhythmic treatment of patients with severe cardiac conduction system disease, one can predict an increased likelihood of unwanted effects at "therapeutic" concentrations, and in these patients low initial dosages are especially important.

## CLASSIFICATION OF ANTIARRHYTHMIC DRUGS

Antiarrhythmic drugs are frequently grouped according to prominent electrophysiologic effects. The most widely used classification scheme is that of Vaughan Williams,[51] who proposed the following scheme:

Class I ("membrane-stabilizing" or "local anesthetic")—Drugs acting primarily by blocking the rapid sodium channel, with resultant decrease in the maximum rate of depolarization ($\dot{V}$max) of the action potential and slowing of intracardiac conduction. Examples include quinidine, lidocaine, and flecainide. (These drugs and those with similiar properties are sometimes subclassified as Class Ia, Ib, and Ic respectively on the basis of effects on intracardiac conduction and refractoriness.)

Class II—Beta-adrenergic blockers.

Class III—Drugs whose predominant effect is prolongation of the cardiac action potential duration. Examples are amiodarone and bretylium.

Class IV—Calcium antagonists.

Although these classifications provide a useful shorthand for characterizing a prominent characteristic of a drug, further utility is limited. Drugs frequently possess properties of more than one class. Also, drugs within a class can have important differences, so that response or lack thereof to one drug in a given class does not necessarily predict success or failure of another.

## REVIEW OF INDIVIDUAL DRUGS

Basic pharmacokinetic, electrophysiologic, and clinical information about the drugs discussed in this review is outlined in Tables 3, 4, and 5. These drugs will be presented in more detail in this section.

### Quinidine

Cinchona alkaloids were used in treatment of arrhythmias as early as 1749, when Jean-Baptiste de Senac reported improvement in patients with "rebellious palpitations" (atrial fibrillation).[52] Quinidine itself was first prepared in 1853 for use as an antimalarial and was incidentally noted to correct atrial fibrillation in some patients.[53] Since its first systematic study in 1918 for treatment of atrial fibrillation,[54] quinidine has been widely used and has been found to be effective in treatment of a wide variety of ventricular and supraventricular arrhythmias including atrial fibrillation, atrial flutter, paroxysmal supraventricular tachycardia, ventricular premature beats, and ventricular tachycardia. The structure of quinidine is shown in Figure 3.

#### Electrophysiologic Effects

Quinidine, like other Class I antiarrhythmic drugs, decreases $\dot{V}$max. This inhibition is rate-, pH-, and voltage-dependent, and most marked at increased heart rate or less negative membrane potential.[55-58] This results in slowed conduction, more marked in the His-Purkinje system than in the atria. The effective refractory period and, to a lesser degree, action potential duration are increased by quinidine.[55-58] These effects on conduction velocity and effective refractory period are probably responsible for the effectiveness of quinidine in re-entrant arrhythmias. Quinidine decreases automaticity by decreasing the slope of phase 4 depolarization and by raising the diastolic excitation threshold.[59] In denervated hearts, quinidine slows conduction, increases the effective refractory period (ERP) in the AV node, and decreases automaticity of the SA node.[60] However, in patients these effects are countered by vagolytic (anticholinergic) properties[61] and changes in sympathetic tone.[62] On the surface ECG, quinidine causes dose-related increases in P–R, QRS, and Q–$T_c$ intervals.[63]

**Table 3.** Pharmacokinetics of antiarrhythmic drugs

| Drug | Inactivation or route of elimination[a] | Active metabolites | Vd (l/kg) | Protein binding | Elimination half-life (hr)[b] | Oral bioavailability | Oral clearance (ml/min) |
|---|---|---|---|---|---|---|---|
| Quinidine | Liver (50–90%) Kidney (10–30%) | Probable | 2–4 | 70–95% | 7–18 | 70% | 200–400 |
| Procainamide | Kidney (30–60%) Liver (40–70%) | Yes | 1.5–2.5 | 15% | 2.5–4.7[c] | 75% | 400–700[d] |
| Acecainide | Kidney | No | 1–1.5 | | 7–11 | 85% | 100–150 |
| Disopyramide | Kidney (36–77%) Liver (11–37%) | Yes | 1 | 20–60%[c] | 7–9 | 80% | 95 |
| Lidocaine | Liver (90%) | Yes | Vc = 1–1.5 | 40–70% | 1.5–4[f] | 35% | 700–1000 |
| Phenytoin | Liver (95%) | No | 0.64 | 85% | 24 | 70–100%[c] | 50[e] |
| Mexiletine | Liver (90%) | No | 10 | 70% | 8–12[g]; 12–24[h] | 90% | 400–700 |
| Tocainide | Liver (50–60%) Kidney (40–50%) | No | 3 | 50% | 12–15 | 100% | 150–200[d] |
| Imipramine | Liver | Yes | 15 | 76–96% | 4–15 | 29–77% | 1400 |
| Moricizine | Liver (90%) | Probable | | 40% | 6–13 | ?(Good) | 200–800 |
| Flecainide | Liver (70%) | No | 10 | | 11–30 | 95% | 200–12,000 |
| Encainide | Liver (90%)[b,c] | Yes | 8–10 | 85% | 2.7[i]; 8.7[k] | 26%; 89%[k] | 1100 |
| Lorcainide | Liver (98%) | Yes | | 85% | 7.6 | 80–100%[d,j] | 800–50,000[c,e] |
| Propafenone | Liver (99%) | Yes | 3–4 | 90% | 2–24[c] | 10–50%[c,e] | 150 |
| Sotalol | Kidney (90%) | No | 2.5 | 0% | 10–20 | 100% | 1300[d] |
| Bretylium | Kidney (70–80%) | No | 3.4 | ?(low) | 4–16 | 20% | 6500–11,000 |
| Amiodarone | Liver (99%) | Unknown | 20–200 | ?(high) | 3–15 wks | 20–50% | |

a"Kidney" refers to renal elimination of unchanged drug
bHalf-lives of normals and patients; shorter half-lives are those reported in normal volunteers
cInherited differences in metabolism
dReduced by renal insufficiency
eDose- or concentration-dependent
fHalf-life increases during prolonged infusion
gIn normal volunteers
hIn patients
iIn "extensive metabolizers" (see text)
jAt steady state
kIn "poor metabolizers" (see text)
Vc = volume of central compartment

**Table 4.** Electrophysiologic effects of antiarrhythmic drugs

| | Cellular electrophysiology (canine Purkinje fiber) | | | Intracardiac electrophysiology | | | | Surface ECG | | |
|---|---|---|---|---|---|---|---|---|---|---|
| | APD | Vmax | Automaticity | A–H | H–V | ERP-AVN | ERP-V | P–R | QRS | Q–T |
| Quinidine | 1 | D | D | D,O,1 | 1 | | 1 | D,O,1 | 1 | 1 |
| Procainamide | 1 | D | D | O,1 | 1 | O,1 | 1 | O | 1 | 1 |
| Acecainide | 1 | O | O,D[a] | O | O | O | 1 | O | O | 1 |
| Disopyramide | 1 | D | D | D,O,1 | 1 | | O,1 | O,1 | 1 | O,1 |
| Lidocaine | D | O,D[a] | D | O,1[a] | O | O,1 | D | O | O | O |
| Mexiletine | D | D[a] | D | O,1 | O | | D | O | O | O |
| Tocainide | D | O,D[a] | D | O,1[a] | O,1[a] | O | O | U,1[a] | O | O,D |
| Phenytoin | D | O,D[a] | D | O,1[a] | O | O,D | D | O,1[a] | O | O |
| Imipramine | D | D | D | O | 1 | O | O | 1 | 1 | 1 |
| Moricizine | D | D | O,D[a] | O | 1 | O | O | 1 | 1 | 1[c] |
| Flecainide | D | D | D | O | 1 | O | 1 | 1 | 1 | 1[c] |
| Encainide | D | D | D | O | 1 | 1[b] | 1[b] | O | 1 | 1[c] |
| Lorcainide | D | D | D | O | 1 | 1[b] | 1[b] | 1 | 1 | 1[c] |
| Propafenone | D | D | D | 1 | 1 | 1 | 1 | 1 | 1 | 1[c] |
| Propranolol | O,[d]D[e] | O,[d]D[e] | O,[d]D[e] | O,[f]1[g] | O | O,[f]1[g] | O | O,[f]1[g] | O | O,1 |
| Sotalol | 1 | O | O | 1 | O | 1 | 1 | 1 | O | 1 |
| Bretylium | 1 | O,[d]1,[h]D[e] | O,1[h] | O,1,O[h] | O | O | 1 | O | O | O |
| Amiodarone | 1 | D | D | 1 | 1[a] | 1 | 1 | 1 | O | 1 |

1 = Increase; D = decrease; O = no change; APD = action potential duration; Vmax = maximum rate of depolarization in phase 0; A–H = A–H interval; H–V = H–V interval; ERP = effective refractory period of AV node (AVN) or ventricle (V).

[a] More marked in abnormal tissue or in patients with conduction system disease.
[b] In chronic treatment.
[c] Q–T prolongation largely due to increased QRS; little or no increase in J–T interval.
[d] Low concentrations.
[e] High concentrations.
[f] Direct effect.
[g] Due to beta blockade.
[h] Transient effect due to catecholamine release.

**Table 5.** Dosages and plasma concentrations of drugs used in treatment of ventricular arrhythmias[a]

| | Usual initial dosage[b] | Range of dosages | Maximum single dose (mg) | Therapeutic range (mc/ml) |
|---|---|---|---|---|
| Quinidine (sulfate) | 200 mg q 6h | 800–2400 mg/day | 600 | 2–5 |
| Procainamide (sustained-release) | 500 mg q 6h | 2000–6000 mg/day | 1500 | 4–10[c] |
| Acecainide | 500 mg q 6h | 2000–8000 mg/day | 2000 | 5–19 |
| Disopyramide | 150 mg q 6h | 400–800 mg/day | 300 | 2–4 |
| Lidocaine | See Fig 2 | 1–4 mg/min IV | — | 1.5–5.0 |
| Mexiletine | 200 mg q 8h | 450–1200 mg/day | 4000 | 0.75–2.0 |
| Tocainide | 400 mg q 8h | 1200–2400 mg/day | 400 | 3–19 |
| Phenytoin | 100 mg q 8h | 200–400 mg/day | 200 | 10–20 |
| Imipramine | 50 mg q 8h | 75–400 mg/day | 100 | 0.07–0.38[d] |
| Moricizine | 200 mg q 8h | 600–750 mg/day | 2500 | .03–? |
| Flecainide | 100 mg q 8h | 300–600 mg/day | 300 | 1.0 |
| Encainide | 25 mg q 6h | 75–300 mg/day | 75 | — |
| Lorcainide | 100 mg q 12h | 200–450 mg/day | 150 | 0.15–0.40 |
| Propafenone | 300 mg q 12h | 450–900 mg/day | 300 | 70.40 |
| Propranolol | 40 mg q 6h | 40–640 mg/day | 160 | 0.05–0.60 |
| Sotalol | 80 mg q 12h | 160–960 mg/day | 480 | 1–3 |
| Bretylium | See text | 1–4 mg/min IV | — | — |
| Amiodarone | 800–2000 mg/day (load) | 200–800 mg/day | 600–1000 | 1–2.5 |

[a]These dosages and concentrations should be considered to be general guidelines only. Dosage should be determined in light of clinical response, plasma concentrations, and adverse effects.

[b]Initial dosages of many drugs must be reduced in the presence of congestive heart failure.

[c]Some authors recommend higher plasma concentrations (see text).

[d]Imipramine + desipramine.

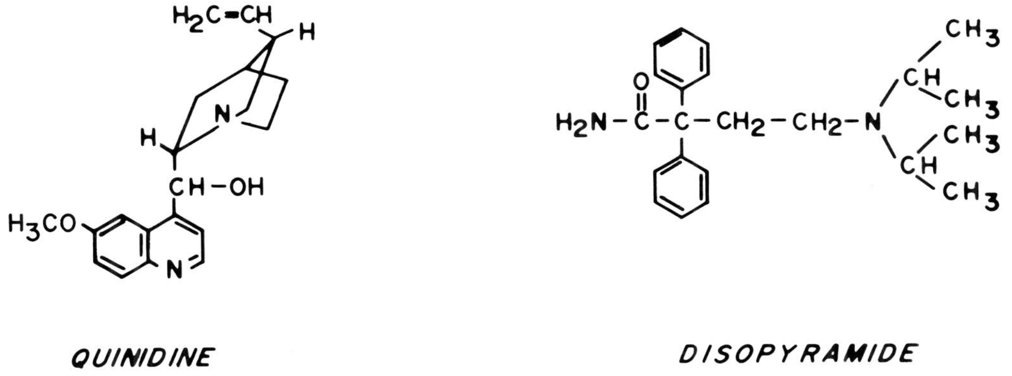

**Figure 3.** Structures of quinidine and disopyramide.

## Hemodynamic Effects

Quinidine is a vasodilator, acting via alpha-adrenergic blockade.[64] It has mild negative inotropic effects,[65] which are countered by the vasodilator effect during oral therapy. In excessive doses or after rapid intravenous administration, quinidine can cause hypotension, primarily due to vasodilation.

## Indications

Quinidine has been successfully used in a wide variety of arrhythmias including conversion of atrial fibrillation or flutter,[66,67] supraventricular tachycardia,[63,68] ventricular extrasystoles,[69–71] ventricular tachycardia, and ventricular fibrillation.[72,73] It has been used successfully in treatment of tachycardia related to Wolff-Parkinson-White syndrome,[74] although there are reports of arrhythmia worsening that may be due to quinidine's vagolytic effects.[75] Quinidine has been used in combination with mexiletine,[76] aprindine,[77] or amiodarone[78] for treatment of arrhythmias refractory to single-agent therapy. The combination of quinidine with amiodarone has been reported to cause torsades de pointes in some patients and should be avoided.[79] Although it is reported to have an abortifacient effect at high concentrations, quinidine is believed by some investigators to be the agent of choice for arrhythmias during pregnancy.

## Disposition

Quinidine undergoes extensive hepatic metabolism. Indirect human evidence and data from animal studies suggest the presence of cardioactive metabolites, but their clinical role is unclear.[80,81]

## Dosage, Plasma Concentrations

Because of possible arrhythmogenic effects of quinidine, treatment should be started at a low dosage (equivalent to 200 mg of quinidine sulfate every 6 hours) and carefully titrated. We recommend continuous monitoring of the rhythm of patients at least during the early portion of the dose titration period (see Adverse Effects section below). Dosage ranges and the generally accepted therapeutic concentration range are outlined in Table 5. Elderly patients have been reported to require smaller dosages of quinidine than other patients because of reduced clearance and volume of distribution. Because of changes in assay methods to better differentiate quinidine from its metabolites, the minimum effective concentration range (using EMIT, double extraction, or HPLC method) has been lowered.[82-84] The minimum effective concentration of quinidine measured by newer assays ranges from 0.7 to 1.5 $\mu$g/ml, whereas toxic side effects are encountered with increased frequency at concentrations greater than 5 $\mu$g/ml. The concentration–response relationship for quinidine has not been well studied, however, and therapy must be individualized. Because of decreased protein binding in patients with liver failure,[85] efficacy and toxicity can occur at lower than usual total plasma concentrations. Dosage does not appear to be altered in the presence of renal failure. Specific recommendations for dosage in hepatic failure are not available.

## Adverse Effects

In some patients, marked Q–T$_c$ prolongation can be encountered. The risk of torsades de pointes is markedly increased in these patients. It is this arrhythmia that is probably responsible for many cases of "quinidine syncope" and quinidine-induced sudden death. Typically, torsades de pointes occurs early in treatment (although it can occur later) and at a time when plasma quinidine concentration is less than 3.5 $\mu$g/ml.[86-89] We have estimated the incidence of this problem among patients started on quinidine at our institution at 1 to 2 percent per year.[89] The Q–T$_c$ prolongation and associated arrhythmia are aggravated in the presence of hypokalemia or bradycardia.[89] The recognition of this arrhythmia is critical because its treatment is very different from that of other arrhythmias. An example of a typical run of torsades de pointes is shown in Figure 4. Successful management requires discontinuation of quinidine, correction of hypokalemia, and maneuvers to increase heart rate and shorten Q–T intervals (isoproterenol, temporary pacing).[90,91] Such maneuvers must be continued until the Q–T$_c$ interval returns to the normal range and the ventricular tachycardia has resolved. If further antiarrhythmic treatment is needed for patients with a history of torsades de pointes, drugs with potential for prolonging Q–T$_c$ should be avoided.

In patients with sinus node dysfunction or AV block, quinidine, like other Class I drugs, can have marked depressant effects, resulting in sinus bradycardia or high-grade AV block.

A common side effect of quinidine is diarrhea, which has been anecdotally reported to be improved in some cases by changing to a different form of the drug, for example from quinidine sulfate to quinidine gluconate. Whether such improvement is due to the drug preparation itself or a reduced dosage of quinidine base is not clear. Other reported side effects include nausea, vomiting, and cinchonism. Quinidine can cause antibody-mediated thrombocytopenia.[92] Patients with such a history should be instructed to avoid taking quinidine,

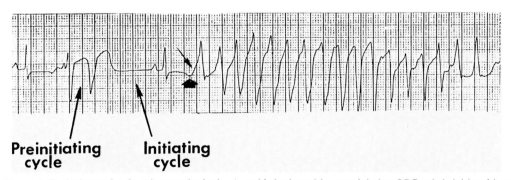

**Preinitiating cycle**    **Initiating cycle**

**Figure 4.** Typical torsades de pointes arrhythmia. A rapid rhythm with an undulating QRS axis is initiated by a premature ventricular contraction (small arrow) falling on the T wave (large arrow) of the preceding beat. Note the long Q–T interval of the first complex on the strip. The short "preinitiating" cycle followed by a long "initiating" cycle accentuates Q–T prolongation of the initiating complex. This sequence of cycle length changes is encountered in many cases of torsades de pointes.[89]

quinine, or quinine-containing products (e.g., tonic water). When given intravenously, quinidine induces vasodilation and hypotension by alpha-adrenergic blockade.[64] For this reason, parenteral administration of quinidine should be avoided or, if unavoidable, should be at a rate no faster than 16 mg/min under carefully monitored conditions, and discontinued if hypotension or greater than 25 percent QRS prolongation is observed.

There have been reports of abrupt increases in ventricular response in patients treated with quinidine for atrial flutter without prior AV nodal blockade.[93] This is due to a slight reduction of the flutter rate and enhanced AV nodal conduction via quinidine's anticholinergic effects, allowing 1:1 conduction through the AV node, often at a rate of 200 to 250 beats per min. On theoretical grounds, one would predict this possibility to be particularly of concern in patients concomitantly administered drugs that increase AV nodal conduction, such as beta-adrenergic agonists.

## Drug Interactions

Quinidine increases plasma digoxin concentrations by up to 100 percent, primarily by displacement of digoxin from tissue binding sites and reduced renal elimination.[94–97] There are also reports of elevation of digitoxin concentrations by quinidine.[98] For this reason, digoxin dosage should be decreased by 50 percent in patients beginning quinidine therapy, and plasma levels followed closely. Guidelines for digitoxin dosage are less well defined. Phenytoin, phenobarbital, and rifampin can markedly enhance hepatic quinidine metabolism, with resultant decrease in plasma concentrations and efficacy.[15–17] Cimetidine has been reported to reduce quinidine clearance.[99] Hypokalemia potentiates quinidine-related $Q-T_c$ prolongation,[89,100] whereas hyperkalemia accentuates quinidine's negative dromotropic and chronotropic effects. The combination of quinidine and organic nitrates sometimes causes orthostatic hypotension, presumably related to the additive vasodilator effects of both.[101] Quinidine worsens neuromuscular blockade in patients with myasthenia gravis,[102] and may prolong the effects of succinylcholine.[103]

## Procainamide and N-acetylprocainamide (Acecainide)

Procaine was noted in 1936 to raise myocardial excitability threshold.[104] Because of unacceptable side effects of procaine, a systematic search for a clinically useful congener was initiated. This led to the discovery of procainamide (Pronestyl and others),[105] which has been in clinical use for the treatment of arrhythmias for three decades. Its major metabolite, N-acetylprocainamide (acecainide, NAPA), was found to be cardioactive with electrophysiologic, antiarrhythmic, and toxic profile different from that of the parent drug.[106–109] Procainamide has served as a prototype for the development of several newer antiarrhythmic drugs. The structures of procainamide and similar newer drugs are shown in Figure 5.

## Electrophysiologic Effects

Like quinidine, procainamide slows conduction, prolongs refractoriness, and decreases automaticity and excitability of atrial and ventricular myocardium and Purkinje fibers, and decreases conduction in bypass tracts.[63,74,110–112] In contrast to quinidine, procainamide has little vagolytic activity in man, and it causes less marked action potential duration (APD) and $Q-T_c$ prolongation.[63] Hypotension and bradycardia observed in some patients after intravenous administration may be due to the ganglionic blocking action of procainamide observed in animal studies.[113] N-acetylprocainamide prolongs action potential duration and refractoriness in atrial and ventricular myocardium and prolongs the Q–T interval on the surface electrocardiogram.[106–109,114,115] It has no effect on $\dot{V}$max in Purkinje fibers and ventricular muscle and does not alter His-Purkinje conduction velocity in man.

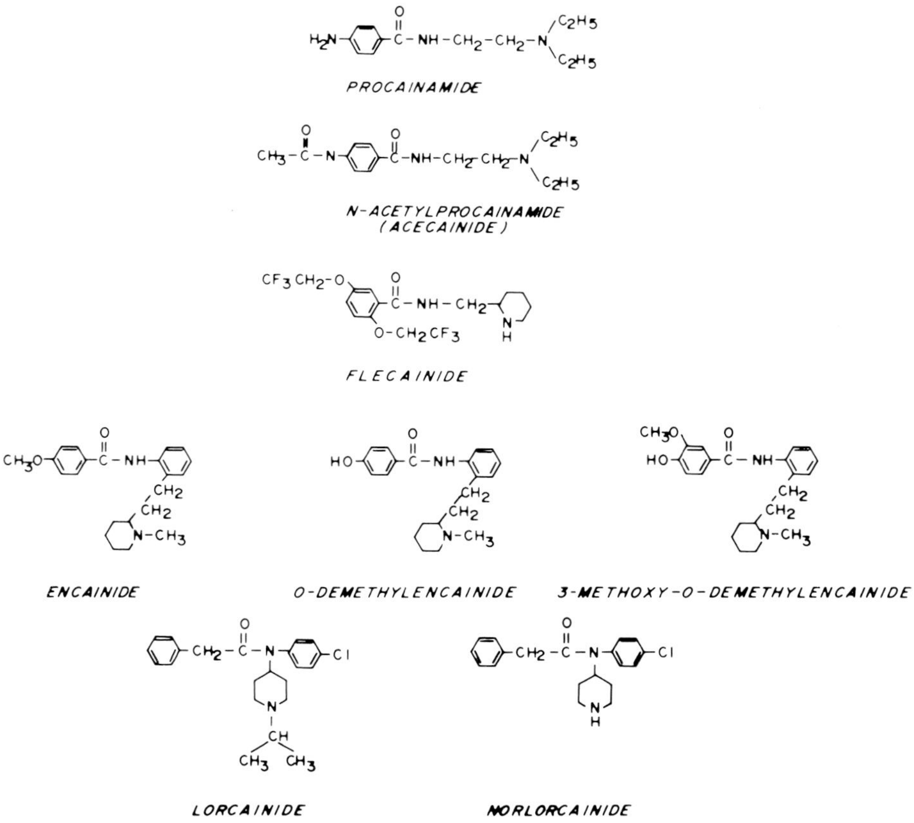

**Figure 5.** Structures of procainamide and its amide "descendents."

## Hemodynamic Effects

Procainamide, like quinidine, has minimal negative inotropic effects and causes clinically apparent decreased myocardial contractility only in patients with poor ventricular function or when given intravenously at a rapid rate.[116,117]

## Indications

Procainamide is effective for the same broad spectrum of arrhythmias treated with quinidine, and one may be effective where the other fails.[74,118-125] Procainamide is useful in acute management of re-entrant supraventricular tachycardia and atrial fibrillation and flutter associated with Wolff-Parkinson-White syndrome.[106,107,128,129] N-acetylprocainamide has been shown to be effective in treatment of stable ventricular arrhythmias, but its use is limited by a narrow therapeutic index.

## Disposition

Procainamide is well absorbed after oral administration.[130-132] Approximately 50 to 70 percent of procainamide is eliminated unchanged in the urine, while 20 to 40 percent undergoes hepatic conversion to N-acetylprocainamide, which is eliminated unchanged in the urine.[133-135] Acetylation of procainamide is dependent on the activity of the liver enzyme, N-acetyltransferase. This action is genetically influenced, with 45 percent of white and black populations and 10 to 20 percent of orientals carrying the "slow acetylator" trait.[136] Both procainamide and N-acetylprocainamide can accumulate to high concentrations in renal failure, even at low procainamide dosages.[35,137]

### Dosage, Plasma Concentrations

Oral use of procainamide has been made more convenient with the development of sustained-release preparations (Procan SR, Pronestyl SR) allowing 6- to 8-hour dosing intervals. There remains some variation in bioavailability of these formulations, however, and therapy must be individualized. The range of plasma concentrations of procainamide usually accepted for treatment of arrhythmias is 4 to 10 $\mu$g/ml.[138] Some investigators advocate use of procainamide at dosages producing plasma concentrations of 10 to 20 $\mu$g/ml for malignant ventricular arrhythmias.[139-142] Such treatment frequently leads to side effects and must be carefully monitored to ensure that excessive negative chronotropic and dromotropic effects and QRS widening do not occur. Also, at these high concentrations of procainamide, the metabolite N-acetylprocainamide can reach toxic concentrations in rapid acetylators or patients with renal insufficiency.

Onset of antiarrhythmic effect can be hastened by intravenous or oral "loading" of procainamide. We use an infusion of 275 $\mu$g/kg/min for 25 to 40 minutes as an intravenous load (not to exceed 1.5 g in the loading infusion). Other investigators have successfully used a similar regimen of 100-mg boluses, each given over 2 to 3 minutes at 5-minute intervals, to a maximum dosage of 15 mg/kg.[38] The usual maintenance intravenous infusion rate is 20 to 80 $\mu$g/kg/min.[138]

When N-acetylprocainamide is administered to patients with ventricular arrhythmias, it is effective at concentrations of 5 to 19 $\mu$g/ml, and frequently causes side effects at concentrations greater than 15 $\mu$g/ml. Concentrations in this range can be encountered in rapid acetylators or patients with renal insufficiency who are taking procainamide, and can contribute to adverse effects.[35]

As mentioned previously, the electrophysiologic effects of procainamide and N-acetylprocainamide are quite dissimilar, and, in theory, alterations of their relative concentrations could lead to changes in therapeutic and toxic effects. For this reason, monitoring of patients receiving procainamide should include measurement of plasma concentrations of both procainamide and N-acetylprocainamide.

### Adverse Effects

A frequent adverse effect encountered in patients receiving procainamide is the lupus syndrome. The development of positive antinuclear antibodies (ANA) and lupus syndrome appears to be related to cumulative dose of procainamide as well as duration of administration. Antinuclear antibodies can be found in more than 80 percent of patients taking procainamide for 1 year, and patients with positive ANA need not be withdrawn from therapy unless they become symptomatic.[143-146] ANA and the lupus syndrome appear more rapidly in slow acetylators than in rapid acetylators, with median times to positive ANA of 2.9 and 7.3 months, respectively.[146] Mean duration of treatment in slow and rapid acetylators developing the lupus syndrome is 12 and 48 months, respectively.[146] The mechanism by which the lupus syndrome and positive ANA develop is not fully understood, but enhanced helper T cell function,[147] impaired suppressor T cell function,[148] and hapten formation via covalent linkage of procainamide metabolites to nuclear macromolecules have all been postulated.[149] N-acetylprocainamide causes positive ANA very rarely and has not been found to cause lupus; in fact, patients with procainamide-induced lupus have noted symptomatic improvement after switching to N-acetylprocainamide treatment.[150] This fact and the prolonged time to ANA positivity in rapid acetylators suggests that acetylation may have a protective role against development of lupus. The lupus syndrome resolves with discontinuation of procainamide, but ANA positivity resolves only slowly.

Other reported side effects of procainamide include nausea, anorexia, rash, insomnia, and rarely agranulocytosis, fever, hallucinations, and psychosis. Like quinidine, procainamide can cause torsades de pointes (although apparently less frequently).[151] Heart block and sinus node dysfunction also can occur in patients with pre-existing conduction system abnormalities.[152] Reported side effects of N-acetylprocainamide include nausea, anorexia, marked Q–T prolongation, and torsades de pointes.[128,153–155] The possible contribution of N-acetylprocainamide to torsades de pointes during procainamide administration is fascinating, particularly in view of its APD-prolonging effect. However, torsades de pointes has also been reported following acute intravenous procainamide administration (when little of the metabolite would be present), implying a more complex mechanism.[151]

## Disopyramide

Disopyramide (Norpace, Rhythmodan) was first synthesized 20 years ago, and has been marketed in France since 1969 and in the United States since 1977. It is effective in treatment of a wide spectrum of arrhythmias. Disopyramide's structure is shown in Figure 3.

### Electrophysiologic Effects

Disopyramide produces changes in automaticity, conduction, and refractoriness of atrial and ventricular tissue similar to those of quinidine and procainamide.[61,156–158] Q–$T_c$ prolongation is less marked with clinically achieved concentrations of disopyramide than with quinidine, although cases of disopyramide-induced torsades de pointes have been reported.[159] The stereoisomers of disopyramide do not have identical pharmacologic activity. Anticholinergic effects are predominatly due to l-disopyramide and the metabolite l-nordisopyramide.[160–162] Q–$T_c$ prolongation is caused only by the d- isomer.[162] The lack of clinically apparent depression of AV nodal conduction by disopyramide in normal individuals may be due to its anticholinergic effects.[61,156]

### Hemodynamic Effects

Disopyramide has significant concentration-dependent negative inotropic effects in patients with and without pre-existing left ventricular dysfunction.[163,164] The high incidence of disopyramide-induced congestive heart failure relative to quinidine and procainamide may be due to disopyramide's vasoconstrictor effect, which causes increased afterload and left ventricular decompensation.[165,166]

### Indications

Disopyramide has been reported to be effective in a wide variety of supraventricular and ventricular arrhythmias, and is similar to quinidine in efficacy.[167–179] Disopyramide has been reported to slow conduction in atrioventricular bypass tracts, and has been successfully used in patients with pre-excitation syndrome to supress re-entrant tachycardia and to slow ventricular response to atrial fibrillation.[180,181]

### Disposition

Disopyramide is usually well absorbed after oral administration, but its absorption and elimination are decreased after an acute myocardial infarction.[173,182] It is excreted by the kidney unchanged (50 percent), as the cardioactive monodealkylated metabolite (20 percent), or as other metabolites.[183,185] There is variability in plasma protein binding within the therapeutic range, with a threefold increase in total disopyramide concentration leading to as much as a sixfold increase in the concentration of unbound disopyramide.[186-188] This effect is complicated still further by differences in protein-binding characteristics of the two steroisomers, and their binding interaction with each other.[189] Determinations of free or unbound disopyramide concentrations may improve patient management, but their application to clinical situations is still only theoretical.

## Dosage, Plasma Concentrations

Dosages and desired plasma concentrations[190] are listed in Table 5. Dosage must be decreased in the presence of renal or hepatic failure. A slow-release dosage form is now available for disopyramide phosphate (Norpace CR). Dosage recommendations for this preparation are preliminary, and patients should be monitored closely at the time of switching from one dosage form to another.

## Adverse Effects

The most frequent side effects of disopyramide are anticholinergic and include dry mouth, urinary retention, blurred vision, worsening of glaucoma, and constipation.[170,171,173,175,178] As already mentioned, disopyramide causes a decrease in ejection fraction in both normal and abnormal hearts leading to worsening of congestive heart failure. Because of these negative inotropic and anticholinergic effects, disopyramide should be avoided if possible in patients with congestive heart failure,[191,192] a history of prostatism, urinary hesitancy, or glaucoma. Disopyramide in usual doses rarely causes advanced heart block in patients with pre-existing conduction abnormalities.[193] Disopyramide has been reported to cause torsades de pointes.[194] Disopyramide can cause accelerated ventricular response in atrial flutter by decreasing flutter rate and increasing AV nodal conduction, allowing 1:1 conduction.[195]

## Drug Interactions

Clearance of disopyramide is markedly increased by concomitant administration of phenytoin or rifampin, leading to a fall in plasma concentration and reported loss of antiarrhythmic effect.[196,197] The combination of disopyramide with beta-adrenergic blockers or calcium-channel antagonists may cause marked depression of contractility, and should be avoided in patients with any impairment of ventricular function.[198] Disopyramide does not alter digoxin plasma concentrations.[199] Disopyramide may potentiate the effect of warfarin.[200]

## Lidocaine, Phenytoin, Mexiletine, Tocainide

Lidocaine was first introduced in 1946 for use as an anesthetic,[201] and was first used as an antiarrhythmic agent in the 1950s, initially for the treatment of arrhythmias arising during cardiac catheterization.[202] In the 1960s, it was increasingly used in a variety of settings, and became the most widely used intravenous antiarrhythmic drug. Extensive first-pass metabolism limited its oral use, leading to a search for congeners with antiarrhythmic potency. Tocainide (Tonocard) and mexiletine (Mexitil) were products of that search. Their structures are shown in Figure 6. Phenytoin (Dilantin) is an antiepileptic drug with structural similarities to the barbiturates. In 1950, it was reported to have antiarrhythmic properties in dogs,[203] and subsequently it was shown to be effective for arrhythmias in humans,[204-214] particularly those associated with digitalis intoxication.[207] The structure of phenytoin is shown in Figure 7, along with some other antiarrhythmic drugs with suspected neurologic contribution to their effectiveness.

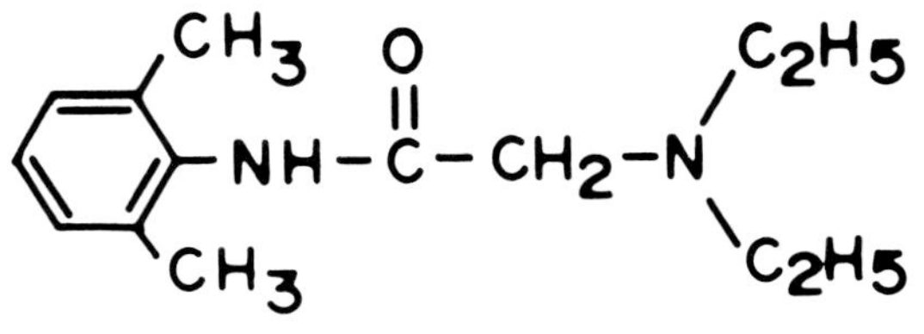

**Figure 6.** Structures of lidocaine and its congeners.

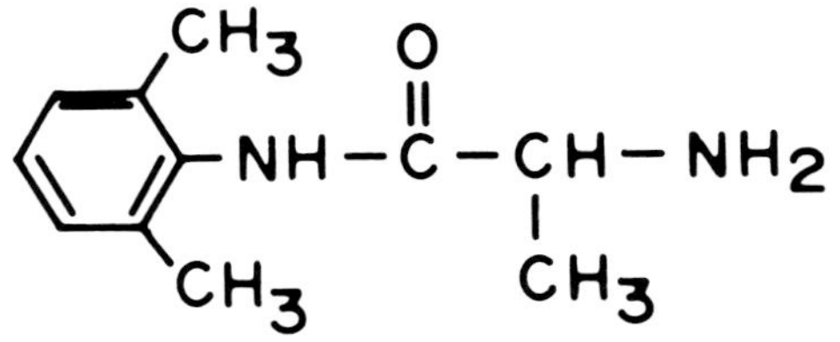

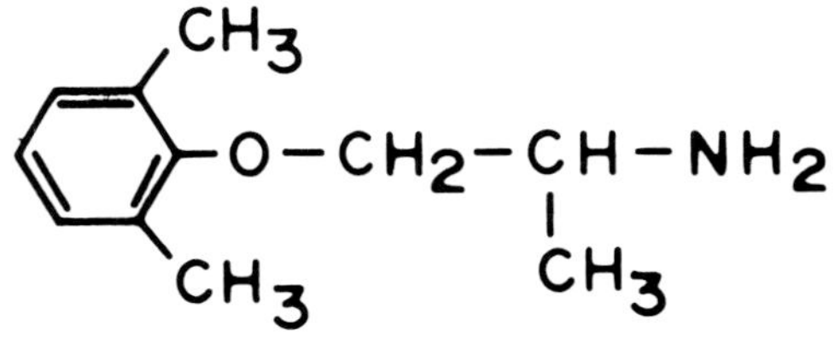

## Electrophysiologic Effects

Lidocaine depresses $\dot{V}$max and impulse conduction velocity in a rate- and voltage-dependent manner. Although clinically achieved concentrations of lidocaine produce no change in $\dot{V}$max and conduction in normal Purkinje fibers at normal cycle lengths,[215] they depress these parameters in partially depolarized or rapidly firing cells.[56,58,59,216–218,219] This effect may account for its effectiveness in arrhythmias associated with ischemia and for its greater effectiveness in rapid than in "slow" ventricular tachycardia. Lidocaine decreases automaticity of normal Purkinje fibers,[217,218] but has less effect on automaticity in ischemic tissue.[59,219] Lidocaine has little or no effect on atrial myocardium.[220] It does not alter sinus node function or His-Purkinje conduction in normal hearts,[220,221] but can markedly depress these parameters in patients with sick sinus syndrome or conduction abnormalities.[222–228] Unlike quinidine, lidocaine shortens action potential duration and, to a lesser degree, effective refractory period in Purkinje fibers and ventricular myocardium.[59,215,220]

Phenytoin's electrophysiologic effects are similar to those of lidocaine.[229,230] In addition, it appears to depress digitalis-induced sympathetic activity and may depress vagal stimulation as well.[229,231–235] These effects appear to be mediated by the central nervous system, and may

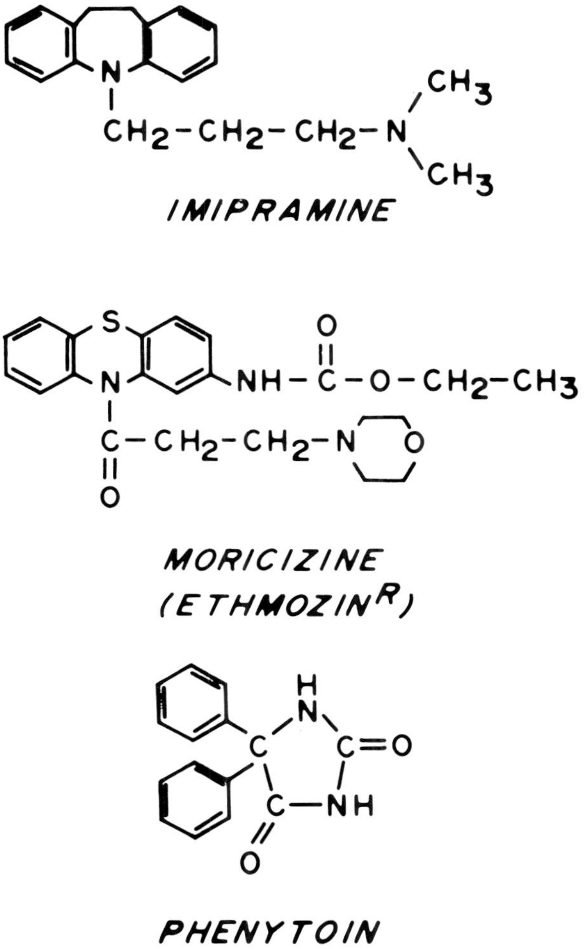

**Figure 7.** Structures of antiarrhythmic agents with possible CNS effects or structural similarities to CNS-active drugs: imipramine (a tricyclic antidepressant), moricizine (a phenothiazine), and phenytoin (an anticonvulsant).

be largely responsible for the effectiveness of phenytoin in arrhythmias caused by digitalis intoxication. This hypothesis is supported by experimental evidence in animals that phenytoin administered intrathecally prevents digoxin-induced arrhythmias without achieving detectable concentrations in plasma.[235]

Mexiletine and tocainide also share many electrophysiologic effects with lidocaine. $\dot{V}$max and the depolarization threshold of both atrial and ventricular myocardium are decreased by mexiletine in animal studies.[236,237] In man, AV nodal conduction time and refractoriness, and His-Purkinje conduction time (H–V interval) are either increased or unchanged.[238] Ventricular effective refractory period has been reported to be consistently increased by the drug.[238,239] The rate-dependence of mexiletine's effects is different from that of lidocaine in that mexiletine has more marked effects at slower pacing rates.[240]

Tocainide also shares many of its electrophysiologic properties with lidocaine.[241–243] Tocainide, in contrast to lidocaine, produces slight concentration-dependent slowing of AV nodal conduction.[241] Effects on sinus node function or His-Purkinje conduction in patients with conduction system disease have not been studied.

**Hemodynamic Effects**

These drugs cause little hemodynamic change in normal subjects, although a slight negative inotropic effect may be encountered in patients with left ventricular dysfunction.[46,244-254] Phenytoin can cause hypotension when given intravenously at rates exceeding 25 mg/min.[253]

**Indications**

This group of drugs has been used primarily for ventricular arrhythmias.[46,203-214,250,251,254-264] However, phenytoin, mexiletine, and tocainide have been reported to be effective in some cases of supraventricular tachycardia.[268] Lidocaine is ineffective for most supraventricular arrhythmias, and is contraindicated in patients with atrial fibrillation or flutter and an uncontrolled ventricular response because of the risk of increasing AV nodal conduction and thereby increasing ventricular response.[93,269] The use of lidocaine in pre-excitation-related tachycardias is not recommended because of reports of increased tachycardia rate following lidocaine.[270] Phenytoin is considered by many to be the drug of choice for arrhythmias associated with digitalis intoxication or long Q–T syndromes,[271,272] and in vitro data suggest that several drugs in this group may be effective in these situations. Although phenytoin, mexiletine, and tocainide can control ventricular arrhythmias as single-drug regimens, they appear less potent in this regard than the other drugs mentioned here. Mexiletine's efficacy has been reported to be much greater when used in combination therapy with quinidine,[76] propranolol,[273] disopyramide,[274] or procainamide.[275]

**Disposition**

Lidocaine undergoes extensive first-pass metabolism after oral administration, producing metabolites with CNS toxicity additive to that of the parent drug.[276,277] Hence, lidocaine is unsatisfactory for oral use because of unacceptable CNS side effects at antiarrhythmic lidocaine concentrations. After intravenous injection, lidocaine is cleared at a rate dependent on liver blood flow.[278-281] Factors decreasing liver blood flow (e.g., low cardiac output, cimetidine, beta-adrenergic blockers) or impairing hepatic metabolism (e.g., liver disease, cimetidine) can lead to decreased clearance.[20-22,282-285] In acute myocardial infarction or congestive heart failure, lidocaine clearance may be decreased by reduction in free lidocaine concentration owing to increased lidocaine binding by the acute phase reactant alpha-1-acid glycoprotein.[50] This binding change also alters the relationship between total lidocaine concentration and antiarrhythmic effect. Lidocaine clearance is increased by enzyme induction with agents such as phenobarbital, phenytoin, and rifampin.[287,288] It decreases during prolonged intravenous infusions,[289,290] necessitating careful monitoring for side effects and measurement of plasma levels and, if necessary, decrease in infusion rate. As mentioned previously, decreases in central volume of distribution and hepatic blood flow in patients with congestive heart failure necessitate reduction of bolus dosage in those patients.

Tocainide is rapidly and completely absorbed, with oral bioavailability approaching 100 percent.[251,252,264,291,292] Approximately 30 percent is excreted unchanged in the urine, with most of the remainder being metabolized in the liver to form glucuronides and other conjugates.[293,294] Renal clearance is decreased by as much as 75 percent if urine is alkalinized.[291] No active metabolites of tocainide have been identified.[295]

Mexiletine is well absorbed, with bioavailability of nearly 90 percent.[296] Less than 10 percent is excreted unchanged in the urine, with the rest undergoing hepatic metabolism.[297,298] Kinetics are not modified by renal failure.[299] Clearance is reduced in congestive heart failure.[300] Increased mexiletine clearance has been reported following hepatic enzyme induction.[301]

Phenytoin is slowly and unpredictably absorbed.[302-304] It is extensively metabolized in the liver, with less than 10 percent excreted unchanged in the urine.[305] The enzyme systems metabolizing phenytoin are saturable, leading to a disproportionate increase in plasma concentration with high dosages.[305] Protein binding is decreased in uremia,[36,306] hyperbilirubinemia, and late pregnancy, leading to potentially toxic concentrations of unbound phenytoin despite "therapeutic" total phenytoin concentrations.[307,308] These binding changes do not consistently alter dosage requirements.

## Dosage, Plasma Concentrations

In order to achieve rapid antiarrhythmic effectiveness, lidocaine must be given with a loading dose. Several loading regimens have been used successfully. All represent a trade-off between complexity and reliability of the regimen. Some of these are illustrated in Figure 2. Two recently proposed innovative means of simplifying loading are use of a microprocessor-controlled pump and use of a 2-bottle dilution-infusion apparatus.[48] These two techniques deliver lidocaine at an exponentially decreasing rate designed to rapidly achieve and maintain a given plasma concentration.

Mexiletine and tocainide should be started at low dosage and increased at 2- to 3-day intervals until efficacy or intolerable side-effects (usually tremor or other CNS symptoms) are encountered. The "therapeutic" dosage of each is broad, and side effects occur frequently at higher dosages.[252,254,309] Because peak plasma concentration of tocainide is decreased but total bioavailability is unchanged when the drug is taken with meals, a postprandial dosage regimen may reduce side effects.

The usual therapeutic range of unbound phenytoin is 1 to 2 $\mu$g/ml,[309] corresponding to 10 to 20 $\mu$g/ml total phenytoin in nonuremic patients. In patients with renal failure, monitoring of total drug concentration can be misleading, and therefore unbound concentrations should be measured and dosage adjustments made accordingly. The dosage change in patients with renal or hepatic failure is variable. If arrhythmias are not controlled at total concentrations of phenytoin greater than 20 $\mu$g/ml, further increase in dosage is unlikely to produce a response and frequently will cause side effects.

## Adverse Effects

This group of drugs has a high frequency of dose-related side effects. Most of these untoward effects are neurologic, including tremor, visual blurring, dizziness, dysphoria, depersonalization, and nausea. At extremely high concentrations, lidocaine can cause seizures and respiratory depression.[310] As mentioned previously, pre-existing His-Purkinje conduction abnormalities can be worsened by lidocaine, as can ventricular response to atrial fibrillation and flutter. At high concentrations, mexiletine can cause worsening of heart block.[254]

Phenytoin, in addition to the potential adverse effects listed above, has a long list of well-recognized side effects[311] including nystagmus, psychosis, peripheral neuropathy, and gingival hyperplasia. Idiopathic reactions include rash, lupus syndrome, Stevens-Johnson syndrome, cytopenias (any or all blood cell lines), and lymphadenopathy. Two potentially fatal adverse effects of phenytoin are hypotension and high-grade heart block.[271,311] The latter effects most frequently occur during rapid intravenous administration, and for this reason phenytoin should be given at infusion rates no greater than 25 to 50 mg/min and only with careful hemodynamic and electrocardiographic monitoring.

## Drug Interactions

Phenytoin has been reported to have many drug interactions. It increases clearance of theophylline, prednisolone, thyroxine, lidocaine, quinidine, mexiletine, disopyramide, and other drugs, primarily resulting from hepatic enzyme induction.[15–33,287,301,307] The clearance of phenytoin is decreased by isoniazid, chloramphenicol, dicumarol, disulfiram, and some sulfonamides.[307] Absorption of phenytoin is impaired by antacids. Clearance of lidocaine, phenytoin, and mexiletine can be decreased by cimetidine and increased by hepatic enzyme induction. As mentioned previously, clearance of lidocaine and probably mexiletine is reduced by propranolol and other beta blockers via reduction in liver blood flow.

## Imipramine

Imipramine is a tricyclic antidepressant introduced for the treatment of depressive illness in the late 1950s. Its structure is shown in Figure 7. In the first few years after its introduction, several fatalities and near-fatalities were reported. Although most of these complications were due to overt drug overdose, some occurred in patients taking only small excesses of the drug.[312-314] These patients had prominent electrocardiographic abnormalities, including tachycardia, QRS and Q-T widening, second-degree AV block, ventricular tachycardia, and sudden death. Because of this, some physicians have considered imipramine potentially unsafe for patients with cardiovascular disease. In 1977, imipramine was reported to decrease arrhythmias in depressed patients.[315]

### Electrophysiology

Imipramine decreases action potential duration, effective refractory period, $\dot{V}$max, conduction velocity, and membrane responsiveness in canine Purkinje fibers, while it prolongs APD in ventricular muscles.[316-318] The effect of $\dot{V}$max and conduction velocity is more marked in partially depolarized or ischemic tissues than in normal tissues.[319] In man, imipramine causes increases in heart rate and P-R, QRS, and Q-$T_c$ interval durations.[319-321] Imipramine's antiarrhythmic effects are believed to be due to its effect on impulse conduction, although CNS-mediated mechanisms have not been excluded.

### Hemodynamic Effects

Imipramine has been reported to cause no change in ejection fraction in patients with normal or abnormal baseline ejection fraction.[319-323] Although recent studies do not report congestive heart failure in patients taking imipramine, there are sketchy reports from the early 1960s.[315] Imipramine is known to cause orthostatic hypotension in some patients, and commonly causes a slight increase in heart rate.[319-324]

### Indications

Imipramine has been shown to effectively suppress ventricular ectopic depolarizations and ventricular tachycardia.[319-323] Experience with supraventricular arrhythmias is limited.

### Disposition

Imipramine is well absorbed after oral administration.[325] It undergoes variable, extensive first-pass metabolism, leaving a mean oral bioavailability of 47 to 21 percent (but with a wide range of the degree of first-pass clearance).[325] The primary metabolite of imipramine is desmethylimipramine (desipramine), which appears to have cardiovascular effects similar to those of imipramine.[326,327] Other metabolism is via hydroxylation of either imipramine or desmethylimipramine.[327] This oxidation appears to be genetically determined and to follow the debrisoquin pathway.[327] There is some evidence that hydroxylated metabolites of imipramine have CNS activity.[327] The cardiovascular effect of these metabolites is not known.

### Administration, Plasma Concentrations

Imipramine is usually antiarrhythmic at doses of 75 mg t.i.d. or higher.[319] We have found fewer side effects if the initial dosage is somewhat lower and titrated upward over several days. The therapeutic range is reported to be similar to that for the antidepressant effect; that is, total imipramine plus desmethylimipramine concentration greater than 225 $\mu$g/ml.

### Adverse Effects

Adverse effects reported include fatigue, dry mouth, tremor, orthostatic dizziness, hallucinations, sedation, restlessness, dysphoria, nightmares, insomnia, heart block, and hypotension.[319–324]

## Moricizine

Moricizine (Ethmozin) is a phenothiazine derivative synthesized in the Soviet Union and found to be effective for treatment of a variety of arrhythmias. Its structure is shown in Figure 7.

### Electrophysiologic Effects

The electrophysiology of moricizine is similar to that of lidocaine.[328,329] In isolated Purkinje fibers, moricizine slows $\dot{V}$max and shortens action potential (ERP was not measured). Although it has no effect on phase 4 automaticity in normal Purkinje fibers, it markedly reduces phase 4 depolarization and automaticity in fibers injured by barium chloride and ischemia. In animal studies, moricizine does not acutely depress SA node automaticity or AV nodal conduction.[328] On the surface ECG, moricizine produces no change in P–R, Q–T, or R–R intervals and either no change or an increase in QRS duration.[330–334] In limited experience with patients having first- and second-degree heart block or bundle branch block, no increased block was noted. There are reports of a delay of at least 24 hours between initiation of treatment and onset of antiarrhythmic effect and of unexpected persistence of antiarrhythmic activity, suggesting either slow accumulation of drug or the presence of active metabolites.[331]

### Hemodynamic Effects

In limited studies, moricizine has had no effect on heart rate or blood pressure when given orally, although mild hypotension has been noted after intravenous administration. Further hemodynamic evaluation of moricizine is required.

### Disposition

Moricizine is well absorbed after oral administration. It is apparently extensively metabolized, with only 1 percent of a dose found unchanged in urine or feces.[331] The identity and pharmacologic activity of its metabolites are not known. Elimination half-life is 2 to 5 hours in normal subjects, 6 to 13 hours in cardiac patients, and 47.5 hours in one reported patient with renal insufficiency.[330,331]

### Indications

Moricizine has been shown to effectively suppress atrial and ventricular ectopic depolarizations (VEDs) and ventricular tachycardia, with greater than 60 percent mean suppression of VEDs in patients taking 750 mg/day.[330,331,335] Moricizine was as effective as disopyramide, and better tolerated, in one study.[335]

### Dosage, Plasma Concentrations

Moricizine appears to be effective in the majority of patients taking 200 to 250 mg every 8 hours. Correlation between plasma concentration and effect has not been well elucidated. Most responders have had plasma concentrations greater than 0.3 $\mu$g/ml.

### Adverse Effects

Adverse effects have been reported in approximately 15 percent of patients during short-term studies and have included pruritus, headache, nausea, disorientation, and seizures.[330,331]

### Drug Interactions

No data are available on drug interactions of moricizine.

## Flecainide, Encainide, Lorcainide

These three drugs are currently undergoing clinical trial in the United States. They are grouped because of some similarities in electrophysiologic effects, indications, and toxicity. Their structures are illustrated in Figure 5.

### Electrophysiologic Effects

Flecainide reduces V̇max and decreases action potential duration of isolated canine Purkinje fibers.[336−338] In intact hearts, it slows conduction in atrium, AV node, and His-Purkinje system, and increases refractory period of atrium and AV node in dogs.[339] In patients with normal conduction systems, flecainide prolongs ventricular ERP relative to monophasic action potential duration, and to a lesser extent prolongs refractoriness of the atrium and AV node.[340] Flecainide slows conduction throughout the heart, with resultant increases in P–A, A–H, and H–V intervals on electrophysiologic studies and marked increase in P–R and QRS intervals on surface ECGs.[340−347] QRS increases of 25 percent are common and in stable patients do not appear to carry a bad prognosis, although the significance in other patients is not yet clear. Q–T$_c$ is slightly increased in some patients, primarily due to the increase in QRS duration. There is little change in the J–T interval. Flecainide prolongs ERP relative to APD in atrium and ventricle, with a smaller increase in ERP of the AV node. Flecainide prolongs refractoriness in accessory pathways.[340] Flecainide raises pacing threshold in the ventricle, which may be of concern in patients requiring pacemakers.[348] It markedly increases sinus node recovery time in patients with symptomatic sinus node dysfunction without altering sino-atrial conduction time.[342]

Electrophysiologic effects of encainide and lorcainide are somewhat complicated because of a prominent effect of active metabolites with properties different from those of the parent drug.[349−351] The active metabolites of encainide (O-desmethylencainide [ODE] and 3-methoxy-O-demethylencainide [MODE]) and lorcainide (norlorcainide) appear to have electrophysiologic properties similiar to those of flecainide, whereas parent encainide and lorcainide appear to have little effect on AV nodal conduction or atrial and ventricular refractoriness.[351−353] In a study of the electrophysiologic effects of intravenous and chronic oral administration of lorcainide, it was shown that decreases in AV nodal conduction and prolongation of atrial and ventricular ERP were present only after chronic oral treatment, suggesting that metabolies were responsible for these effects.[351] These metabolites would be present, if at

**Table 6.** Change in electrophysiologic parameters during acute and chronic administration of encainide and lorcainide

| | Encainide | | Lorcainide | |
|------|------------------------|---------------------------|------------------------|---------------------------|
| | Acute IV[388] | Chronic oral[386] | Acute IV[388] | Chronic oral[388] |
| A–H | +8% | +41.6% | 0 | +22.6% |
| H–V | +7% | +41.3% | +25.1% | +21.2% |
| AERP | +6% | +21% | +1.6% | +13.2% |
| VERP | −1% | +13.3% | +2.9% | +17.3% |

all, only in very small concentrations immediately after an intravenous dose. The electrophysiologic effects of these drugs in acute and chronic treatment (sugggesting parent drug alone and parent plus metabolites) are listed in Table 6.

## Hemodynamic Effects

Flecainide has a mild negative inotropic effect, which becomes clinically apparent only in patients with poor ventricular function or following rapid intravenous administration of the drug.[354] Negative inotropic effects of encainide and lorcainide appear to be minimal, although use of these drugs in patients with congestive heart failure is limited.[355,356]

## Indications

These drugs are primarily used for ventricular arrhythmias, but have been successfully used for treatment of supraventricular tachycardia, atrial fibrillation and flutter, and arrhythmias associated with pre-excitation syndromes.[39,343–346,349,351,357–363] Flecainide and encainide have been reported to cause worsened arrhythmias in some patients, both in terms of increased complexity of arrhythmia and increased difficulty in resuscitation, and some deaths have been reported.[364,364] Lorcainide, which has had less extensive clinical use, has not been reported to be proarrhythmic in man, but in vitro experiments indicating proarrhythmic potential have been described.[366] Patients at particularly high risk for proarrhythmic effects appear to be those with poor left ventricular function and a history of sustained ventricular tachycardia. The mechanism of worsened arrhythmias in these patients may be marked slowing of conduction in abnormal tissues, allowing development of a re-entrant circuit. This characterization is preliminary and remains to be validated in a larger population. Because of their profound depressant effects on cardiac conduction, flecainide, encainide, and lorcainide should be used with caution in patients with bundle branch block or AV block.

## Disposition

Flecainide is well absorbed orally and undergoes minimal first-pass metabolism.[367] It is eliminated in the urine unchanged (25 percent) or as apparently inactive metabolites.

Encainide is well absorbed and extensively metabolized after oral administration.[39] Bioavailability is highly variable, perhaps related to genetic differences in hepatic oxidation of the drug. O-demethylation of encainide appears to parallel the hydroxylation of debrisoquin.[13] After an oral dose, in poor metabolizers, encainide reaches high concentrations and is slowly metabolized by N-demethylation. In extensive metabolizers, the maximum concentration of encainide is lower, and large quantities of the cardioactive metabolites ODE and MODE are found. Despite these differences in metabolism, the range of dosages of encainide is usually the same for both groups.[39]

Like encainide, lorcainide is well absorbed, and undergoes extensive first-pass metabolism.[368–371] Only a small amount of drug enters the systemic circulation unchanged, while most of the remainder is present as the cardioactive metabolite norlorcainide. There is evidence of saturable first-pass metabolism.[371] Lorcainide is extensively metabolized, and has an elimination half-life of approximately 10 hours. Norlorcainide achieves plasma concentrations more than twice as high as those of lorcainide at steady state, and has an elimination half-life of approximately 27 hours. Possibly because of the long half-life of the active metabolite, once- or twice-daily dosing can be used.

### Dosage, Plasma Concentrations

Usual dosages for these three drugs are listed in Table 5. As with any Class I drug, treatment should be initiated at a low dosage, with careful upward titration if an adequate antiarrhythmic effect does not occur within 3 or 4 days of a change in dosage.

### Adverse Effects

These three drugs are generally well tolerated. Minor side effects are primarily neurologic, and include transient blurred vision, dizziness, and paresthesias. Lorcainide causes insomnia in many patients.[360] All these drugs can potentially precipitate bundle branch block or complete heart block in patients with pre-existing conduction system disease. Flecainide, and perhaps encainide and lorcainide, can cause worsened congestive heart failure in susceptible patients.

## Propafenone

Propafenone was first synthesized in 1971 and has been marketed in West Germany since 1977. It has reportedly been relatively free of serious side effects and has been used for a wide variety of arrhythmias. It has some structural similarity to propranolol (Fig. 8).

### Electrophysiologic Effects

Propafenone slows conduction in the atrium, AV node, and ventricle, and prolongs effective refractory periods in those tissues.[372,373] It produces no consistent change in action potential duration. On the surface ECG, propafenone causes prolongation of the P–R interval proportional to the plasma concentration in a given individual and increases the QRS interval with little or no prolongation of the $Q-T_c$ interval. In microelectrode studies, propafenone decreases $\dot{V}$max and reduces automaticity of Purkinje fibers by decrease in the slope of phase 4 depolarization.[374, 375]

Propafenone has been shown both in vitro and in human studies to possess beta-adrenergic blocking activity with approximately one fortieth the potency of propranolol.[375–378] When the difference in clinically achieved concentrations of these drugs is taken into account, this beta-blocking action could theoretically become significant, particularly at high propafenone concentrations, although clinically significant beta blockade has not been reported. Propafenone also appears to possess mild calcium-channel antagonist properties, with a potency approximately one one-hundredth that of verapamil.[375,379,380] This property also has not been shown to be clinically important.

### Indications

Propafenone has been reported to be effective in the treatment of atrial fibrillation and flutter with a reported 45 percent success rate in conversion to sinus rhythm.[381] It has also

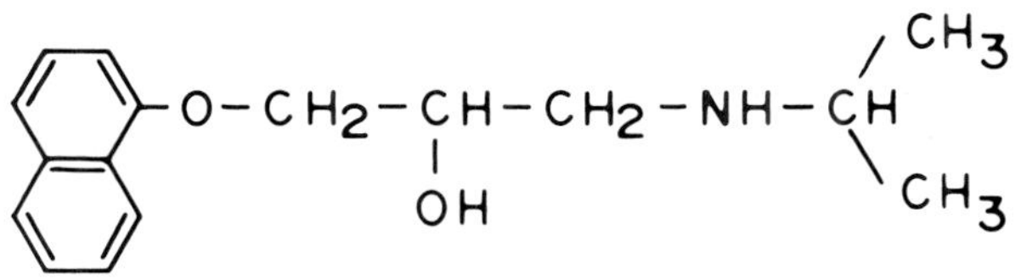

**PROPRANOLOL**

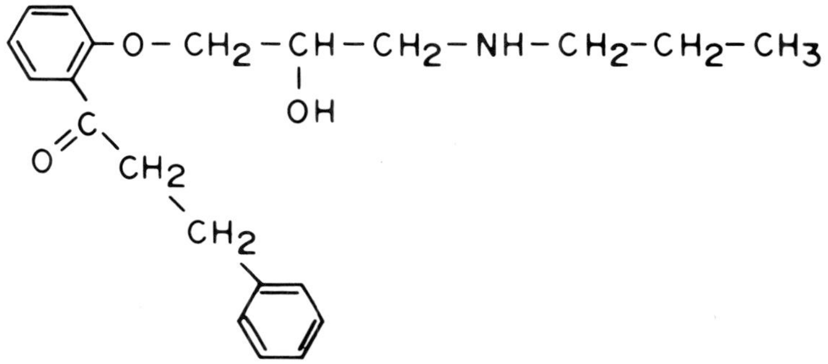

**PROPAFENONE**

**Figure 8.** Structures of propranolol and propafenone. Note marked similarities of the alkylamine side chains of the two drugs.

been used in treatment and prophylaxis of supraventricular tachycardias, for treatment of WPW-related arrhythmias, and for suppression of ventricular arrhythmias.[255,373,382–390] Electrophysiologic testing is predictive of long-term arrhythmia control.[388]

### Disposition

Propafenone is slowly absorbed, with maximum plasma concentrations reached 3 or 4 hours after a dose.[11,372] It undergoes extensive dose-related first-pass metabolism, with the oral bioavailability ranging from 10 to 50 percent,[11] and less than 1 percent is excreted unchanged. The primary metabolite, 5-hydroxypropafenone, appears to have antiarrhythmic and beta-blocking activity in animal models.[389] There is some evidence that the metabolism of propafenone is polymorphic, with a fraction of patients excreting propafenone at a much slower rate than others.[28] This metabolic trait appears to coinherit with that for the oxidation of debrisoquin. Patients who metabolize propafenone slowly develop high plasma concentrations and could theoretically reach high enough plasma concentrations for clinically significant beta blockade to become apparent.

### Dosage, Plasma Concentrations

The usual dosages of propafenone are 450 to 900 mg/day divided into fractions of 150 or 300 mg. The dosage requirement does not appear to be altered by genetic differences in drug metabolism.[28] The therapeutic range is poorly defined, with a poor correlation between concentrations and effect in a population, although a good correlation can be shown for a given individual. Most patients require plasma concentrations greater than 400 ng/ml for therapeutic effect.[373]

## Adverse Effects

The most common adverse effects related to propafenone treatment are a metallic taste in the mouth (owing to the bitter taste of the drug itself) and constipation.[373,390] Other reported problems are dose-related and include visual blurring, dizziness, paresthesias, nausea, and anorexia. The drug has been reported to cause worsening of arrhythmia in approximately 3 percent of patients.[373,390] An infrequent side effect is psychosis. Because of its marked effects on conduction, propafenone can increase the degree of atrioventricular block.

## Beta-adrenergic Blockers

Beta-adrenergic blockers have been used clinically for a variety of arrhythmias for more than a decade. The discovery of a reduction in sudden cardiac death following myocardial infarction in patients receiving practolol, metoprolol, timolol, propranolol, or sotalol has further increased interest in these drugs. The mechanism of reduction of sudden cardiac death by beta blockers is not known. Possible mechanisms include (1) anti-ischemic effects due to beta-adrenergic blockade itself, (2) direct antiarrhythmic effects, or (3) indirect effects on the central nervous system, platelet aggregation, or metabolism.

### Electrophysiologic Effects

Electrophysiologic properties of these drugs can be divided into beta-adrenergic blockade, intrinsic sympathomimetic activity (weak beta stimulation), cardioselectivity, and other effects (e.g., Class I and Class III effects). Table 7 describes these properties of several drugs marketed in the United States or Europe. Beta blockade causes decrease in sinus rate, decreased conduction and prolonged refractoriness in the AV node, and increased fibrillation threshold (this response appears to be less with drugs possessing intrinsic sympathomimetic activity). All beta blockers appear to effectively control stable ventricular arrhythmias in approximately 40 percent of patients.[391] However, response rates of 50 to 75 percent can be achieved with some drugs, including propranolol, acebutolol, and sotalol.[392-395]

Antiarrhythmic efficacy of propranolol can be demonstrated to improve at levels above those associated with physiologic beta-adrenergic blockade.[395] This may be due to previously described "Class I" effects of the drug. In cellular electrophysiologic studies, propranolol decreases action potential duration in canine Purkinje fibers.[396] In man, clinical plasma con-

**Table 7.** Electrophysiologic properties of beta-adrenergic blockers

| Drug | Cardioselective | ISA | Other effects |
|------|-----------------|-----|---------------|
| Propranolol | No | No | "Class I" (see text) |
| Metoprolol | Yes | No | Weak "Class I" |
| Nadolol | No | No | No |
| Atenolol | Yes | No | No |
| Timolol | No | No | No |
| Pindolol | No | Yes | Weak "Class I" |
| Sotalol | No | No | "Class III" (see text) |
| Alprenolol | No | Yes | Weak "Class I" |
| Oxprenolol | No | Yes | Weak "Class I" |
| Acebutolol | Yes | Yes | Weak "Class I" |

centrations of 40 to 120 ng/ml produce slowing of sinus rate and prolongation of A–H interval, which is not augmented by further increase in concentration.[397] These effects are expected with beta blockade. However, action potential duration decreased slightly at low concentrations and still further at high plasma concentrations (400 to 600 ng/ml), suggesting this effect was not mediated by beta blockade. Other evidence indicating the antiarrhythmic importance of propranolol's non-beta-mediated effect comes from studies of d-propranolol. Propranolol is marketed as a racemic mixture of equal amounts of d- and l-propranolol. Both isomers appear equipotent in terms of the effects on the Purkinje action potential, but the d- isomer has only very weak beta-blocking properties.[397] In animal models, the d- isomer has antiarrhythmic and antifibrillatory properties.[398] In man, high concentrations of d-propranolol significantly prolong the H–V interval and decrease action potential duration.[399] These effects are not encountered with concentrations of racemic propranolol producing equivalent degrees of beta blockade, suggesting it is not beta mediated. Thus, antiarrhythmic effects of propranolol observed only at high concentrations may be due to propranolol's direct membrane effect, whereas antiarrhythmic activity at low concentrations may be due to beta blockade, direct membrane effect, or both.

Sotalol is another beta blocker with prominent "other" properties. It produces concentration-related increases in action potential duration and $Q–T_c$ similar to that found with amiodarone.[395,400] As with propranolol, antiarrhythmic effectiveness is further enhanced by dosage increase beyond those required for beta blockade.[395]

## Hemodynamic Effects

Beta blockers reduce heart rate and blood pressure. The mechanism of antihypertensive effect is not well understood. Beta blockers can produce marked negative inotropic effects in patients with pre-existing left ventricular dysfuntion and reduce the force of concentration (dp/dt) in all patients. Beta blockers can cause vasoconstriction via unopposed alpha-adrenergic effects, with resultant worsening of claudication or vasospastic angina.

## Indications

Beta blockers have been reported to be effective in treatment of a wide array of arrhythmias.[401] For many of these arrhythmias, the mode of action appears to be beta blockade, and might be expected with any beta blocker. Examples are paroxysmal supraventricular tachycardia (via AV nodal conduction slowing); reduction of ventricular rate in atrial fibrillation/flutter; symptomatic sinus tachycardia; catecholamine-related ventricular arrhythmias (such as those induced by halothane); and ischemia-related arrhythmias. Beta blockers also reduce arrhythmias in patients with long Q–T syndromes (sotalol should be avoided in this disorder). As previously mentioned, a minority of patients with chronic stable ventricular arrhythmias will respond to beta blockers, with an improved response rate to drugs with additional non-beta-mediated activity. Propranolol in combination with quinidine has been reported to control re-entrant supraventricular tachycardia associated with Wolff-Parkinson-White syndrome (although either drug can worsen WPW arrhythmias when given alone).[402–404]

## Disposition

Disposition of these drugs is well reviewed in a recent paper, and will not be further discussed here.[405]

## Administration, Plasma Concentrations

Usual dosage regimens are outlined in Table 5. Plasma concentration monitoring has limited value in beta-blocker therapy.

## Adverse Effects

Many of the reported adverse effects appear to be due to beta blockade: fatigue, malaise, congestive heart failure, bronchospasm, claudication, cold extremities, and heart block. Worsening of congestive heart failure appears to be mediated by increased peripheral vascular resistance and reduction of sympathetic tone. The beta blockers have negligible direct negative inotropic effects. CNS side effects (nightmares, dysphoria, poor concentration) appear to be more marked with drugs achieving high CNS concentrations, such as propranolol.[405]

## Drug Interactions

Negative dromotropic effects are accentuated by coadministration of digitalis or Class I drugs, and can lead to complete heart block. Beta blockers reduce liver blood flow and can lead to increased concentrations of extensively metabolized drugs such as lidocaine.[19]

## Bretylium

Bretylium is a halogenated quaternary ammonium compound that was first introduced in the 1950s for the treatment of hypertension, an indication for which it was used only briefly because of adverse side effects and unreliable oral absorption.[406] In 1965, it was found to be protective against arrhythmias in a hypokalemic dog model.[407] It has been marketed in the United States in intravenous form and has been widely used for refractory ventricular arrhythmias and in the treatment of arrhythmias complicating myocardial infarction. Its structure is shown in Figure 9.

Other similar compounds with better oral bioavailability are undergoing clinical trials in the United States now. These drugs, which include bethanidine, meobentine, and clofilium, are electrophysiologically similar to bretylium and will not be further discussed here.

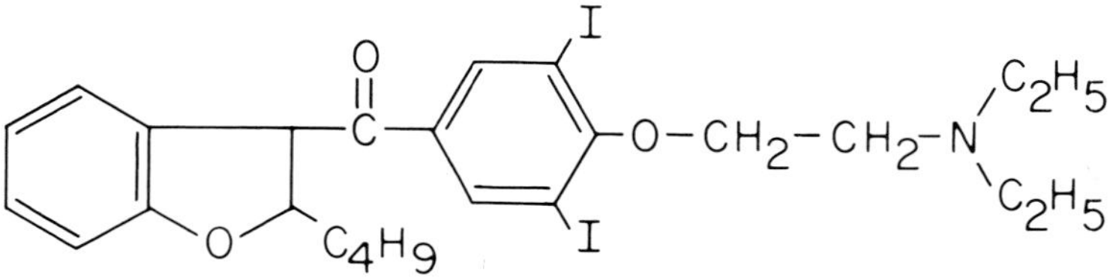

*AMIODARONE*

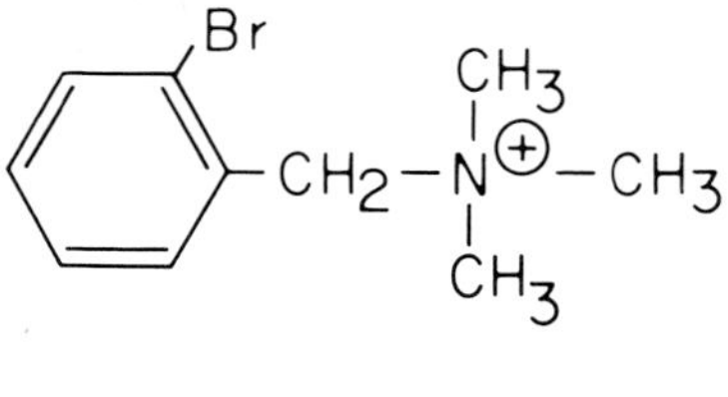

*BRETYLIUM*

**Figure 9.** Structures of the Class III antiarrhythmic agents, bretylium and amiodarone.

### Electrophysiologic and Hemodynamic Effects

Bretylium is taken up by the presynaptic nerve terminal, with initial transient catecholamine release followed by ganglionic blockade.[408] In addition to these adrenergic effects, it also has direct cardiac effects.[408] In mammalian cellular electrophysiologic studies, bretylium prolongs APD and ERP in ventricular muscle and Purkinje fibers with no change in the ratio of ERP/APD.[409] In normal tissue, maximum diastolic potential, $\dot{V}$max, and conduction velocity are either unchanged or decreased at very high concentrations.[409] There is a transient hyperpolarization and increase in $\dot{V}$max following bretylium administration, presumed to be related to catecholamine release. In animal models, bretylium increases ventricular fibrillation threshold.[410] In man,[411] bretylium initially causes a transient increase in sinus rate, automaticity, blood pressure, peripheral vascular resistence, contractility, and arrhythmias, presumably due to catecholamine release. This is followed shortly by blockade of peripheral norepinephrine release from presynaptic nerve endings. Concurrent with this, peripheral vascular resistance and blood pressure may decrease, with particularly notable orthostatic changes. This postural hypotension can be inhibited by concurrent treatment with the tricyclic antidepressant protryptyline.[412] The sinus rate then slows to below baseline (an adrenergic blockade effect), and the action potential duration and effective refractory period of atrial and ventricular muscle and Purkinje fibers increase (a direct effect). After the sympathomimetic phase, bretylium has little effect on myocardial contractility or conduction at clinically achieved concentrations.

### Indications

Bretylium has not been shown to be effective in supraventricular arrhythmias. Its primary efficacy is for treatment of ventricular tachycardia and ventricular fibrillation, and it is considered by some to be the drug of choice for treatment of ventricular fibrillation.[413-418] Bretylium has been reported to be particularly useful in treatment of arrhythmias complicating acute myocardial infarction.

### Disposition

Bretylium is poorly and variably absorbed after oral administration, with bioavailability of less than 25 percent.[419] More than 85 percent of intravenously administered bretylium is excreted unchanged in the urine, with a good correlation between creatinine clearance and bretylium elimination. Clearance is decreased in patients with renal insufficiency.

### Dosage, Therapeutic Concentrations

The usual dose of bretylium given intravenously is 5 mg/kg administered over 5 to 10 minutes. This dose may be repeated after 20 minutes if an adequate antiarrhythmic effect does not occur, and again, if necessary, in 1 to 2 hours. Doses of up to 9 g in 24 hours have been given without serious adverse effects,[413] although the risk of bradyarrhythmias is increased at high dosage, and loading doses beyond a total of 20 mg/kg should be given only with very careful monitoring of ECG and blood pressure. After the initial bolus doses are given, a maintenance infusion may be continued at a rate of 1 to 4 mg/minute. The dosage should be decreased in the presence of renal failure.

### Adverse Effects

The most common adverse effect of bretylium is postural hypotension, which can be quite severe in patients with impaired left ventricular function or volume depletion. It appears that this effect is primarily mediated via vasodilation, with no evidence of a direct negative inotropic effect.[420,421] As mentioned previously, the hypotensive effect of bretylium can be prevented by administration of a tricyclic antidepressant. Other reported side effects include nausea and vomiting, diarrhea, abdominal cramps, and bradyarrhythmias. Parotitis has been reported during chronic oral treatment. During the initial catecholamine-release phase, a proarrhythmic effect can occur in some patients

## Amiodarone

Amiodarone is an iodinated benzofuran with vasodilating properties, first introduced in Europe in the 1960s for treatment of angina pectoris.[422] It was subsequently found to have unusual electrophysiologic effects, and in 1974 was first reported to be effective for treatment of arrhythmias.[423] Amiodarone bears some structural resemblance to thyroxine. Its structure is shown in Figure 9.

### Electrophysiologic Effects

In cellular studies using tissues obtained from rabbits chronically administered amiodarone, there is prolongation of action potential duration and refractory period of atrial and ventricular myocardium, sinus and AV nodal tissues, and Purkinje fibers.[424] Amiodarone has no effect on resting membrane potential but decreases $\dot{V}$max. It slows phase 4 depolarization of sinus nodal tissue, and slows conduction through the AV node.[425] In man, chronic administration of amiodarone slows the heart rate, and prolongs sinoatrial conduction time without significantly changing sinus node recovery time.[426] It prolongs effective and functional refractory periods of atrium and AV node, and increases ventricular ERP. Amiodarone greatly prolongs ERP in bypass tracts in Wolff-Parkinson-White syndrome.[427] In chronic treatment amiodarone prolongs A–H and H–V intervals, and on surface ECG causes increase in P–R and Q–T$_c$ without significantly altering the QRS duration.[424, 426] These effects of amiodarone are encountered at intervals ranging from 2 to 30 days after initiation of treatment, depending partly on the dosage administered. Acute intravenous administration of amiodarone in man produces electrophysiologic findings discordant from those observed with chronic treatment.[428] Although prolongation of A–H interval and increase of AV nodal and bypass tract refractory periods occur, there is no acute effect on sinus rate or atrial or ventricular ERP. There are some data to suggest that some of the acute changes after intravenous amiodarone are due to the vehicle polysorbate 80 (Tween 80), a detergent that in animal studies causes decreased AV nodal conduction.[429]

The mechanism by which amiodarone produces its electrophysiologic effects is not well understood. It has been described as a noncompetitive blocker of both alpha- and beta-adrenergic stimuli.[430,431] The changes in cardiac action potentials are similar to those found in hypothyroid states,[432] and in one study administration of thyroxine was found to blunt the electrophysiologic changes induced by amiodarone.[424] However, in man, systemic hypothyroidism need not be present to produce amiodarone's characteristic effects. This does not preclude the possibility that amiodarone produces selective "cardiac hypothyroidism" as its mode of action.

### Hemodynamic Effects

Amiodarone reduces sinus rate and systemic blood pressure. Orally, it produces little change in myocardial contractility, but after intravenous bolus administration of dosages greater than 5 mg/kg it significantly decreases contractility and peripheral vascular resistance, resulting in severe hypotension in some patients.[433] Some of this effect may be due to the vehicle.

## Indications

Amiodarone has been shown to be effective in the treatment of a wide array of arrhythmias, including atrial fibrillation (both to slow ventricular response and to convert to sinus rhythm), pre-excitation-related tachycardias, paroxysmal supraventricular tachycardia, ventricular ectopic depolarization, and recurrent ventricular tachycardia and fibrillation.[434-438] A major disadvantage is a relatively high incidence of unusual adverse effects, some of which can be fatal. Another disadvantage is the delay between initiation of teatment and onset of antiarrhythmic effect. Because of these problems, amiodarone should be reserved only for life-threatening or severely disabling arrhythmias refractory to other available drugs.

## Disposition

Amiodarone is slowly absorbed and oral bioavailability varies from 20 to 80 percent, presumably due to variable absorption.[430] Amiodarone is extensively metabolized, with 1 percent excreted unchanged. A metabolite, desethylamiodarone, is found at concentrations similar to those of amiodarone during chronic treatment.[440] The elimination half-life of amiodarone is long, reportedly ranging from 3 to 15 weeks. The drug has a very large volume of distribution, reflecting concentration of large amounts of drug in fat and some other tissues. Loading doses of amiodarone are therefore required to achieve a therapeutic effect more rapidly.[441]

## Dosage, Plasma Concentrations

Optimum dosage regimens for amiodarone have not been thoroughly worked out. In order to decrease latency of antiarrhythmic effect, the drug must initially be given at high "loading" dosages. Such regimens have varied from 600 to 1400 mg daily for 2 to 21 days.[441] In order to preserve effect, dosage should be tapered slowly over a period of several weeks. Maintenance dosages have been less variable, with supraventricular arrhythmias usually well controlled by dosages of 200 to 400 mg daily.[434] Most ventricular arrhythmias are suppressed chronically with dosages of 400 to 600 mg/day, although some patients require higher dosages. Although the relationship between dosage and serious side effects is not proven, it would seem prudent to reduce dosage to the minimum effective level. Because of the slow offset of effects, patients should be supervised for as long as reasonably possible after a dosage reduction. In situations in which life-threatening arrhythmias are present, it may be necessary to add a second drug. Plasma concentrations of amiodarone have not yet proven to be helpful in general clinical monitoring, especially early in therapy.

## Adverse Effects

Amiodarone has been reported to produce several unusual adverse effects.[442-446] The most frequent is corneal microdeposits, which can occasionally interfere with vision. Both hypothyroidism and hyperthyroidism have been reported. Blue-gray skin discoloration sometimes occurs in patients taking large doses of the drug for long periods of time. The most serious adverse effect is pulmonary interstitial fibrosis, which has been reported to occur in up to 10 percent of patients and to lead to death in some instances. It is notable that pulmonary toxicity has been encountered with other benzofurans (e.g., nitrofurantoin), suggesting that this moiety in amiodarone may contribute to its lung toxicity. Pulmonary fibrosis has resolved in some cases with discontinuation of the drug. Amiodarone can cause torsades de pointes either alone or in combination with quinidine.[446]

## Drug Interactions

Amiodarone interferes with clearance of several drugs[447] including warfarin, digoxin, quinidine, procainamide, disopyramide, mexiletine, and propafenone. This results in accumulation

231

of these drugs and enhancement of their pharmacologic effects, which can lead to excessive bleeding, heart block, or torsades de pointes. This effect on clearance is not always predictable and may vary over time. For example, prothrombin time can vary greatly without a warfarin dosage change in patients taking amiodarone. It is likely that concentrations of other drugs can also be affected by amiodarone. Therefore, the clinician must be vigilant to the possibility of toxic accumulation of virtually any drug taken concomitantly with amiodarone. In addition to those interactions mediated by effects on clearance, the additive effects of amiodarone and other drugs can cause deleterious effects. For example, the combination of quinidine and amiodarone can cause torsades de pointes, and procainamide and amiodarone can cause heart block. Also, the combination of amiodarone with beta blockers or calcium antagonists can precipitate severe bradycardia or heart block, and anesthetic agents may cause excessive hypotension and bradycardia in the presence of amiodarone.

## SUMMARY

The number of antiarrhythmic drugs available in the United States is increasing, with the discovery of antiarrhythmic properties of drugs previously marketed for other indications (phenytoin, imipramine) and the development of several new drugs, many of which are likely to become commercially available in the next 5 years. The currently available drugs and several promising investigational drugs are reviewed in this report. Their optimal use is dependent on an understanding of their electropharmacologic effects, pharmacokinetics, drug interactions, and clinical pharmacology. Such use may allow better attempts to reduce arrhythmia-related death and morbidity.

## ACKNOWLEDGMENTS

The authors would like to express their deepest appreciation to Drs. Katherine A. Thompson, R. Kirby Primm, and Alastair J. J. Wood for review and commentary during the preparation of this manuscript; and to Shawn Henderson Underwood and Janice Thomas Neely for excellent clerical assistance.

## REFERENCES

1. LINDENBAUM, J, MELLOW, MH, BLACKSTONE, MO, ET AL: *Variability in biological availability of digoxin from four preparations.* N Engl J Med 285:1344, 1971.

2. HARTER, JG, SKELLY, JP, AND STEERS, AW: *Digoxin—the regulatory viewpoint.* Circulation 49:395, 1974.

3. FLANAGAN, AD: *Pharmacokinetics of a sustained release procainamide preparation.* Angiology 33:71, 1982.

4. DOLLERY, CT, EMSLIE-SMITH, D, AND MCMICHAEL, J: *Bretylium tosylate in the treatment of hypertension.* Lancet 1:296, 1960.

5. SPIRO, HM: *Regional enteritis.* In *Clinical Gastroenterology.* Macmillan, New York, 1977.

6. ROWLAND, M AND TOZER, TN: *Clinical Pharmacokinetics: Concepts and Applications.* Lea & Febiger, Philadelphia, 1980.

7. BAAR, WH, ADIR, J, AND GARNETSON, L: *Decrease of tetracycline absorption in man by sodium bicarbonate.* Clin Pharmacol Ther 12:779, 1971.

8. LINDENBAUM, J, RUND, DG, BUTLER, VP, ET AL: *Inactivation of digoxin by the gut flora: Reversal by antibiotic therapy.* N Engl J Med 305:789, 1981.

9. COMMITTEE ON NUTRITION, AMERICAN ACADEMY OF PEDIATRICS: *Vitamin K supplementation for infants receiving milk substitute infant formulas and for those with fat malabsorption.* Pediatrics 48:483, 1971.

10. OCHS, HR, GREENBLATT, DJ, WOO, E, ET AL: *Single and multiple dose pharmacokinetic of oral quinidine sulfate and gluconate.* Am J Cardiol 41:770, 1978.

11. HOLLMANN, M, BRODE, E, HOTZ, D, ET AL: *Investigations of the pharmacokinetics of propafenone in man.* Arzneim-Forsch/Drug Res 33:763, 1983.

12. TILSTONE, WJ, LAWSON, DH, CAMPBELL, W, ET AL: *The pharmacokinetics of slow-release procainamide.* Eur J Clin Pharmacol 14:261, 1978.

13. WOOSLEY, RL, RODEN, DM, DUFF, HJ, ET AL: *Co-inheritance of deficient oxidative metabolism of encainide and debrisoquine.* Clin Res 29:501A, 1981.

14. WANG, T, RODEN, DM, WOLFENDEN, HT, ET AL: *Pharmacokinetics of encainide and its metabolites in man.* Clin Pharmacol Ther 31:278, 1982.

15. DATA, JL, WILKINSON, GR, AND NIES, AS: *Interaction of quinidine with anticonvulsant drugs.* N Engl J Med 294:699, 1976.

16. TWUM-BARIMA, Y AND CARRUTHERS, SG: *Quinidine-rifampin interaction.* N Engl J Med 304:1466, 1981.

17. FORMAN, MB, SIDDOWAY, LA, CAIN, MA, ET AL: *Effects of enzyme induction on quinidine pharmacodynamics.* Clin Res 31:247A, 1983.

18. GIBSON, DG: *Pharmacodynamic properties of beta-adrenergic receptor blocking drugs in man.* Drugs 7:8, 1974.

19. OCHS, HR, CARSTENS, G, AND GREENBLATT, DJ: *Reduction in lidocaine clearance during continuous infusion and by coadministration of propranolol.* N Engl J Med 303:373, 1980.

20. FEELY, J, WILKINSON, GR, MCALLISTER, CB, ET AL: *Increased toxicity and decreased clearance of lidocaine by cimetidine.* Ann Intern Med 96:592, 1982.

21. FEELY, J, WILKINSON, GR, AND WOOD, AJJ: *Reduction of liver blood flow and propranolol metabolism by cimetidine.* N Engl J Med 304:692, 1981.

22. KNAPP, AB, MAGUIRE, W, KEREN, G, ET AL: *The cimetidine lidocaine interaction.* Ann Intern Med 98:174, 1983.

23. LEBREC, D, GOLDFARB, G, AND BENHAMOU, JP: *Reduction of liver blood flow by cimetidine.* N Engl J Med 305:100, 1981.

24. WEBER, WW: *Acetylating, deacetylating, and amino acid conjugating enzymes.* In BRODIE, BB AND GILLETTE, JR (EDS): *Handbook of Pharmacology.* Springer, Berlin, 1971.

25. SILAS, JH, LENNARD, MS, TUCKER, GT, ET AL: *Why hypertensive patients vary in their response to oral debrisoquine.* Br J Clin Pharmacol 5:27, 1977.

26. PRICE EVANS, DA, MAHGOUB, A, SLOAN, TP, ET AL: *A family and population study of the genetic polymorphism of debrisoquine oxidation in a white British population.* J Med Genetics 17:102, 1980.

27. DAYER, P, BALANT, L, COURVOISIER, F, ET AL: *The genetic control of bufuralol metabolism in man.* Eur J Drug Metab Pharmacokinet 7:73, 1982.

28. SIDDOWAY, LA, MCALLISTER, CB, WANG, T, ET AL: *Polymorphic oxidative metabolism of propafenone in man.* Circulation 68(Suppl III):III-64, 1983.

29. VASKO, MR, BELL, RD, DALY, DD, ET AL: *Inheritance of phenytoin hypometabolism: A kinetic study of one family.* Clin Pharmacol Ther 27:96, 1979.

30. BERTILSSON, L, EICHELBAUM, M, MELLSTROM, B, ET AL: *Nortriptyline and antipyrine clearance in relation to debrisoquine hydroxylation in man.* Life Sci 27:1673, 1980.

31. OATES, NS, SHAH, RR, IDLE, JR, ET AL: *Genetic polymorphism of phenformin 4-hydroxylation.* Clin Pharmacol Ther 32(1):81, 1982.

32. SLOAN, TP, IDLE, JR, AND SMITH, RL: *Influence of $D^H/D^L$ alleles regulating debrisoquine oxidation on phenytoin hydroxylation.* Clin Pharmacol Ther 29:493, 1981.

33. HANSTEN, PD: *Drug Interactions.* Lea & Febiger, Philadelphia, 1979.

34. KOUP, JR, JUSKO, WJ, ELWOOD, CM, ET AL: *Digoxin pharmacokinetics: Role of renal failure in dosage regimen design.* Clin Pharmacol Ther 18:9, 1975.

35. DRAYER, DE, LOWENTHAL, DT, WOOSLEY, RL, ET AL: *Cumulation of N-acetylprocainamide, an active metabolite of procainamide, in patients with impaired renal function.* Clin Pharmacol Ther 22:63, 1977.

36. HOOPER, WD, BOCHNER, F, EADIE, MJ, ET AL: *Plasma protein binding of diphenylhydantoin: Effects of sex hormones, renal and hepatic disease.* Clin Pharmacol Ther 15:276, 1974.

37. KALOW, W AND GUNN, DR: *Some statistical data on atypical cholinesterase of human serum.* Ann Human Genet 23:239, 1959.

38. ZAROSLINSKI, J, BORGMAN, RJ, O'DONNELL, JP, ET AL: *Ultra-short acting beta-blockers: A proposal for the treatment of the critically ill patient.* Life Sci 31:899, 1982.

39. RODEN, DM, REELE, SB, HIGGINS, SB, ET AL: *Total suppression of ventricular arrhythmias by encainide.* N Engl J Med 302:877, 1980.

40. FRISHMAN, W: *Clinical pharmacology of the new beta-adrenergic blocking drugs: Part I. Pharmacodynamic and pharmacokinetic properties.* Am Heart J 97:633, 1979.

41. CONWAY, FJ, FITZGERALD, JD, MCAINSH, J, ET AL: *Human pharmacokinetic and pharmacodynamic studies on atenolol (ICI 66082)—a new cardioselective beta-adrenoceptor blocking drug.* Br J Clin Pharmacol 3:267, 1976.

42. JOHNSSON, G, REGARDH, C-G, AND SOLVELL, L: *Combined pharmacokinetic and pharmacodynamic studies in man of the adrenergic beta₁ receptor antagonist metoprolol.* Acta Pharmacol Toxicol 36(Suppl V):31, 1975.

43. BUHLER, FR, LARAGH, JH, VAUGHAN, ED, ET AL: *Antihypertensive action of propranolol.* Am J Cardiol 32:511, 1973.

44. SHEINER, LB, STANSKI, DR, VOZEH, S, ET AL: *Simultaneous modeling of pharmacokinetics and pharmacodynamics: Application to d-tubocurarine.* Clin Pharmacol Ther 25:358, 1979.

45. MCMARTIN, C, RONDEL, RK, VINTER, J, ET AL: *The fate of guanethidine in two hypertensive patients.* Clin Pharmacol Ther 11:523, 1970.

46. COLLINSWORTH, KA: *The clinical pharmacology of lidocaine as an antiarrhythmic drug.* Circulation 50:1217, 1974.

47. STARGEL, WW, SHAND, DG, ROUTLEDGE, PA, ET AL: *Clinical comparison of rapid infusion and multiple injection method for lidocaine loading.* Am Heart J 102:872, 1981.

48. RIDDELL, JG, MCALLISTER, CB, WILKINSON, GR, ET AL: *Constant plasma drug concentrations—a new technique with application to lidocaine.* Ann Intern Med 100:25, 1984.

49. ODAR-CEDARLÖF, I AND BORGÅ, O: *Kinetics of diphenylhydantoin in uraemic patients: Consequences of decreased plasma protein binding.* Eur J Clin Pharmacol 7:31, 1974.

50. BARCHOWSY, A, SHAND, DG, STARGEL, WW, ET AL: *On the role of αl-acid glycoprotein in lignocaine accumulation following myocardial infarction.* Br J Clin Pharmacol 13:411, 1982.

51. VAUGHAN WILLIAMS, EM: *Electrophysiological basis for a rational approach to antidysrhythmic drug therapy.* In HARPER, NJ AND SIMMONDS, AB (EDS): *Advances in Drug Research.* Academic Press, London, 1974.

52. WILLIUS, FA AND KEYS, TE: *A remarkably early reference to the use of cinchona in cardiac arrhythmia.* Proc Staff Meet Mayo Clin 17:294, 1942.

53. WENCKEBACH, KF: *Die unregelmässige Herztätigkeit und ihre klinische Bedeutung.* W Engelmann, Leipzig, 1914.

54. FREY, W: *Weitere Erfährungen mit Chinidin bei absoluter Herzunregelmässigkeit.* Wien Klin Wochenschr 55:849, 1918.

55. HONDEGHEM, LM AND KATZUNG, BG: *Time- and voltage-dependent interactions of antiarrhythmic drugs with cardiac sodium channels.* Biochem Biophys Acta 474:373, 1977.

56. CHEN, CM, GETTES, LS, AND KATZUNG, BG: *Effects of lidocaine and quinidine on steady-state characteristics and recovery kinetics $(dV/dT)_{max}$ in guinea pig ventricular myocardium.* Circ Res 37:20, 1975.

57. JOHNSON, EA AND MCKINNON, MG: *The differential effect of quinidine and pyrilamine on the myocardial action potential at different rates of stimulation.* J Pharmacol Exp Ther 120:460, 1957.

58. NATTEL, S, ELHARRAR, V, ZIPES, D, ET AL: *pH-dependent electrophysiologic effects of quinidine and lidocaine on canine cardiac Purkinje fibers.* Circ Res 48:55, 1981.

59. CARMELIET, E AND SAIKAWA, T: *Shortening of the action potential and reduction of pacemaker activity by lidocaine, quinidine, and procainamide in sheep cardiac Purkinje fibers: An effect on Na or K currents?* Circ Res 50:257, 1982.

60. MASON, JW, WINKLE, RA, RIDER, AK, ET AL: *The electrophysiologic effects of quinidine in the transplanted human heart.* J Clin Invest 59:481, 1977.

61. MIRRO, MJ, MANALAN, AS, BAILEY, JC, ET AL: *Anticholinergic effects of disopyramide and quinidine on guinea pig myocardium: Mediation by direct muscarinic receptor blockade.* Circ Res 47:855, 1980.

62. ROBERTS, J, STADLER, RP, CAIROLI, V, ET AL: *Relationship between adrenergic activity and cardiac actions of quinidine.* Circ Res 11:758, 1962.

63. HOFFMAN, BF, ROSEN, MR, AND WIT, AL: *Electrophysiology and pharmacology of cardiac arrhythmias: VII. Cardiac effects of quinidine and procaine amide.* Am Heart J 89:804, 1975.

64. SCHMID, PG, NELSON, LD, MARK, AL, ET AL: *Inhibition of adrenergic vasoconstriction by quinidine.* J Pharmacol Exp Ther 188:124, 1974.

65. PARMLEY, WW AND BRAUNWALD, E: *Comparative myocardial depressant and antiarrhythmic properties of d-propranolol, dl-propranolol, and quinidine.* J Pharmacol Exp Ther 158:11, 1967.

66. SODERMARK, T, EDHAG, O, SJOGREN, A, ET AL: *Effect of quinidine on maintaining sinus rhythm after conversion of atrial fibrillation or flutter: A multicentre study from Stockholm.* Br Heart J 37:486, 1975.

67. LEVI, GF AND PROTO, C: *Combined treatment of atrial fibrillation with quinidine and beta-blockers.* Br Heart J 34:911, 1972.

68. WU, D, HUNG, J, KUO, C, ET AL: *Effects of quinidine on atrioventricular nodal reentrant paroxysmal tachycardia.* Circulation 64:823, 1981.

69. BLOOMFIELD, SS, ROMHILT, DW, CHOU, T, ET AL: *Natural history of cardiac arrhythmias and their prevention with quinidine in patients with acute coronary insufficiency.* Circulation 47:967, 1973.

70. YOUNT, EH, ROSENBLUM, M, AND MCMILLAN, RL: *Use of quinidine in treatment of chronic auricular fibrillation.* Arch Intern Med 89:63, 1952.

71. WEISMAN, SA: *Do's and don'ts in the treatment of auricular fibrillation with quinidine.* Am J Cardiol 3:333, 1959.

72. CARLINER, NH, CROUTHAMEL, WG, FISHER, ML, ET AL: *Quinidine therapy in hospitalized patients with ventricular arrhythmias.* Am Heart J 98:708, 1979.

73. WINKLE, RA, GRADMAN, AH, AND FITZGERALD, JW: *Antiarrhythmic drug effect assessed from ventricular arrhythmia reduction in the ambulatory electrocardiogram and treadmill test: Comparison of propranolol, procainamide, and quinidine.* Am J Cardiol 42:473, 1978.

74. WELLENS, HJJ AND DURRER, D: *Effect of procainamide, quinidine,and aprindine in the Wolff-Parkinson-White syndrome.* Circulation 50:114, 1974.

75. CAIN, ME AND JOSEPHSON, ME: *Quinidine.* In GOULD, LA (ED): *Drug Treatment of Cardiac Arrhythmias.* Futura, Mount Kisco, N Y, 1983.

76. DUFF, HJ, RODEN, DM, PRIMM, RK, ET AL: *Mexiletine for resistant ventricular tachycardia: Comparison with lidocaine and enhancement of efficacy by combination with quinidine.* Am J Cardiol 47:438, 1981.

77. FASOLA, AF, NOBLE, RJ, AND ZIPES, DP: *Treatment of recurrent ventricular tachycardia and fibrillation with aprinidine.* Am J Cardiol 39:903, 1977.

78. HEGER, JJ, PRYSTOWSKY, EN, RINKENBERGER, RL, ET AL: *Amiodarone: Clinical efficacy and electrophysiology during long-term therapy for recurrent ventricular tachycardia or ventricular fibrillation.* N Engl J Med 305:539, 1981.

79. TARTINI, R, STEINBRUNN, W, KAPPENBERGER, L, ET AL: *Dangerous interaction between amiodarone and quinidine.* Lancet 1:1327, 1982.

80. DRAYER, DE, LOWENTHAL, DT, RESTIVO, KM, ET AL: *Steady-state serum levels of quinidine and active metabolites in cardiac patients with varying degrees of renal function.* Clin Pharmacol Ther 24:31, 1978.

81. HOLFORD, NHG, COATES, PE, GUENTERT, TW, ET AL: *The effect of quinidine and its metabolites on the elctrocardiogram and systolic time intervals: Concentration-effect relationships.* Br J Clin Pharmacol 11:187, 1981.

82. SOKOLOW, M AND EDGAR, AL: *Blood quinidine concentrations as a guide in the treatment of cardiac arrhythmias.* Circulation 1:576, 1950.

83. CRAMER, G AND ISAKSSON, B: *Quantitative determination of quinidine in plasma.* Scand J Clin Lab Invest 15:553, 1963.

84. DRAYER, DE, LORENZO, B, AND REIDENBERG, MM: *Liquid chromatography and fluorescence spectroscopy compared with a homogeneous enzyme immunoassay technique for determining quinidine in serum.* Clin Chem 27:308, 1981.

85. OCHS, HR, GREENBLATT, DJ, AND WOO, E: *Clinical pharmacokinetics of quinidine.* Clin Pharmacokinet 5:150, 1980.

86. JENZER, HR AND HAGEMEIJER, F: *Quinidine syncope: Torsade de pointes with low quinidine plasma concentration.* Eur J Cardiol 4:447, 1976.

87. SMITH, WM AND GALLAGHER, JJ: *Les Torsades de Pointes: An unusual ventricular arrhythmia.* Ann Intern Med 93:578, 1980.

88. TZIVONI, D, KEREN, A, AND STERN, S: *Torsades de pointes versus polymorphous ventricular tachycardia.* Am J Cardiol 52:639, 1983.

89. RODEN, DM, WOOSLEY, RL, BOSTICK, D, ET AL: *Quinidine-induced long QT syndrome: Incidence and presenting features.* Circulation 68 (Suppl. III):III-276, 1983.

90. KEREN, A, TZIVONI, D, GAVISH, D, ET AL: *Etiology, warning signs and therapy of torsade de pointes.* Circulation 64:1167, 1981.

91. ANDERSON, JL AND MASON, JW: *Successful treatment by overdrive pacing of recurrent quinidine syncope due to ventricular tachycardia.* Am J Med 64:715, 1978.

92. NAIR, MRS, DEWERNOY, WFC, AND LEICHTMAN, DA: *Severe leukopenia and thrombocytopenia secondary to quinidine.* Clin Cardiol 4:247, 1981.

93. DANAHY, DT AND ARONOW, WS: *Lidocaine-induced cardiac rate changes in atrial fibrillation and flutter.* Am Heart J 95:474, 1978.

94. LEAHEY, EB, REIFFEL, JA, DRUSIN, RE, ET AL: *Interaction between quinidine and digoxin.* JAMA 240:533, 1978.

95. LEAHEY, EB, REIFFEL, JA, GIARDINA, EGV, ET AL: *The effect of quinidine and other oral antiarrhythmic drugs on serum digoxin: A prospective study.* Ann Intern Med 92:605, 1980.

96. BIGGER, JT, JR: *The quinidine-digoxin interaction.* Mod Concepts Cardiovasc Dis 51:73, 1982.

97. DOHERTY, JE, STRAUB, KD, MURPHY, ML, ET AL: *Digoxin-quinidine interaction: Changes in canine tissue concentration from steady state with quinidine.* Am J Cardiol 45:1196, 1980.

98. GARTZ, M, SOOD, P, AND ROLLINS, D: *Digitoxin elimination reduced during quinidine therapy.* Ann Intern Med 94:35, 1981.

99. HARDY, BG, ZADOR, IT, GOLDEN, L, ET AL: *Effect of cimetidine on the pharmacokinetics and pharmacodynamics of quinidine.* Am J Cardiol 52:172, 1983.

100. WATANABE, Y, DREIFUS, L, AND LIKOFF, W: *Electrophysiological antagonism and synergism and potassium and antiarrhythmic agents.* Am J Cardiol 12:702, 1963.

101. BIGGER, JT AND HOFFMAN, BF: *Antirrhythmic drugs.* In GILMAN, AG, GOODMAN, LS, AND GILMAN, A (EDS): *The Pharmacological Basis of Therapeutics.* Macmillan, New York, 1980.

102. KORNFELD, P, HOROWITZ, SH, GENKINS, G, ET AL: *Myasthenia gravis unmasked by antiarrhythmic agents.* Mt Sinai J Med 43:10, 1976.

103. GROGONO, AW: *Anesthesia for atrial fibrillation: Effect of quinidine on muscle relaxation.* Lancet 2:1039, 1963.

104. MAUTZ, FR: *The reduction of cardiac irritability by the epicardial and systemic administration of drugs as a protection in cardiac surgery.* J Thorac Surg 5:612, 1936.

105. MARK, LC, KAYDEN, HJ, STEELE, JM, ET AL: *The physiologic disposition and cardiac effects of procaine amide.* J Pharmacol Exp Ther 102:5, 1951.

106. ELSON, J, STRONG, JM, LEE, WK, ET AL: *Antiarrhythmic potency of N-acetylprocainamide.* Clin Pharmacol Ther 17:134, 1975.

107. DANGMAN, KH AND HOFFMAN, BF: *In vivo and in vitro antiarrhythmic and arrhythmogenic effects of N-acetylprocainamide.* J Pharmacol Exp Ther 217:851, 1981.

108. JAILLON, P, RUBENSON, D, PETERS, F, ET AL: *Electrophysiologic effects of N-acetylprocainamide in human beings.* Am J Cardiol 47:1134, 1981.

109. JAILLON, P AND WINKLE, RA: *Electrophysiologic comparative study of procainamide and N-acetylprocainamide in anesthetized dogs: Concentration-response relationships.* Circulation 60:1385, 1979.

110. ROSEN, MR, GELBAND, H, AND HOFFMAN, BF: *Canine electrocardiographic and cardiac electrophysiologic changes induced by procainamide.* Circulation 46:528, 1972.

111. ROSEN, M, GELBAND, H, MERKER, C, ET AL: *Effects of procaine amide on the electrophysiologic properties of the canine ventricular conducting system.* J Pharmacol Exp Ther 185:438, 1973.

112. ARNSDORF, MF AND BIGGER, JT: *The effect of procainamide on components of excitability in long mammalian cardiac Purkinje fibers.* Circ Res 38:115, 1976.

113. SCHMID, PG, NELSON, LD, HEISTAD, DD, ET AL: *Vascular effects of procainamide in the dog: Predominance of the inhibitory effect on ganglionic transmission.* Circ Res 35:948, 1974.

114. LEE, WK, STRONG, JM, KEHOE, RF, ET AL: *Antiarrhythmic efficacy of N-acetylprocainamide in patients with premature ventricular contractions.* Clin Parmacol Ther 19:508, 1976.

115. WINKLE, RA, JAILLON, P, KATES, RE, ET AL: *Clinical pharmacology and antiarrhythmic efficacy of N-acetylprocainamide.* Am J Cardiol 47:123, 1981.

116. LIMA, JJ, GOLDFARB, AL, CONTI, DR, ET AL: *Safety and efficacy of procainamide infusions.* Am J Cardiol 43:98, 1979.

117. GIARDINA, EGV, HEISSENBUTTEL, RH, AND BIGGER, JT, JR: *Intermittent intravenous procainamide to treat ventricular arrhythmias: Correlation of plasma concentration with effect on arrhythmias, electrocardiogram, and blood pressure.* Ann Intern Med 78:183, 1973.

118. BIGGER, JT, JR AND HEISSENBUTTEL, RH: *The use of procaine amide and lidocaine in the treatment of cardiac arrhythmias.* Prog Cardiovasc Dis 11:515, 1969.

119. BIGGER, JT, JR AND GIARDINA, EGV: *The pharmacology and clinical uses of lidocaine and procainamide.* Med Coll Va Q 9:65, 1973.

120. WELLENS, HJJ, BÄR, FWHM, LIE, KI, ET AL: *Effect of procainamide, propranolol, and verapamil on mechanisms of tachycardia in patients with chronic recurrent ventricular tachycardia.* Am J Cardiol 40:579, 1977.

121. WYNDHAM, CR, MEERAN, MK, WU, D, ET AL: *Recent insights into paroxysmal supraventricular tachycardia: An integrated approach to diagnosis and therapy.* Aust NZ J Med 7:212, 1977.

122. BERRY, K, GARLETT, EL, BELLET, S, ET AL: *Use of Pronestyl in the treatment of ectopic rhythms—treatment of ninety-eight episodes in seventy-eight patients.* Am J Med 11:431, 1951.

123. KAYDEN, HJ, BRODIE, BB, AND STEELE, JM: *Procaine amide: A review.* Circulation 15:118, 1957.

124. MILLER, G, WEINBERG, SL, AND PICK, A: *The effect of procaine amide in clinical auricular fibrillation and flutter.* Circulation 6:41, 1952.

125. SCHACK, JA, HOFFMAN, I, AND VESSELL, H: *The response of arrhythmias and tachycardias of supraventricular origin to oral procaine amide.* Br Heart J 14:465, 1952.

236

126. SELLERS, TD, JR, CAMPBELL, RF, BASHORE, TM, ET AL: *Effects of procainamide and quinidine sulfate in the Wolff-Parkinson-White syndrome.* Circulation 55:15, 1977.

127. MANDEL, W, LAKS, M, OBAYASHI, K, ET AL: *Electrophysiologic features of the Wolff-Parkinson-White syndrome: Modification by procainamide.* Circulation 48(Suppl IV):IV-195, 1973.

128. RODEN, DM, REELE, SB, HIGGINS, SB, ET AL: *Antiarrhythmic efficacy, pharmacokinetics and safety of N-acetylprocainamide in human subjects: Comparison with procainamide.* Am J Cardiol 46:463, 1980.

129. KLUGER, J, DRAYER, D, REIDENBERG, M, ET AL: *The clinical pharmacology and antiarrhythmic efficacy of acetylprocainamide in patients with arrhythmias.* Am J Cardiol 45:1250, 1980.

130. KOCH-WESER, J AND KLEIN, SW: *Procainamide dosage schedules, plasma concentrations and clinical effects.* JAMA 215(9):1454, 1971.

131. MARION, CV, LALKA, D, BAER, DT, ET AL: *Absorption kinetics of procainamide in humans.* J Pharm Sci 66:981, 1977.

132. GRAFFNER, C, JOHNSSON, G, AND SJOGREN, J: *Pharmacokinetics of procainamide intravenously and orally as conventional and slow-release tablets.* Clin Pharmacol Ther 17:414, 1975.

133. GIARDINA, EGV, DREYFUSS, J, BIGGER, JT, JR, ET AL: *Metabolism of procainamide in normal and cardiac subjects.* Clin Pharmacol Ther 19:339, 1976.

134. KARLSSON, E, MOLIN, L, NORLANDER, B, ET AL: *Acetylation of procainamide in man studied with a new gas chromatographic method.* Br J Clin Pharmacol 1:467, 1974.

135. REIDENBERG, MM, DRAYER, DE, LEVY, M, ET AL: *Polymorphic acetylation of procainamide in man.* Clin Pharmacol Ther 17:722, 1975.

136. ELLARD, GA: *Variations between individuals and populations in the acetylation of isoniazid and its significance for the treatment of pulmonary tuberculosis.* Clin Pharmacol Ther 19:610, 1976.

137. GIBSON, TP, LOWENTHAL, DT, NELSON, HA, ET AL: *Elimination of procainamide in end-stage renal failure.* Clin Pharmacol Ther 17:321, 1975.

138. GIARDINA, EGV, HEISSENBUTTEL, RH, AND BIGGER, JT: *Intermittent intravenous procainamide to treat ventricular arrhythmias.* Ann Intern Med 78:183, 1973.

139. GREENSPAN, AM, HOROWITZ, LN, SPIELMAN, SR, ET AL: *Large dose procainamide therapy for ventricular tachyarrhythmias.* Am J Cardiol 46:453, 1980.

140. MATTIASSON, I, HANSON, A, AND JOHANSSON, BW: *Massive doses of procainamide for ventricular arrhythmias due to myocardial infarction.* Acta Med Scand 204:27, 1978.

141. EMBREE, LJ AND LEVINE, SA: *Ventricular tachycardia: A case requiring massive doses of procaine amide (Pronestyl) for reversion.* Ann Intern Med 50:222, 1959.

142. MYERBURG, RJ, KESSLER, KM, KIEM, I, ET AL: *Relationship between plasma levels of procainamide, suppression of premature ventricular complexes and prevention of recurrent ventricular tachycardia.* Circulation 64:280, 1981.

143. DAVIES, DM, BEEDIE, MA, AND RAWLINS, MD: *Antinuclear antibodies during procainamide treatment and drug acetylation.* Br Med J 3:682, 1975.

144. BLOMGREN, SE, CONDEMI, JJ, AND VAUGHN, JH: *Procainamide-induced lupus erythematosus—clinical and laboratory observations.* Am J Med 52:338, 1972.

145. BLOMGREN, SE, CONDEMI, JJ, BIGNALL, MC, ET AL: *Antinuclear antibody induced by procainamide: A prospective study.* N Engl J Med 281:64, 1969.

146. WOOSLEY, RL, DRAYER, DE, REIDENBERG, MM, ET AL: *Effect of acetylator phenotype on the rate at which procainamide induces antinuclear antibodies and the lupus syndrome.* N Engl J Med 298:1157, 1978.

147. MILLER, KB AND SALEM, D: *Immune regulatory abnormalities produced by procainamide.* Am J Med 73:487, 1982.

148. OCHI, T, GOLDINGS, EA, LIPSKY, PE, ET AL: *Immunomodulatory effect of procainamide in man: Inhibition of human suppressor T-cell activity in vitro.* J Clin Invest 71:36, 1983.

149. FREEMAN, RW, UETRECHT, JP, WOOSLEY, RL, ET AL: *Covalent binding of procainamide in vitro and in vivo to hepatic protein in mice.* Drug Metab Disp 9:188, 1981.

150. STEC, GP, LERTORA, JJL, ATKINSON, AJ, ET AL: *Remission of procainamide-induced lupus erythematosus with N-acetylprocainamide therapy.* Ann Intern Med 90:799, 1979.

151. STRASBERG, B, SCLAROVSKY, S, ERDBERG, A, ET AL: *Procainamide-induced polymorphous ventricular tachycardia.* Am J Cardiol 47:1309, 1981.

152. WYSE, DG, McANULTY, JH, AND RAHIMTOOLA, SH: *Influence of plasma drug level and the presence of conduction disease on the electrophysiologic effects of procainamide.* Am J Cardiol 43:619, 1979.

153. OLSHANSKY, B, MARTINS, J, AND HUNT, S: *N-acetylprocainamide causing torsades de pointes.* Am J Cardiol 50:1439, 1982.

154. ATKINSON, AJ, JR, LERTORA, JJL, KUSHNER, W, ET AL: *Efficacy and safety of N-acetylprocainamide in long-term treatment of ventricular arrhythmias.* Clin Pharmacol Ther 33:565, 1983.

155. KLUGER, J, DRAYER, DE, REIDENBERG, MM, ET AL: *Acetylprocainamide therapy in patients with previous procainamide-induced lupus syndrome.* Ann Intern Med 95:18, 1981.

156. MIRRO, MJ, WATANABE, AM, AND BAILEY, JC: *Electrophysiological effects of disopyramide and quinidine on guinea pig atria and canine Purkinje fibers.* Circ Res 46:660, 1980.

157. DANILO, P, HORDOF, AM, AND ROSEN, MR: *Effects of disopyramide on electrophysiologic properties of canine cardiac Purkinje fibers.* J Pharmacol Exp Ther 201:701, 1977.

158. KUS, T AND SASYNIUK, BI: *The electrophysiologic effects of disopyramide phosphate on canine ventricular muscle and Purkinje fibers in normal and low potassium.* Can J Physiol Pharmacol 56:139, 1978.

159. NICHOLSON, WJ, MARTIN, CE, GRACEY, JG, ET AL: *Disopyramide-induced ventricular fibrillation.* Am J Cardiol 43:1053, 1979.

160. GIACOMINI, KM, COX, BM, AND BLASCHKE, TF: *Comparative anticholinergic potencies of R-and S-disopyramide in longitudinal muscle strips from guinea pig ileum.* Life Sci 27:1191, 1980.

161. NELSON, WL, SNEED, CK, GIACOMINI, KM, ET AL: *Synthesis and anticholinergic properties of the enantiomers of 4-(disopropylamino)-2-(2-pyridyl)-2-phenylbutamide, the mono-N-dealkylated metabolite of disopyramide.* J Med Chem 24:614, 1981.

162. BURKE, TR, JR, NELSON, WL, MANGION, M, ET AL: *Resolution, absolute configuration, and antiarrhythmic properties of the enantiomers of disopyramide, 4-(diisopropylamino)-2-(2-pyridyl)-2-phenylbutyramide.* J Med Chem 23:1044, 1980.

163. MATHUR, PP: *Cardiovascular effects of a newer antiarrhythmic agent—disopyramide phosphate.* Am Heart J 84:764, 1972.

164. GOTTDIENER, JS, DIBIANCO, R, BATES, R, ET AL: *Effects of disopyramide on left ventricular function: Assessment by radionuclide cineangiography.* Am J Cardiol 51:1554, 1983.

165. KÖTTER, V, LINDERER, T, AND SCHRÖDER, R: *Effects of disopyramide on systemic and coronary hemodynamics and myocardial metabolism in patients with coronary artery disease—comparison with lidocaine.* Am J Cardiol 46:469, 1980.

166. WALSH, RA AND HORWITZ, LD: *Adverse hemodynamic effects of intravenous disopyramide compared with quinidine in conscious dogs.* Circulation 60:1053, 1979.

167. GALLAGHER, JJ, PRITCHETT, ELC, BENDITT, DG, ET AL: *High dose disopyramide phosphate: An effective treatment for refractory ventricular tachycardia.* Circulation 56:225, 1977.

168. HULTIAG, J AND ROSENHAMER, G: *Disopyramide in ventricular tachycardia.* Acta Med Scand 200:209, 1976.

169. JENNINGS, G, JONES, MBS, BESTERMAN, EMM, ET AL: *Oral disopyramide in prophylaxis of arrhythmias following myocardial infarction.* Lancet 1:51, 1976.

170. VISMARA, LA, MASON, DT, AND AMSTERDAM, EA: *Disopyramide phosphate: Clinical efficacy of a new oral antiarrhythmic drug.* Clin Pharmacol Ther 16:330, 1974.

171. SBARBARO, JA, RAWLING, DA, AND FOZZARD, HA: *Suppression of ventricular arrhythmias with intravenous disopyramide and lidocaine: Efficacy comparison in a randomized trial.* Am J Cardiol 44:513, 1979.

172. LERMAN, BB, WAXMAN, HL, BUXTON, AE, ET AL: *Disopyramide: Evaluation of electrophysiologic effects and clinical efficacy in patients with sustained ventricular tachycardia or ventricular fibrillation.* Am J Cardiol 51:759, 1983.

173. KUMANA, CR, RAMBIHAR, VS, TANSER, PH, ET AL: *A placebo-controlled study to determine the efficacy of oral disopyramide phosphate for the prophylaxis of ventricular dysrhythmias after acute myocardial infarction.* Br J Clin Pharmacol 14:519, 1982.

174. DEBACKER, M, STOUPEL, E, AND KAHN, RJ: *Efficacy of intravenous disopyramide in acute cardiac arrhythmias.* Eur J Clin Pharmacol 19:11, 1981.

175. KIMURA, E, MASHIMA, S, AND TANAKA, T: *Clinical evaluation of antiarrhythmic effects of disopyramide by multiclinical controlled double-blind methods.* Int J Clin Pharmacol Ther Toxicol 18:338, 1980.

176. NICHOLLS, DP, HAYBYRNE, T, AND BARNES, PC: *Intravenous and oral disopyramide after myocardial infarction.* Lancet 2:936, 1980.

177. GREEN, AGH: *Disopyramide—an effective treatment for lignocaine-resistant ventricular dysrhythmias.* Scot Med J 24:21, 1979.

178. VISMARA, LA, VERA, Z, MILLER, RR, ET AL: *Efficacy of disopyramide phosphate in the treatment of refractory ventricular tachycardia.* Am J Cardiol 39:1027, 1977.

179. HÄRTEL, G, LOUHIJA, A, AND KONTTINEN, A: *Disopyramide in the prevention of recurrence of atrial fibrillation after electroconversion.* Clin Pharmacol Ther 15:551, 1974.

180. BENNETT, DH: *Disopyramide in patients with the Wolff-Parkinson-White syndrome and atrial fibrillation.* Chest 74:624, 1978.

181. SPURRELL, RAJ, THORBURN, CW, CAMM, J, ET AL: *Effects of disopyramide on electrophysiological properties of specialized conduction system in man on an accessory atrioventricular pathway in Wolff-Parkinson-White syndrome.* Br Heart J 37:861, 1975.

182. ILETT, KF, MADSEN, BW, AND WOODS, JD: *Disopyramide kinetics in patients with acute myocardial infarction.* Clin Pharmacol Ther 26:1, 1979.

183. RANGNO, RE, WANUCH, W, AND OGILVIE, RI: *Correlation of disopyramide pharmacokinetics with efficacy in ventricular tachyarrhythmias.* J Intern Med Res 4(Suppl 1):54, 1976.

184. HINDERLING, PH AND GARRETT, ER: *Pharmacodynamics of the antiarrhythmic disopyramide in healthy humans: Correlation of the kinetics of the drug and its effects.* J Pharmacokinet Biopharm 4:231, 1976.

185. KARIM, A: *The pharmacokinetics of Norpace.* Angiology 26:85, 1975.

186. DAVID, BM, MADSEN, BW, AND ILETT, KF: *Plasma binding of disopyramide.* Br J Clin Pharmacol 9:614, 1980.

187. MEFFIN, PJ, ROBERTS, EW, WINKLE, RA, ET AL: *Role of concentration-dependent plasma protein binding in disopyramide disposition.* J Pharmacokinet Biopharm 7:29, 1979.

188. GIACOMINI, KM, SWEZEY, SE, TURNER-TAMIYASU, K, ET AL: *The effect of saturable protein binding to plasma proteins on the pharmacokinetic properties of disopyramide.* J Pharmacokinet Biopharm 10:1, 1982.

189. VALDIVIESO, L, BLASCHKE, T, AND GIACOMINI, K: *Disopyramide enantiomers bind stereoselectively to human plasma protein.* World Conf on Clin Pharmacol Ther II:116, 1983.

190. NIARCHOS, AP: *Disopyramide: Serum level and arrhythmia conversion.* Am Heart J 92:57, 1976.

191. PODRID, PJ, SCHOENEBERGER, A, AND LOWN, B: *Congestive heart failure caused by oral disopyramide.* N Engl J Med 302:614, 1980.

192. LEACH, AJ, BROWN, JE, AND ARMSTRONG, PW: *Cardiac depression by intravenous disopyramide in patients with left ventricular dysfunction.* Am J Med 68:839, 1980.

193. DESAI, JM, SCHEINMAN, M, PETERS, RW, ET AL: *Electrophysiologic effects of disopyramide in patients with bundle branch block.* Circulation 59:215, 1979.

194. DHURANDAR, RW, NADEMANEE, K, AND GOLDMAN, AM: *Ventricular tachycardia-flutter associated with disopyramide therapy: A report of three cases.* Heart Lung 7:783, 1978.

195. ROBERTSON, CE AND MILLER, HC: *Extreme tachycardia complicating the use of disopyramide in atrial flutter.* Br Heart J 44:602, 1980.

196. AITIO, ML, MANSURY, L, TALA, E, ET AL: *The effect of enzyme induction on the metabolism of disopyramide in man.* Br J Clin Pharmacol 11:279, 1981.

197. AITIO, ML AND VUORENMAA, T: *Enhanced metabolism and diminished efficacy of disopyramide by enzyme induction?* Br J Clin Pharmacol 9:149, 1980.

198. CUMMING, AD AND ROBERTSON, C: *Interaction between disopyramide and practolol.* Br Med J 2:1264, 1979.

199. WELLENS, HJJ, GORGELS, AP, BRAAT, SJ, ET AL: *Effect of oral disopyramide on serum digoxin levels.* Am Heart J 100:934, 1980.

200. HAWORTH, E AND BURROUGHS, AK: *Disopyramide and warfarin interaction.* Br Med J 2:866, 1977.

201. LOGGREN, N: *Studies on local anesthetics: Xylocaine, a new synthetic drug.* Ivar Haeggstroms, Stockholm, 1948.

202. SOUTHWORTH, JL, MCKUSICK, VA, PIERCE, EC, ET AL: *Ventricular fibrillation precipitated by cardiac catheterization.* JAMA 143:717, 1950.

203. HARRIS, S AND KOKERNOT, RH: *Effects of diphenylhydantoin sodium (Dilantin sodium) upon ectopic ventricular tachycardia in acute myocardial infarction.* Am J Physiol 163:505, 1950.

204. LEONARD, WA: *Use of diphenylhydantoin (Dilantin) sodium in the treatment of ventricular tachycardia.* Arch Intern Med 101:714, 1958.

205. CONN, RD: *Diphenylhydantoin sodium in cardiac arrhythmias.* N Engl J Med 272:277, 1965.

206. ROSEN, MR, LISAK, R, AND RUBIN, IL: *Diphenylhydantoin in cardiac arrhythmias.* Am J Cardiol 20:674, 1967.

207. LANG, TW, BERNSTEIN, MD, BARHIERI, F, ET AL: *Digitalis toxicity: Treatment with dyphenylhydantoin.* Arch Intern Med 116:563, 1965.

208. BIGGER, JT, JR, SCHMIDT, DH, AND KUTT, H: *Relationship between the plasma level of diphenylhydantoin sodium and its cardiac antiarrhythmic effects.* Circulation 38:363, 1968.

209. STONE, N, KLEIN, MD, AND LOWN, B: *Diphenylhydantoin in the prevention of recurring ventricular tachycardia.* Circulation 43:420, 1971.

210. MATHUR, KS, WAHAL, PK, SETH, HC, ET AL: *Diphenylhydantoin sodium in cardiac arrhythmias.* J Indiana Med Assoc 57:256, 1971.

211. KEMP, GL: *Treatment of ventricular ectopic rhythm with diphenylhydantoin.* J Am Geriatr Soc 20:265, 1972.

212. O'REILLY, MV AND MACDONALD, RT: *Efficacy of phenytoin in the management of ventricular arrhythmias induced by hypokalemia.* Br Heart J 35:631, 1973.

213. GARSON, A, JR, KUGLAR, JD, GILLETTE, PC, ET AL: *Control of late postoperative ventricular arrhythmias with phenytoin in young patients.* Am J Cardiol 46:290, 1980.

214. KAVEY, RW, BLACKMAN, MS, AND SONDHEIMER, HM: *Phenytoin therapy for ventricular arrhythmias occurring late after surgery for congenital heart disease.* Am Heart J 104:794, 1982.

215. DAVIS, LD AND TEMTE, JV: *Electrophysiological actions of lidocaine on canine ventricular muscle and Purkinje fibers.* Circ Res 24:639, 1969.

216. GINTANT, GA AND HOFFMAN, BF: *Different local anesthetic characteristics of charged and uncharged forms of lidocaine and other antiarrhythmic drugs in canine Purkinje fibers.* Am J Cardiol 49:1044, 1982.

217. HONDEGHEM, LM AND KATZUNG, BG: *Test of a model of antiarrhythnmic drug action: Effects of quinidine and lidocaine on myocardial conduction.* Circulation 61:1217, 1980.

218. BIGGER, JT, JR AND MANDEL, WT: *Effect of lidocaine on transmembrane potentials of ventricular muscle and Purkinje fibers.* J Clin Invest 49:63, 1970.

219. IMANISHI, S, MCALLISTER, RG, JR, AND SURAWICZ, B: *The effects of verapamil and lidocaine on the automatic depolarization in guinea-pig ventricular myocardium.* J Pharmacol Exp Ther 207:294, 1978.

220. MANDEL, WJ AND BIGGER, JT, JR: *Electrophysiologic effects of lidocaine on isolated canine and rabbit atrial tissues.* J Pharmacol Exp Ther 178:81, 1971.

221. ROSEN, KM, LAU, SH, WEISS, MB, ET AL: *The effect of lidocaine on atrioventricular and intraventricular conduction in man.* Am J Cardiol 25:1, 1970.

222. LIPPESTAD, CT AND FORGANS, K: *Production of sinus arrest by lignocaine.* Br Med J 1:537, 1971.

223. JERSATZ, R, KAHN, A, AND LANDRY, A: *Sinoatrial arrest due to lidocaine in a patient receiving quinidine.* Chest 61:683, 1972.

224. CHENG, TO AND WADHIVA, N: *Sinus standstill following intravenous lidocaine administration.* JAMA 223:790, 1973.

225. AGRAWAL, BU, SINGH, RB, AND VAISH, SK: *Cardiac asystole due to lidocaine in patients with digitalis toxicity.* Acta Cardiol 29:341, 1974.

226. JOSEPHSON, ME, CARCACTA, AR, LAU, SH, ET AL: *Effects of lidocaine on refractory periods in man.* Am Heart J 84:778, 1972.

227. GUPTA, PK, LICHSTEIN, E, AND CHADDA, KD: *Lidocaine-induced heart block in patients with bundle branch block.* Am J Cardiol 33:487, 1974.

228. LICHSTEIN, E, CHEDDA, KD, AND GUPTA, PK: *Atrioventricular block with lidocaine therapy.* Am J Cardiol 31:277, 1973.

229. ROSEN, MR, DANILO, P, JR, ALONSO, MB, ET AL: *Effects of therapeutic concentrations of diphenylhydantoin on transmembrane potentials of normal and depressed Purkinje fibers.* J Pharmacol Exp Ther 197:594, 1974.

230. STRAUSS, HC, BIGGER, JT, BASSETT, AL, ET AL: *Actions of diphenylhydantoin on the electrical properties of isolated rabbit and canine atria.* Circ Res 23:463, 1968.

231. HELFANT, RH, SCHERLAG, BJ, AND DAMATO, AN: *The electrophysiological properties of diphenylhydantoin sodium as compared to procaine amide in the normal and digitalis-intoxicated heart.* Circulation 36:108, 1967.

223. ROSATI, RA, ALEXANDER, JA, SCHAAL, SF, ET AL: *Influence of diphenylhydantoin on electrophysiological properties of the canine heart.* Circ Res 21:757, 1967.

233. GARAN, H, RUSKIN, JN, AND POWELL, WJ, JR: *Centrally mediated effects of phenytoin on digoxin-induced ventricular arrhythmias.* Am J Physiol 241:H67, 1981.

234. EVANS, DE AND GILLIS, RA: *Effects of diphenylhydantoin and lidocaine on cardiac arrhythmias induced by hypothalamic stimulation.* J Pharmacol Exp Ther 191:506, 1974.

235. GILLIS, RA, MCCLELLAN, JR, AND SAUER, T: *Depression of cardiac sympathetic nerve activity by diphenylhydantoin.* J Pharmacol Exp Ther 179:599, 1971.

236. YAMAGUCHI, I, SINGH, B, AND MANDEL, W: *Electrophysiological action of mexiletine on isolated rabbit atria and canine ventricular muscle Purkinje fiber.* Cardiovasc Res 13:288, 1979.

237. WELD, FM, BIGGER, JT, SWISTEL, D, ET AL: *Electrophysiological effects of mexiletine (K01173) on bovine cardiac Purkinje fibers.* J Pharmacol Exp Ther 210:222, 1979.

238. Roos, JC, Paalman, DCA, and Dunning, AJ: *Electrophysiological effects of mexiletine in man.* Postgrad Med J 53(Suppl I):92, 1977.

239. McConvish, M, Robinson, C, Kitson, D, et al: *Clinical electrophysiological effects of mexiletine.* Postgrad Med J 53(Suppl I):85, 1977.

240. Frame, L, Grintant, G, and Hoffman, B: *Mexiletine and tocainide differ from lidocaine in their use-dependent kinetics.* Circulation 66(Suppl II):II-292, 1982.

241. Moore, EN, Spear, JF, Horowitz, LN, et al: *Electrophysiologic properties of a new antiarrhythmic drug—tocainide.* Am J Cardiol 41:703, 1978.

242. Oshita, S, Soda, H, Kajima, M, et al: *Effects of tocainide and lidocaine on the transmembrane action potentials as related to external potassium and calcium concentrations in guinea-pig papillary muscles.* Naunyn-Schmiedeberg's Arch Pharmacol 314:67, 1980.

243. Anderson, JL, Mason, JW, Winkle, RA, et al: *Clinical electrophysiologic effects of tocainide.* Circulation 57:685, 1978.

244. Binnion, PF, Murtheh, G, Pollock, AM, et al: *Relation between plasma lignocaine levels and induced hemodynamic changes.* Br Med J 3:390, 1969.

245. Grossman, JI, Cooper, JA, and Frieden, J: *Cardiovascular effects of infusion of lidocaine in patients with heart disease.* Am J Cardiol 24:191, 1969.

246. Stannard, M, Slowman, G, and Sangster, L: *Hemodynamic effects of lignocaine in acute myocardial infarction.* Br Med J 2:468, 1968.

247. Heger, JJ, Nattel, S, Rinkenberger, RL, et al: *Mexiletine therapy in fifteen patients with drug resistant ventricular tachycardia.* Am J Cardiol 45:627, 1980.

248. Waspe, LE, Waxman, HL, Buxton, AE, et al: *Mexiletine for control of drug resistant ventricular tachycardia: Clinical and electrophysiologic results in 44 patients.* Am J Cardiol 51:1175, 1983.

249. Mehta, J and Conti, CR: *Mexiletine, a new antiarrhythmic agent, for treatment of premature ventricular complexes.* Am J Cardiol 49:455, 1982.

250. Podrid, PJ and Lown, B: *Mexiletine for ventricular arrhythmias.* Am J Cardiol 47:895, 1981.

251. Klein, ND, Levine, PA, and Ryan, TJ: *Antiarrhythmic efficacy, pharmacokinetics and clinical safety of tocainide in convalescent myocardial infarction patients.* Chest 77:726, 1980.

252. Winkle, RA, Anderson, JL, Peters, F, et al: *The hemodynamic effects of intravenous tocainide in patients with heart disease.* Circulation 57:787, 1978.

253. Mixter, GC, III, Moran, JN, and Austen, WG: *Cardiac and peripheral vascular effects of diphenylhydantoin sodium.* Am J Cardiol 17:332, 1966.

254. Campbell, RWF, Dolder, MA, Prescott, LF, et al: *Comparison of procainamide and mexiletine in prevention of ventricular arrhythmias after acute myocardial infarction.* Lancet 1:1257, 1975.

255. Klempt, H-W, Nayebagha, A, and Fabry, E: *Antiarrhythmic efficacy of mexiletine, propafenone and flecainide in ventricular premature beats: A comparative study in patients after myocardial infarction.* Z Kardiol 71:340, 1982.

256. Horowitz, JD, Anavekar, SN, Morris, PM, et al: *Comparative trial of mexiletine and lignocaine in the treatment of early ventricular tachyarrhythmias after acute myocardial infarction.* J Cardiovasc Pharmacol 3:409, 1981.

257. DiMarco, JP, Garan, H, and Ruskin, JN: *Mexiletine for refractory ventricular arrhythmias: Results using serial electrophysiologic testing.* Am J Cardiol 47:131, 1981.

258. Wang, RYC, Lee, PK, Wong, KL, et al: *Mexiletine in the treatment of recurrent ventricular tachycardia: Prediction of long term arrhythmia suppression from acute and short term response.* J Clin Pharmacol 23:89, 1983.

259. Esterbrooks, D, Mohiuddin, SM, Aronow, WS, et al: *Effect of oral mexiletine versus quinidine on premature ventricular complexes.* Curr Ther Res 33:1070, 1083.

260. Rehnqvist, N, Earhardt, L, Ericsson, C-G, et al: *Comparative study of tocainide and lidocaine in patients admitted for suspected acute myocardial infarction.* Acta Med Scand 214:21, 1983.

261. Haffajee, CI, Alpert, JS, and Dalen, JE: *Tocainide for refractory ventricular arrhythmias of myocardial infarction.* Am Heart J 100:1013, 1980.

262. Wasenmiller, JE and Aronow, WS: *Effect of tocainide and quinidine on premature ventricular contractions.* Clin Pharmacol Ther 28:431, 1980.

263. Engler, R, Ryan, W, LeWinter, M, et al: *Assessment of long-term antiarrhythmic therapy: Studies on the long-term efficacy and toxicity of tocainide.* Am J Cardiol 43:612, 1979.

264. Woosley, RL, McDevitt, DG, Nies, AS, et al: *Suppression of ventricular ectopic depolarizations by tocainide.* Circulation 56:980, 1977.

265. KARLINER, JS: *Intravenous diphenylhydantoin sodium (Dilantin) in cardiac arrhythmias.* Dis Chest 51:256, 1967.

266. EDDY, JD AND SINGH, SP: *Treatment of cardiac arrhythmias with phenytoin.* Br Med J 4:270, 1969.

267. SALEM, HH: *Persistent supraventricular tachycardia treated with mexiletine.* Lancet 2:94, 1977.

268. WALEFFE, A, BRUNINX, R, MARY-RABINE, L, ET AL: *Effects of tocainide studied with programmed electrical stimulation of the heart in patients with re-entrant tachyarrhythmias.* Am J Cardiol 43:292, 1979.

269. SINATRA, ST AND JERESATY, RM: *Enhanced atrial conduction in atrial fibrillation after lidocaine administration.* JAMA 237:1356, 1977.

270. AKHTAR, M, GILBERT, CJ, AND SHENASA, M: *Effect of lidocaine on atrioventricular response via the accessory pathway in patients with Wolff-Parkinson-White syndrome.* Circulation 63:435, 1981.

271. ATKINSON, AJ AND DAVISON, R: *Diphenylhydantoin as an antiarrhythmic drug.* Annu Rev Med 25:99, 1974.

272. ANDERSON, JL, HARRISON, DC, MEFFIN, PJ, ET AL: *Antiarrhythmic drugs: Clinical pharmacology and therapeutic uses.* Drugs 15:271, 1978.

273. LEAHEY, EB, HEISSENBUTTEL, RJ, AND BIGGER, JD: *Combined mexiletine and propranolol for resistant ventricular arrhythmias.* Circulation 62(Suppl III):III-181, 1980.

274. BREITHARDT, G, SEIPEL, L, AND ABENDROTH, RR: *Comparative cross-over study of the effects of disopyramide and mexiletine on stimulus induced ventricular tachycardia.* Circulation 62(Suppl III):III-153, 1980.

275. RUSKIN, JN, DIMARCO, JP, AND GARAN, H: *Out-of-hospital cardiac arrest: Electrophysiologic observations of selection of long-term antiarrhythmic therapy.* N Engl J Med 303:607, 1980.

276. BOYES, RN, SCOTT, DP, JEBSON, TJ, ET AL: *Pharmacokinetics of lidocaine in man.* Clin Pharmacol Ther 12:105, 1971.

277. BLUMER, J, STRONG, JM, AND ATKINSON, AJ, JR: *The convulsant potency of lidocaine and its N-dealkylated metabolites.* J Pharmacol Exp Ther 186:31, 1973.

278. BENOWITZ, N, FORSYTH, RP, MELMON, KL, ET AL: *Lidocaine disposition kinetics in monkey and man.* Clin Pharmacol Ther 16:87, 1974.

279. STENSON, RE, CONSTANTINO, RT, AND HARRISON, DC: *Interrrelationship of hepatic blood flow, cardiac output and blood levels of lignocaine in man.* Circulation 43:205, 1971.

280. NATION, RL, TRIGGS, EJ, AND SELIG, M: *Lignocaine kinetics in cardiac patients and aged subjects.* Br J Clin Pharmacol 4:439, 1977.

281. NIES, AS, SHAND, DG, AND WILKINSON, GR: *Altered hepatic blood flow and drug disposition.* Clin Pharmacokinet 1:135, 1976.

282. THOMPSON, PD, MELMON, KL, RICHARDSON, JA, ET AL: *Lidocaine pharmacokinetics in advanced heart failure, liver disease and renal failure in humans.* Ann Intern Med 78:499, 1973.

283. BRANCH, RA, SHAND, DG, WILKINSON, GR, ET AL: *Reduction of lidocaine clearance by dl-propranolol: An example of a hemodynamic drug interaction.* J Pharmacol Exp Ther 184:515, 1973.

284. COLLINSWORTH, AK, STRONG, JM, ATKINSON, AJ, JR, ET AL: *Pharmacokinetics and metabolism of lidocaine in patients with renal failure.* Clin Pharmacol Ther 18:59, 1975.

285. PRESCOTT, LF, ADJEPOM-YAMOAH, KK, AND TALBOT, RG: *Impaired lignocaine metabolism in patients with myocardial infarction and cardiac failure.* Br Med J 1:939, 1976.

286. FORREST, JAH, FINLAYSON, NDC, ADJEPOM-YOMOAH, KK, ET AL: *Antipyrine, paracetamol, and lignocaine elimination in chronic liver disease.* Br Med J 1:1384, 1977.

287. HEINONEN, J, TAKKI, S, AND JARHO, L: *Plasma lidocaine levels in patients treated with potential inducers of microsomal enzymes.* Acta Anesthesiol Scand 14:89, 1970.

288. DIFAZIO, LA AND BROWN, RD: *Lidocaine metabolism in normal and phenobarbital pre-treated dogs.* Anesthesiology 36:238, 1972.

289. LELORIER, J, GRENON, D, LATOUR, Y, ET AL: *Pharmacokinetics of lidocaine after prolonged intravenous infusions in uncomplicated myocardial infarction.* Ann Intern Med 87:700, 1977.

290. DAVISON, R, PARKER, M, AND ATKINSON, AJ, JR: *Excessive serum lidocaine levels during maintenance infusions: Mechanisms and prevention.* Am Heart J 104:203, 1982.

291. LALKA, D, MEYER, NB, DUCE, BR, ET AL: *Kinetics of the oral antiarrhythmic lidocaine congener, tocainide.* Clin Pharmacol Ther 19:757, 1976.

292. MCDEVITT, DG, NIES, AS, WILKINSON, GR, ET AL: *Antiarrhythmic effects of a lidocaine congener, tocainide, 2-amino-2',6'-propionoxylidide, in man.* Clin Pharmacol Ther 19:396, 1976.

293. ELVIN, AT, KEENAGHAN, JB, BYRNES, EW, ET AL: *Conjugation of tocainide in man: Evidence for a novel pathway of biotransformation for a primary amine.* Pharmacologist 18:114, 1976.

294. ELVIN, AT, KEENAGHAN, JB, BYRNES, EW, ET AL: *Tocainide conjugation in humans: Novel biotransformation pathway for a primary amine.* J Pharm Sci 69:47, 1980.

242

295. RONFELD, RA, WOLSHIN, EM, AND BLOCK, AJ: *On the kinetics and dynamics of tocainide and its metabolites.* Clin Pharmacol Ther 31:384, 1982.

296. PRESCOTT, LF, POTTAGE, A, AND CLEMENTS, JA: *Absorption, distribution and the elimination of mexiletine.* Postgrad Med J 53(Suppl 1):50, 1977.

297. CAMPBELL, NPS, KELLY, JG, ADJEE, AAG, ET AL: *The clinical pharmacology of mexiletine.* Br J Clin Pharmacol 6:103, 1978.

298. BECKETT, AH AND CHIDOMERE, EC: *The distribution, metabolism and excretion of mexiletine in man.* Postgrad Med J 53(Suppl 1):60, 1977.

299. EL ALLAF, D, HENRARD, L, CROCHELET, L, ET AL: *Pharmacokinetics of mexiletine in renal insufficiency.* Br J Clin Pharmacol 14:431, 1982.

300. LEAHEY, EB, GIARDINA, EGV, AND BIGGER, JT, JR: *Effect of ventricular failure on steady state kinetics of mexiletine.* Clin Res 28:239A, 1980.

301. PENTIKÄINEN, PJ, KOIVULA, IH, AND HILTUNEN, HA: *Effect of enzyme induction on pharmacokinetics of mexiletine.* Clin Pharmacol Ther 31:260, 1982.

302. JUSKO, WJ, KOUP, JR, AND ALVAN, G: *Nonlinear assessment of phenytoin bioavailability.* J Pharmacokinet Biopharm 4:327, 1976.

303. ALBERT, KS, SAKMAR, E, HALLMARK, MR, ET AL: *Bioavailability of diphenylhydantoin.* Clin Pharmacol Ther 16:727, 1974.

304. GUGLER, R, MANION, CV, AND AZARNOFF, DL: *Phenytoin pharmacokinetics and bioavailability.* Clin Pharmacol Ther 19:135, 1976.

305. MAYNERT, EW: *The metabolic fate of diphenylhydantoin in the dog, rat and man.* J Pharmacol Exp Ther 130:275, 1960.

306. REIDENBERG, M, ODAR-CEDARLOF, I, VON BAHR, C, ET AL: *Protein binding of DPH and desmethylimipramine in plasma from patients of poor renal function.* N Engl J Med 285:264, 1971.

307. RALL, TW AND SCHLEIFER, LF: *Drugs effective in the therapy of the epilepsies.* In GILMAN, AG, GOODMAN, LS, AND GILMAN, A (EDS): *The Pharmacological Basis of Therapeutics.* Macmillan, New York, 1980.

308. BOOKER, HE AND DARCEY, B: *Serum concentrations of free diphenylhydantoin and their relationship to clinical intoxication.* Epilepsia 14:177, 1973.

309. RODEN, DM, REELE, SB, HIGGINS, SB, ET AL: *Tocainide therapy for refractory ventricular arrhythmias.* Am Heart J 100:15, 1980.

310. PFEIFER, AJ, GREENBLATT, DJ, AND KOCH-WESER, J: *Clinical use and toxicity of intravenous lidocaine.* Am Heart J 92:168, 1976.

311. KUTT, H AND SEHOMAN, GE: *Phenytoin: Relevant side effects.* In GLASER, GH, PENREY, JK, AND WOODBURY, DM (EDS): *Anti-Epileptic Drugs: Mechanism of Action.* Raven Press, New York, 1980.

312. STANNARD, N AND CAPLAN, HL: *Cardiac arrest due to imipramine hydrochloride.* Med J Aust 2:22, 1967.

313. RASMUSSEN, J: *Amitryptiline and imipramine poisoning.* Lancet 2:850, 1965.

314. NAMN, AM, CATTERSON, AG, AND MACPHERSON, AS: *Toxicity of imipramine: Reports of serious side effects and massive overdose.* Can Med Assoc J 81:23, 1959.

315. BIGGER, JT, JR, GIARDINA, EGV, PEREL, JM, ET AL: *Cardiac antiarrhythmic effect of imipramine hydrochloride.* N Engl J Med 296:206, 1977.

316. BRENNAN, FJ: *Electrophysiologic effects of imipramine and doxepin on normal and depressed cardiac Purkinje fibers.* Am J Cardiol 46:599, 1980.

317. WELLS, FM AND BIGGER, JG, JR: *Electrophysiological effects of imipramine on bovine cardiac Purkinje and ventricular muscle fibers.* Circ Res 46:167, 1980.

318. WALLINGS, D AND FOZZARD, HA: *Electrophysiological effects of imipramine on cardiac Purkinje fibers.* J Pharmacol Exp Ther 209:371, 1979.

319. GIARDINA, EGV AND BIGGER, JT, JR: *Antiarrhythmic effect of imipramine hydrochloride in patients with ventricular premature complexes without psychological depression.* Am J Cardiol 50:172, 1982.

320. GIARDINA, EGV, BIGGER, JT, JR, GLASSMAN, AH, ET AL: *The electrocardiographic and antiarrhythmic effects of imipramine hydrochloride at therapeutic plasma concentrations.* Circulation 60:1045, 1979.

321. CONNOLLY, SJ, MITCHELL, LB, SWERDLOW, CD, ET AL: *Clinical efficacy and electrophysiology of impramine for ventricular tachycardia.* Am J Cardiol 53:516, 1984.

322. VEITH, RC, RASKIND, MA, CALDWELL, JH, ET AL: *Cardiovascular effects of tricyclic antidepressants in depressed patients with chronic heart disease.* N Engl J Med 306:954, 1982.

323. RADER, EA, BURCKHARDT, D, NEUBAUER, H, ET AL: *Long-term tri- and tetra-cyclic antidepressants, myocardial contractility, and cardiac rhythms.* Br Med J 2:666, 1978.

324. GLASSMAN, AH, GIARDINA, EGV, PEREL, JM, ET AL: *Clinical characteristics of imipramine-induced orthostatic hypotension.* Lancet 1:468, 1979.

325. GRAN, LS AND CHRISTIANSEN, J: *First-pass metabolism of imipramine in man.* Clin Pharmacol Ther 17:555, 1975.

326. CHRISTIANSEN, J, GRAN, LF, KOFOD, B, ET AL: *Imipramine metabolism in man.* Psychopharmacologia 11:255, 1967.

327. POTTER, WZ, CALIL, HM, SUTFIN, TA, ET AL: *Active metabolites of imipramine and desipramine in man.* Clin Pharmacol Ther 31:393, 1982.

328. RUFFY, R, ROZENSHTRAUKH, LV, ELHARRAR, V, ET AL: *Electrophysiological effects of ethmozin on canine myocardium.* Cardiovasc Res 13:354, 1979.

329. BOYDEN, PA AND WIT, AL: *Pharmacology of the antiarrhythmic drugs.* In ROSEN, MR AND HOFFMAN, BF (EDS): *Cardiac Therapy.* Martinus Nijhoff, Boston, 1983.

330. PODRID, PJ, LYAKISHEV, A, LOWN, B, ET AL: *Ethmozin, a new antiarrhythmic drug for depressing ventricular premature complex.* Circulation 61:450, 1980.

331. MORGANROTH, J, PEARLMAN, AS, DUNKMAN, WB, ET AL: *Ethmozin: A new antiarrhythmic agent developed in the U.S.S.R.: Efficacy and tolerance.* Am Heart J 98:621, 1979.

332. MANN, DE, LUCK, JC, PRATT, CM, ET AL: *Clinical and electrophysiologic effects of ethmozin in man.* Clin Res 30:203A, 1982.

333. PRATT, CM, YEPSEN, SC, TAYLOR AA, ET AL: *Ethmozine suppression of single and repetitive ventricular premature depolarizations during therapy: Documentation of efficacy and long-term safety.* Am Heart J 106:85, 1983.

334. MANN, DE, LUCK, JC, PRATT, CM, ET AL: *Electrophysiologic evaluation of the efficacy of ethmozin in patients with ventricular tachycardia.* J Am Coll Cardiol 3:537, 1984.

335. PRATT, CM, ENGLISH, LJ, YEPSEN, SC, ET AL: *Double-blind placebo-controlled crossover trial of ethmozin and disopyramide in the suppression of complex ventricular arrhythmias.* Circulation 68(Suppl III):III-415, 1983.

336. BORCHARD, U AND BOISTEN, N: *Effect of flecainide on action potentials and alternating current–induced arrhythmias in mammalian myocardium.* J Cardiovasc Pharmacol 4:205, 1982.

337. SCHULZE, JJ AND KNOPOS, J: *Effects of flecainide on contractile force and electrophysiological parameters in cardiac muscle.* Arzneim-Forsch/Drug Res 32:1025, 1982.

338. COWEN, JC AND VAUGHAN WILLIAMS, EM: *Characterization of a new oral antiarrhythmic drug, flecainide (R818).* Eur J Pharmacol 73:333, 1981.

339. HODESS, AB, FOLLANSBEE, WP, SPEAR, JF, ET AL: *Electrophysiological effects of a new antiarrhythmic agent, flecainide, on the intact canine heart.* J Cardiovasc Pharmacol 1:427, 1979.

340. HELLESTRAND, KJ, BECKSTON, RS, MASON, AW, ET AL: *Acute electrophysiologic effects of flecainide acetate on cardiac conduction and refractoriness in man.* Br Heart J 48:140, 1982.

341. OLSSON, SB AND EDVARDSSON, N: *Clinical electrophysiologic study of antiarrhythmic properties of flecainide: Acute intraventricular delayed conduction and prolonged repolarization in regular paced and premature beats using intracardiac monophasic action potentials with programmed stimulation.* Am Heart J 102:864, 1981.

342. VIK-MO, H, OHM, O-J, AND LUND-JOHANSEN, P: *Electrophysiologic effects of flecainide acetate in patients with sinus nodal dysfunction.* Am J Cardiol 50:1090, 1982.

343. THE FLECAINIDE-QUINIDINE RESEARCH GROUP: *Flecainide versus quinidine for treatment of chronic ventricular arrhythmias: A multicenter clinical trial.* Circulation 67:1117, 1983.

344. HODGES, M, HAUGLAND, JM, GRANRUD, G, ET AL: *Depression of ventricular ectopic depolarizations by flecainide acetate, a new anti-arrhythmic agent.* Circulation 65:879, 1982.

345. ANDERSON, JL, STEWART, JR, PERRY, DA, ET AL: *Oral flecainide acetate for the treatment of ventricular arrhythmias.* N Engl J Med 305:473, 1981.

346. DUFF, HJ, RODEN, DM, MAFFUCCI, RJ, ET AL: *Suppression of resistant ventricular arrhythmias by twice daily dosing with flecainide.* Am J Cardiol 48:1133, 1981

347. SALERNO, DM, HODGES, M, GRANRUD, G, ET AL: *Comparison of flecainide with quinidine for suppression of chronic stable ventricular ectopic depolarizations.* Ann Intern Med 98:455, 1983.

348. HELLESTRAND, KJ, NATHAN, AW, BEXTON, RS, ET AL: *Electrophysiologic effects of flecainide acetate on sinus node function, anomalous AV connections, and pacemaker thresholds.* Am J Cardiol 53:30B, 1984.

349. JACKMAN, WM, ZIPES, DP, NACCARRELLI, GV, ET AL: *Electrophysiology of oral encainide.* Am J Cardiol 49:1270, 1982.

350. SAMI, M, MASON, JW, PETERS, F, ET AL: *Clinical electrophysiologic effects of encainide, a newly developed antiarrhythmic agent.* Am J Cardiol 44:526, 1979.

351. ECHT, DS, MITCHELL, LB, KATES, RE, ET AL: *Comparison of the electrophysiologic effects of intravenous and oral lorcainide in patients with recurrent ventricular tachycardia.* Circulation 68:392, 1983.

352. ELHARRAR, V AND ZIPES, DP: *Effects of encainide and metabolites (MJ14030 and MJ9444) on canine cardiac Purkinje and ventricular fibers.* J Pharmacol Exp Ther 220:440, 1982.

353. KEEFE, DL, KATES, RE, AND WINKLE, RA: *Comparative electrophysiology of lorcainide and its major metabolite, norlorcainide, in the dog.* Circulation 64(Suppl IV):IV-127, 1981.

354. CAMPBELL, RWF, HENDERSON, A, BRYSON, LG, ET AL: *Intravenous flecainide: Pharmacokinetics and efficacy.* Circulation 64(Suppl IV):IV-265, 1981.

355. SAMI, MH, DERBEKYAN, VA, AND LISBONA, R: *Hemodynamic effects of encainide in patients with ventricular arrhythmia and poor ventricular function.* Am J Cardiol 52:507, 1983.

356. SHITA, A, BERNARD, R, MOSTINCKX, R, ET AL: *Hemodynamic reactions after intravenous injection of lorcainide hydrochloride in acute myocardial infarction.* Eur J Cardiol 12:237, 1981.

357. COCCO, G AND STROZZI, C: *Initial clinical experience of lorcainide (Ro 13-1042), a new antiarrhythmic agent.* Eur J Clin Pharmacol 14:105, 1978.

358. CARMELIET, E, JANSSEN, PAJ, MARSBOOM, R, ET AL: *Antiarrhythmic, electrophysiologic, and hemodynamic effects of lorcainide.* Arch Int Pharmacodyn 231:104, 1978.

359. KASPER, W, TREESE, N, MEINERTZ, T, ET AL: *Electrophysiologic effect of lorcainide on the accessory pathway in the Wolff-Parkinson-White syndrome.* Am J Cardiol 51:1618, 1982.

360. KEEFE, DL, PETERS, F, AND WINKLE, RA: *A randomized double-blind crossover trial documenting oral lorcainide efficacy in suppression of symptomatic tachyarrhythmias.* Am Heart J 103:511, 1982.

361. SAKSENA, S, ROTHBART, ST, CAPPELLO, G, ET AL: *Clinical and electrophysiologic effects of chronic lorcainide therapy in refractory ventricular tachycardia.* J Am Coll Cardiol 2:538, 1983.

362. CHESNIE, B, PODRID, P, LOWN, B, ET AL: *Encainide for refractory tachyarrhythmias.* Am J Cardiol 52:495, 1983.

363. MASON, JW AND PETERS, FA: *Antiarrhythmic efficacy of encainide in patients with refractory recurrent ventricular tachycardia.* Circulation 63:670, 1981.

364. WINKLE, RA, MASON, JW, GRIFFIN, JC, ET AL: *Malignant ventricular tachyarrhythmias associated with the use of encainide.* Am Heart J 102:857, 1981.

365. MASON, A, HELLESTRAND, K, BEXTON, R, ET AL: *The pro-arrhythmic effects of the new "antiarrhythmic" drug flecainide acetate.* J Am Coll Cardiol 1:709, 1983.

366. SENGES, J, RIZOS, I, BRACKMAN, J, ET AL: *Arrhythmogenic effects of toxic concentrations of the antiarrhythmic drug lorcainide on the isolated canine ventricle.* J Pharmacol Exp Ther 223:547, 1982.

367. CONARD, GJ, CARLSON, GL, FROST, JW, ET AL: *Human plasma pharmacokinetics of flecainide acetate (R-818), a new antiarrhythmic, following single oral and intravenous doses.* Clin Pharmacol Ther 25:218, 1979.

368. KLOTZ, U, MUELLER-SEYDLITZ, P, AND HEIMBURG, P: *Pharmacokinetics of lorcainide in man: A new antiarrhythmic agent.* Clin Pharmacokinet 3:407, 1978.

369. JÄHNCHEN, E, BECHTOLD, H, KASPER, W, ET AL: *Lorcainide: Saturable pre-systemic elimination.* Clin Pharmacol Ther 26:187, 1979.

370. KATZ, RE, KEEFE, DL, AND WINKLE, RA: *Lorcainide disposition kinetics in arrhythmia patients.* Clin Pharmacol Ther 33:28, 1983.

371. AMERY, WK, HEYKANTS, J, BRUYNEEL, K, ET AL: *Bioavailability and saturation of the pre-systemic metabolism of oral lorcainide therapy initiated in three different dose regimens.* Eur J Clin Pharmacol 24:517, 1983.

372. KELLER, K, MEYER-ESTORF, G, BECK, OA, ET AL: *Correlation between serum concentration and pharmacologic effect on atrioventricular conduction time of the antiarrhythmic drug propafenone.* Eur J Clin Pharmacol 13:17, 1978.

373. CONNOLLY, SJ, KATES, RE, LEBSACK, CS, ET AL: *Clinical pharmacology of propafenone.* Circulation 68:589, 1983.

374. KOHLHARDT, N AND SEIFERT, C: *Inhibition of $\dot{V}max$ of the action potential and its voltage-, time-, pH-dependence in mammalian ventricular myocardium.* Arch Pharmacol 315:55, 1980.

375. LEDDA, F, MANTELLI, L, MANZINI, S, ET AL: *Electrophysiological and antiarrhythmic properties of propafenone in isolated cardiac preparation.* J Cardiovasc Pharmacol 3:1162, 1981.

376. SHAND, DG AND MCLEOD, AA: *Human beta-adrenoceptor antagonism by the Class I antiarrhythmic drug propafenone: Clinical study.* II World Conf Clin Pharmacol Ther 1983, p 54.

377. McLeod, AA, Shand, DG, and Stiles, GL: *Human beta-adrenoceptor antagonism by the Class I antiarrhythmic drug propafenone: Radioligand binding studies.* II World Conf Clin Pharmacol Ther 1983, p 68.

378. Kukovetz, WR, Pöch, G, Holzmann, S, et al: *Wirkung von Propafenon auf Phosphodiesterase, Koronärarterien und Herz.* In Hochrein, H, Hapke, H-J and Beck, OA (eds): *Fortschritte in der Pharmakotherapie von Herzrhthmusstörungen.* Fischer, Stuttgart, 1977.

379. Kohlhardt, M: *Der Einfluss von Propafenon auf ben transmembranären Na⁺ und Ca⁺⁺-Strom der Warmblüter-Myokardfasermembran.* In Hochrein, H, Hapke, H-J, and Beck, OA (eds): *Fortschritte in der Pharmakotherapie von Herzrhythmusstörungen.* Fischer, Stuttgart, 1977.

380. Harder, OR and Belandinelli, L: *Effects of propafenone on TEA-induced action potentials in vascular smooth muscle of canine coronary arteries.* Experientia 36:1082, 1980.

381. Beck, OA and Hochrein, H: *Combined use of propafenone and lidoflazine in chronic atrial fibrillation and flutter.* Dtsch Med Wochenschr 105:1243, 1980.

382. Waleffe, A, Mary-Rabine, L, de Rijbel, R, et al: *Electophysiological effects of propafenone: Studies with programmed electrical stimulation of the heart in patients with recurrent PSVT.* Eur Heart J 2:345, 1981.

383. Salerno, D, Granrud, G, Lebens, B, et al: *Efficacy of propafenone for treatment of ventricular ectopic depolarizations.* Circulation 66(Suppl II):II-67, 1982.

384. de Soyza, N, Murphy, N, Sakhii, N, et al: *The safety and efficacy of propafenone in suppressing ventricular ectopy.* Circulation 66(Suppl II):II-67, 1982.

385. Connolly, SJ, Kates, RE, Lebsack, CS, et al: *Clinical efficacy and electrophysiology of oral propafenone for ventricular tachycardia.* Am J Cardiol 52:1208, 1983.

386. Clementy, J, Dallocchio, M, and Brichaud, H: *Comparative study of the therapeutic effect of propafenone and disopyramide in the oral treatment of chronic ventricular premature beats.* In Schlepper, M and Olsson, B (eds) *Cardiac Arrhythmias: Diagnosis, Prognosis, Therapy.* Springer-Verlag, New York, 1983.

387. Asshauer, S and Vorphal, U: *Results of a double-blind comparison of propafenone with a standard drug.* Dev Eval 1:135, 1971.

388. Chilson, DA, Zipes, DP, Heger, JJ, et al: *Propafenone: Discriminant analysis and electrophysiologic results in patients with ventricular tachycardia predicts clinical outcome.* Circulation 68(Suppl III):III-382, 1983.

389. von Philipsborn, G, Gries, J, and Kretzschmar, R: *Antiarrhythmic and beta-sympatholytic effects of the new antiarrhythmic propafenone and its main metabolite 5-hydroxy propafenone.* II World Conf Clin Pharmacol Ther 1983, p 105.

390. Siddoway, LA, Thompson, KA, Bergstrand, RH, et al: *Safety and efficacy of propafenone in treatment of refractory ventricular arrhythmias.* J Am Coll Cardiol 3:474, 1984.

391. Roden, DM, Wang, T, and Woosley, RL: *Antiarrhythmic effects of beta-blocking drugs.* NIH Workshop on Pharmacology of Antiarrhythmic Therapy, September, 1982.

392. Woosley, RL, Kornhauser, D, Smith, R, et al: *Suppression of chronic ventricular arrhythmias with propranolol.* Circulation 60:819, 1979.

393. Gradman, AH, Winkle, RA, Fitzgerald, JW, et al: *Suppression of premature ventricular contractions by acebutolol.* Circulation 55:785, 1977.

394. Singh, SN, DiBianco, R, Davidov, ME, et al: *Comparison of acebutolol and propranolol for treatment of chronic ventricular arrhythmias: A placebo controlled double-blind, randomized crossover study.* Circulation 65:1356, 1982.

395. Wang, T, Bergstrand, RH, Siddoway, LA, et al: *The dissociation of antiarrhythmic and beta-blocking actions of sotalol.* Circulation 68(Suppl III):III-270, 1983.

396. Pruett, JK, Walle, T, and Walle, UK: *Propranolol effects on membrane repolarization time in isolated canine Purkinje fibers: Threshold tissue content and the influence of exposure time.* J Pharmacol Exp Ther 215:529, 1980.

397. Duff, HJ, Roden, DM, Brorson, L, et al: *Electrophysiologic actions of high plasma concentrations of propranolol in human subjects.* J Am Coll Cardiol 2:1134, 1983.

398. Lucchesi, BR, Whitsitt, LS, and Stickney, JL: *Antiarrhythmic effects of beta-adrenergic blocking agents.* Ann NY Acad Sci 139:940, 1967.

399. Duff, HJ, Wood, AJJ, Dawson, AK, et al: *d-Propranolol: Non-adrenergically mediated electrophysiologic actions in man.* Circulation 66(Suppl II):II-372, 1982.

400. Strauss, HC, Bigger, JT, Jr, and Hoffman, BF: *Electrophysiological and beta-receptor blocking effects of MJ1999 on dog and rabbit cardiac tissue.* Circ Res 26:661, 1970.

401. Connolly, NE, Kersting, F, and Dollery, CT: *The clinical pharmacology of beta-adrenoceptor-blocking drugs.* Prog Cardiovasc Dis 19:203, 1976.

402. TONKIN, AM: *New approaches to the management of the Wolff-Parkinson-White syndrome.* Aust NZ J Med 6:441, 1976.

403. TONKIN, AM, MILLER, HC, SVENSON, RH, ET AL: *Refractory periods of the accessory pathway in the Wolff-Parkinson-White syndrome.* Circulation 52:562, 1975.

404. ROSEN, KM, BARWOLF, C, EHSANI, A, ET AL: *Effects of lidocaine and propranolol on the normal and accessory pathways in patients with pre-excitation.* Am J Cardiol 40:801, 1972.

405. SILVERMAN, R AND FRISHMAN, WH: *Drug treatment of cardiac arrhythmia: Propranolol and other beta blockers.* In GOULD, LA (ED): *Drug Treatment of Cardiac Arrhythmias.* Futura, Mt Kisco, New York, 1983.

406. GREEN, AF: *The discovery of bretylium and bethanidine.* Br J Clin Pharmacol 13:25, 1982.

407. LEVEQUE, PD: *Antiarrhythmic action of bretylium.* Nature 207:203, 1965.

408. BOURA, LA AND GREEN, AF: *The actions of bretylium: Adrenergic neuron blocking and other effects.* Br J Pharmacol 14:536, 1959.

409. WIT, AL, STEINER, C, AND DAMATO, AN: *Electrophysiologic effects of bretylium tosylate on single fibers of the canine specialized conducting system and ventricle.* J Pharmacol Exp Ther 173:344, 1970.

410. BACANER, MB: *Bretylium tosylate for suppression of induced ventricular fibrillation.* Am J Cardiol 17:528, 1966.

411. HEISSENBUTTEL, RH AND BIGGER, JT, JR: *Bretylium tosylate: A newly available antiarrhythmic drug for ventricular arrhythmias.* Ann Intern Med 91:229, 1979.

412. WOOSLEY, RL, REELE, SB, RODEN, DM, ET AL: *Pharmacologic reversal of the hypotensive effect that complicates antiarrhythmic therapy with bretylium.* Clin Pharmacol Ther 32:313, 1982.

413. BACANER, MB: *Treatment of ventricular fibrillation and other arrhythmias with bretylium tosylate.* Am J Cardiol 21:530, 1968.

414. TERRY, D, VELLANI, CW, HIGGINS, MR, ET AL: *Bretylium tosylate in the treatment of refractory ventricular arrhythmias complicating myocardial infarction.* Br Heart J 32:21, 1970.

415. DHURANDHAR, RW, TEASDALE, SJ, AND MAHON, WA: *Bretylium tosylate in the management of refractory ventricular fibrillation.* Can Med Assoc J 105:161, 1971.

416. BERNSTEIN, JG AND KOCH-WESER, J: *Effectiveness of bretylium tosylate against refractory ventricular arrhythmias.* Circulation 45:1024, 1972.

417. SANNA, G AND ARCIDIACONO, R: *Chemical ventricular defibrillation of the human heart with bretylium tosylate.* Am J Cardiol 32:982, 1973.

418. HAYNES, RE, CHINN, TL, COPASS, MK, ET AL: *Comparison of bretylium tosylate and lidocaine in management of out-of-hospital ventricular fibrillation: A randomized clinical trial.* Am J Cardiol 48:353, 1981.

419. ANDERSON, JL, PATTERSON, D, WAGNER, JG, ET AL: *Oral and intravenous bretylium disposition.* Clin Pharmacol Ther 28:468, 1980.

420. LUOMANMAKI, K, HEIKKILA, J, AND HARTEL, G: *Bretylium tosylate: Adverse effects in acute myocardial infarction.* Arch Intern Med 135:515, 1975.

421. MARKIS, JE AND KOCH-WESER, J: *Characteristics and mechanisms of inotropic and chronotropic actions of bretylium tosylate.* J Pharmacol Exp Ther 178:94, 1974.

422. CHARLIER, R, DELPOUR, G, TONDEUR, R, ET AL: *Recherches dans la serie des benzofurannes VII.* Arch Int Pharmacodyn Ther 139:255, 1962.

423. ROSENBAUM, MB, CHIALE, PA, RYBA, D, ET AL: *Control of tachyarrhythmias associated with Wolff-Parkinson-White syndrome by amiodarone hydrochloride.* Am J Cardiol 34:215, 1974.

424. SINGH, BM AND VAUGHAN WILLIAMS, EM: *The effect of amiodarone, a new anti-anginal drug, on cardiac muscle.* Br J Pharmacol 39:657, 1970.

425. GOUPIL, N AND LENFANT, J: *The effects of amiodarone on the sinus node activity of the rabbit heart.* Eur J Pharmacol 39:23, 1976.

426. TOUBOUL, P, HUERTA, F, PORTE, J, ET AL: *Bases electrophysiologiques de l'action antiarrhymique l'amiodarone chez l'homme.* Arch Mal Coeur 69:845, 1976.

427. WELLENS, HJJ, LIE, KI, BÄR, FW, ET AL: *Effects of amiodarone in the Wolff-Parkinson-White syndrome.* Am J Cardiol 38:189, 1976.

428 WELLENS, HJJ, BRUGADA, P, ROY, D, ET AL: *The comparison of electrophysiological effects of intravenous and oral amiodarone.* Am J Cardiol 49:1043, 1982.

429. GOUGH, WB, ZEILER, RH, BARRECA, P, ET AL: *Hypotensive action of commercial intravenous amiodarone and polysorbate 80 in dogs.* J Cardiovasc Pharmacol 4:375, 1982.

430. BACQ, AN, BLAKELEY, AGH, AND SUMMERS, RJ: *The effects of amiodarone, an alpha and beta receptor antagonist, on adrenergic transmission in the cat spleen.* Biochem Pharmacol 25:1195, 1976.

431. CHARLIER, R: *Cardiac actions in the dog of a new antagonist of adrenergic excitation which does not produce competitive blockade of adrenoceptors.* Br J Pharmacol 39:668, 1970.

432. BEXTON, RS AND CAMM, AJ: *Drugs with a Class III antiarrhythmic action.* Pharmacol Ther 17:315, 1982.

433. SICART, M, BESSE, P, CHOUSSAT, A, ET AL: *Action hemodynamique be l'amiodarone intravenineuse chez l'homme.* Arch Mal Coeur 70:219, 1977.

434. ROSENBAUM, MB, CHIALE, BA, HALPERN, NS, ET AL: *Clinical efficacy of amiodarone as an antiarrhythmic agent.* Am J Cardiol 38:934, 1976.

435. WARD, DE, CAMM, AJ, AND SPURRELL, RAJ: *Clinical antiarrhythmic effects of amiodarone in patients with resistant paroxysmal tachycardia.* Br Heart J 44:91, 1980.

436. PODRID, PJ AND LOWN, B: *Amiodarone therapy in symptomatic sustained refractory atrial and ventricular tachyarrhythmias.* Am Heart J 101:374, 1981.

437. KASKI, JC, GIROTTI, LA, MESSUTI, H, ET AL: *Long term management of sustained recurrent symptomatic ventricular tachycardia with amiodarone.* Circulation 64:273, 1981.

438. BOPPANA, VK, GREENSPAN, A, SWANSON, BM, ET AL: *Clinical efficacy and serum concentrations of amiodarone.* Clin Pharmacol Ther 33:209, 1983.

439. HOLT, DW, TUCKER, GT, JACKSON, PR, ET AL: *Amiodarone pharmacokinetics.* Am Heart J 106:840, 1983.

440. HARRIS, L, MCKENNA, WJ, ROWLAND, E, ET AL: *Plasma amiodarone and desethyl amiodarone levels in chronic oral therapy.* Circulation 64(Suppl IV):IV-263, 1981.

441. SIDDOWAY, LA, MCALLISTER, CB, WILKINSON, GR, ET AL: *Amiodarone dosing: A proposal based on its pharmacokinetics.* Am Heart J 106:951, 1983.

442. INGRAM, DV: *Ocular effects in long-term amiodarone therapy.* Am Heart J 106:902, 1983.

443. RAKITA, L, SOBEL, SM, MOSTOW, N, ET AL: *Amiodarone pulmonary toxicity.* Am Heart J 106:906, 1983.

444. HARRIS, L, MCKENNA, WJ, ROWLAND, E, ET AL: *Side-effects and possible contraindications of amiodarone use.* Am Heart J 106:916, 1983.

445. HEGER, JJ, PRYSTOWSKY, EN, AND ZIPES, DP: *Relationships between amiodarone dosage, drug concentrations, and adverse side effects.* Am Heart J 106:931, 1983.

446. SINGH, BN AND NADEMANEE, K: *Amiodarone and thyroid function: Clinical implications during antiarrhythmic therapy.* Am Heart J 106:857, 1983.

447. MARCUS, SI: *Drug interactions with amiodarone.* Am Heart J 106:924, 1983.

# Beta-Adrenergic Blockers in the Prevention of Sudden Death

*William H. Frishman, M.D., Lawrence I. Laifer, M.D., and Curt D. Furberg, M.D.*

The introduction of beta-adrenoceptor blocking drugs to clinical medicine 25 years ago ushered in a new era of pharmacologic intervention and revolutionized the management of cardiovascular disease. In addition to becoming a therapeutic mainstay for the treatment of hypertension, angina, and various arrhythmias, beta blockers have now been shown to reduce the risk of mortality after myocardial infarction, and these drugs have numerous applications well beyond the cardiovascular sphere. The use of beta blockers in the treatment of arrhythmias and for the prevention of sudden death will be discussed in this chapter. It is important first to review some basic pharmacologic concepts regarding beta-adrenergic blocking drugs.

## PHARMACOLOGIC CHARACTERISTICS OF BETA BLOCKERS

Based on the observation that the relative potency of a series of sympathomimetic amines varied with the effector organs or systems, Ahlquist,[1] in 1948, postulated that there were two distinct types of adrenergic receptors, which he classified as alpha and beta receptors. Beta receptors were later divided in two groups: beta receptors in the heart, and beta receptors in the bronchi and blood vessels.[2-4]

Ahlquist's theory was viewed with much skepticism until 1958 when Powell and Slater discovered dichloroisoprenaline (DCI), the first beta-blocking agent. The discovery that DCI selectively blocked those responses mediated by beta receptors gave credence to Ahlquist's views and was a pivotal development in human pharmacology. Although DCI was unsuitable for clinical use as a beta blocker because of its excessive beta-stimulant (agonist) activity, the concept that beta blockade of the cardiac receptor might be useful in the therapy of angina led Black and Stephenson[5] and others to develop beta-blocking agents that would become effective antianginal drugs. It soon became evident that their therapeutic efficacy extended well beyond the control of angina to include treatment of arrhythmias and hypertension and management of noncardiovascular disease.

### Pharmacodynamic Properties

#### Beta-Blocking Potency

Beta-blocking drugs competitively inhibit the effects of catecholamines at beta adrenoreceptor sites, thereby diminishing the effect of any concentration of agonist on a sensitive tissue.[6] The dose-response curve is thus shifted to the right, and in the presence of a beta-blocking drug, a higher concentration of agonist is required to evoke a given tissue response. One

**Table 1.** Pharmacodynamic properties and cardiac effects of beta-adrenoceptor blocking drugs

| Drug | Beta$_1$-blockade potency ratio (propranolol = 1.0) | Relative beta$_1$ selectivity | Intrinsic sympathomimetic activity | Membrane stabilizing activity | Resting heart rate | Exercise heart rate | Myocardial contractility | Resting blood pressure | Resting atrioventricular conduction | Anti-arrhythmic effect |
|---|---|---|---|---|---|---|---|---|---|---|
| Acebutolol | 0.3 | + | + | + | → | → | → | → | → | + |
| Atenolol | 1.0 | + | 0 | 0 | → | → | → | → | → | + + |
| Esmolol* | | + + | 0 | 0 | → | NA | → | → | ↕ | + + |
| Labetalol† | 0.3 | 0 | 0 | 0 | ↕ | → | → | → | → | + + |
| Metoprolol | 1.0 | + | 0 | 0 | → | → | → | → | → | + + |
| Nadolol | 1.0 | 0 | 0 | 0 | → | → | → | → | → | + + |
| Oxprenolol | 0.5–1.0 | 0 | + + | + | ↕ | → | ↕ | → | ↕ | + + |
| Penbutolol | 1.0 | 0 | + + | 0 | ↕ | → | ↕ | → | ↕ | + + |
| Pindolol | 6.0 | 0 | + + + | + | ↕ | → | ↕ | → | ↕ | + + |
| Propranolol | | 0 | 0 | + + | → | → | → | → | → | + + |
| LA Propranolol | 0.6–1.0 | 0 | 0 | + + | → | → | → | → | → | + + |
| Sotalol | 0.3 | 0 | 0 | 0 | → | → | → | → | → | + + |
| Timolol | 6.0 | 0 | 0 | 0 | → | → | → | → | → | + + |
| Isomer d-propranolol‡ | | 0 | 0 | + + | ↕ | ↕ | ↕ | ↕ | ↕ | + – |

NA = not available.

*Esmolol is a new ultra–short-acting beta blocker that is available only in intravenous form.

†Labetalol has additional alpha-adrenergic blocking properties and direct vasodilatory activity.

‡Effects of d-propranolol occur with doses in human beings well above the therapeutic level. The isomer also lacks beta-blocking activity.

can assess the relative potency of a beta-blocking agent by its inhibition of isoproterenol-induced tachycardia or by the amount of isoproterenol required to reverse the heart rate slowing effect of a given beta blocker.[7] As shown in Table 1, on a millgram-per-milligram basis, pindolol and timolol are the most potent, and acebutolol, labetalol, and sotalol are the least potent of the beta-blocking drugs.

## Structure-Activity Relationship

The molecular structures of beta-adrenergic blocking agents (Fig. 1) have features in common with isoproterenol, the beta-adrenergic agonist. The affinity for the beta receptor appears to be determined by the size of the alkyl substituted secondary or tertiary amine to the 2-C side chain. The larger the alkyl group, the greater the affinity for the beta receptor. The particular structure attaches to the receptor site, and the nature of the substituents on the aromatic ring determines whether the effects will be predominantly activation or blockade.[8] The configuration of the asymmetric beta carbon of the side chain is crucial for pharmacologic activity. Beta-blocking drugs exist as pairs of optical isomers. However, almost all the beta-blocking activity resides in the levorotatory isomer.[6,9] For example, the (−) levorotatory isomers of propranolol and alprenolol are up to 100 times more active than the (+) dextrorotatory isomers. Only the racemic mixture of each drug, consisting of equal parts of the two isomers, is available for clinical use. The different stereoisomers of beta-adrenergic blocking drugs are useful for differentiating between the effects of beta-receptor blockade and other properties of the drug, but clinically, the (+) dextrorotatory isomers are of no therapeutic value.[6,8]

## Membrane-Stabilizing Activity

Membrane-stabilizing activity, also known as "quinidine-like effect" or "local anesthetic" action, is unrelated to competitive inhibition of catecholamine action. It occurs equally in both optical isomers of the drug.[8] Membrane-stabilizing activity was demonstrated electrophysiologically in propranolol,[9] oxprenolol,[10] and alprenolol[11] by a reduction in the rate of rise of the intracardiac potential without a change in the overall duration of the spike or the resting potential.[9–11] The concentration of propranolol at which this effect has been demonstrated on human ventricular muscle in vitro is approximately 50 to 100 times the blood level associated with inhibition of exercise-induced tachycardia.[12] The difference is even greater with other beta blockers. The antiarrhythmic effect of beta blockers is primarily due to beta blockade and not membrane stabilizing activity;[13] atenolol, metoprolol, nadolol, pindolol, sotalol, and timolol are all devoid of membrane-stabilizing activity, yet they all demonstrate an antiarrhythmic effect.

## Intrinsic Sympathomimetic Activity (ISA)

Certain beta-adrenoreceptor blocking drugs have intrinsic sympathomimetic activity (also known as partial agonist activity). Beta blockers with ISA slightly activate the beta receptor, while preventing the access of natural or synthetic catecholamines to the receptor site. Dichloroisoprenaline, the first beta-adrenoreceptor blocking drug, exhibited such marked partial agonist activity that it was unsuitable for clinical use.[8] However, compounds with less ISA are effective beta-blocking drugs. Acebutolol, oxprenolol, penbutolol, and pindolol cause a very small agonist response, indicating that they partially stimulate as well as block the receptor. Atenolol, metoprolol, nadolol, propranolol, sotalol, and timolol, in contrast, do not produce any agonist response when they interact with beta receptors in the absence of primary agonists such as isoproterenol or epinephrine.

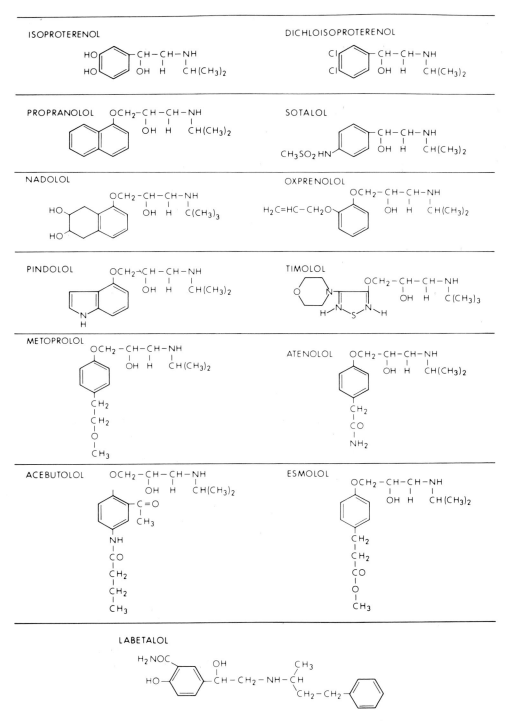

**Figure 1.** Molecular structures of isoproterenol and some beta-adrenergic blocking drugs.

Whether the presence of partial agonist activity in a beta blocker confers any advantage in cardiac therapy is still a matter of some debate.[14-16] Beta blockers with ISA cause less slowing of the heart rate at rest than propranolol or metoprolol, although the exercise-induced increase in heart rate is similarly blunted.[17] They may also depress atrioventricular conduction less than beta blockers without ISA.[18] In general, beta blockers with ISA are as effective as beta blockers without ISA in the treatment of hypertension,[19] effort angina,[17] or arrhythmias.[20] The partial agonist activity in a beta blocker may protect against peripheral vascular complications, bronchial asthma, and myocardial depression, but the evidence for this is preliminary and will require more definitive clinical trials.[17]

## Selectivity

Lands and coworkers[2] suggested that beta adrenoreceptors could be classified into two distinct types: beta$_1$ (lipolysis and cardiac stimulation) and beta$_2$ (bronchodilation and vasodilation). This subclassification has led to the development of agonist or antagonist drugs that are relatively selective at either beta$_1$- or beta$_2$-receptor sites.[3]

Beta$_1$-selective blocking agents (e.g., metoprolol) in low doses inhibit cardiac beta$_1$ receptors but have less effect on vascular and bronchial beta adrenoreceptors. In higher doses, however, this selectivity is overcome and beta$_2$ receptors are blocked as well.[16] Because beta$_1$-selective blockers have little inhibitory effect on the peripheral beta$_2$ receptors, they possess two theoretical advantages. First, beta$_1$-selective agents may be safer than nonselective beta blockers in patients with asthma or chronic obstructive pulmonary disease because adrenergic bronchodilation can still be mediated by the unblocked beta$_2$ receptors. Clinical studies in patients with asthma showed a lower incidence of respiratory side effects with low dose beta$_1$-selective agents than with equivalent doses of propranolol.[6,21] A second advantage of beta$_1$-selective blockers is that they may not block the beta$_2$ receptors that mediate arteriolar dilatation and thus may prove advantageous in the treatment of hypertension.[21] However, beta$_1$ selectivity is a dose-dependent phenomenon that eventually disappears when larger doses, such as those usually required for the treatment of hypertension, are used.[22,23] In contrast, beta-blockers with intrinsic sympathomimetic activity maintain this effect without diminution even at higher doses.[24]

## Alpha-Blocking Activity

Labetalol is a beta blocker with antagonistic properties at both alpha and beta adrenoreceptors.[25] Before labetalol, only antagonists acting at alpha or beta adrenoreceptors, but not both, were available. Labetalol has been shown to be 6 to 10 times less potent than phentolamine at alpha adrenoreceptors, 1.5 to 4 times less potent than propranolol at beta-adrenoreceptors, and is itself 4 to 16 times less potent at alpha than at beta adrenoreceptors.[25]

Labetalol, like other beta blockers, has been shown to be a useful agent in the treatment of arrhythmias, hypertension, and angina pectoris.[26] However, unlike most beta-blocking drugs, the additional alpha-adrenergic blocking actions of labetalol lead to a reduction in peripheral vascular resistance that may maintain cardiac output in patients.[25]

## Pharmacokinetic Properties

### Absorption and Metabolism

All the beta-blocking drugs are well absorbed over a wide portion of the small intestine except for atenolol and nadolol. Absorption is fairly rapid, with peak blood concentrations being achieved 1 to 3 hours after administration.[6]

The beta-adrenergic blocking drugs can be divided by their pharmacokinetic properties into two broad categories: those eliminated by hepatic metabolism, which tend to have relatively short plasma half-lives, and those eliminated by the kidney, which tend to have longer half-lives. Propranolol and metoprolol are both lipid soluble, are almost completely absorbed from the small intestine, and are largely metabolized by the liver. They tend to have highly variable bioavailability and relatively short plasma half-lives,[6,27,28] but because of lack of correlation between plasma half-life and pharmacologic effect, these drugs may be able to be administered twice or even once daily. A sustained-release form of propranolol is now available and approved for once-daily use.[29]

In contrast, drugs like atenolol and nadolol are more water soluble, are incompletely absorbed through the gut, and are eliminated unchanged by the kidney.[6,30–33] They tend to have less variable bioavailability in patients with normal renal function, in addition to longer half-lives allowing once-daily dosing. This latter property may be helpful in patients who are noncompliant with beta-blocker treatment.

Specific pharmacokinetic properties of individual beta-adrenergic blockers (first-pass metabolism, active metabolites, lipid solubility, and protein binding) may be important to the clinician. When drugs with first-pass metabolism are taken orally, they undergo considerable hepatic biotransformation, and relatively little drug may reach the systemic circulation. Depending on the extent of the first-pass effect, an oral dose of a beta blocker must be proportionately larger than an intravenous dose to produce the same clinical effects.[6] Some beta-adrenergic blockers are transformed into pharmacologically active compounds, and the total pharmacologic effect therefore depends on both the amount of drug administered and its active metabolites.[6] Lipid solubility in a beta blocker has been associated with the ability of the drug to concentrate in the brain,[6,15,34] and many side effects of these drugs (lethargy, mental depression, hallucinations, and so on) may be related to actions on the central nervous system.[27] It is still unclear, however, whether drugs that are less lipid soluble cause fewer of these adverse reactions. Some beta-adrenergic blockers are extensively protein-bound in the plasma, and alterations in protein level or binding may influence the pharmacologic effects of these drugs.[6,35]

## ELECTROPHYSIOLOGIC EFFECTS

Beta-adrenoreceptor blocking drugs have two main effects on the electrophysiologic properties of specialized cardiac tissue (Table 2). The first effect of beta blockers results from the specific blockade of adrenergic stimulation of cardiac pacemaker potentials. This is undoubtedly important in the control of arrhythmias caused by enhanced automaticity. In concentrations causing significant inhibition of adrenergic receptors, the beta blockers produce little change in the transmembrane potentials of cardiac muscle. However, by competitively inhibiting adrenergic stimulation, beta blockers decrease the slope of phase 4 depolarization and the spontaneous firing rate of sinus or ectopic pacemakers, and thus decrease automaticity. Arrhythmias occurring in the setting of enhanced automaticity, as encountered in myocardial

**Table 2.** Antiarrhythmic mechanisms for beta blockers

1. Beta blockade
   Electrophysiology: depress excitability; depress conduction
   Prevention of ischemia: decrease automaticity: inhibit re-entrant mechanisms
2. Membrane-stabilizing effects
   Local anesthetic, "quinidine-like" properties: depress excitability; prolong refractory period; delay conduction
3. Special pharmacologic properties (beta$_1$-selectivity, intrinsic sympathomimetic activity) do not appear to contribute to antiarrhythmic effectiveness

infarction, digitalis toxicity, hyperthyroidism, and pheochromocytoma, would therefore be expected to respond well to beta blockade.[36]

The second electrophysiologic effect of beta blockers is membrane-stabilizing action, also known as the "quinidine-like" or "local anesthetic" action. This property is unrelated to inhibition of catecholamine action and is possessed equally by both the d- and l-isomers of the drugs (d-isomers have almost no beta-blocking activity).[37] Characteristic of this effect is a reduction in the rate of rise of the intracardiac action potential without affecting the spike duration of the resting potential.[38] Associated features include an elevated electrical threshold of excitability, delay in conduction velocity, and a significant increase in the effective refractory period. This effect and its attendant changes have been explained by an inhibition of the depolarizing inward sodium current.

Sotalol is unique among the beta blockers in that it alone possesses class III antiarrhythmic properties, causing prolongation of the action potential period and thereby delaying repolarization.[39] Clinical studies have verified the efficacy of sotalol in control of arrhythmias,[40–43] but additional investigation will be required to determine whether its class III antiarrhythmic properties contribute significantly to its efficacy as an antiarrhythmic agent.

The most important mechanism underlying the antiarrhythmic effect of beta blockers (with the possible exclusion of sotalol) is believed to be beta blockade with resultant inhibition of pacemaker potentials. The contribution of membrane-stabilizing action does not appear to be clinically significant. This is borne out by at least two separate lines of evidence. The plasma concentration of propranolol necessary for arrhythmia control is far less than the level required for membrane stabilization to occur. In vitro experiments with human ventricular muscle have shown that the concentration of propranolol required for membrane stabilization is 50 to 100 times the concentration usually associated with inhibition of exercise-induced tachycardia and at which only beta-blocking effects occur.[44] Moreover, d-propranolol, which possesses membrane-stabilizing properties but no beta-blocking action, is a weak antiarrhythmic agent in high doses, whereas beta blockers devoid of membrane-stabilizing action (atenolol, metoprolol, nadolol, pindolol) have been shown to be effective antiarrhythmic drugs.

If, indeed, beta blockade is the major mechanism for antiarrhythmic effect, with the contribution of membrane-stabilizing properties being negligible, then one would expect *all* beta blockers to be similarly effective at a comparable level of beta blockade. In fact, this appears to be the case. No superiority of one beta-blocking agent over another in the therapy of arrhythmias has yet been convincingly demonstrated. Differences in overall clinical usefulness are related to their other associated pharmacologic properties.[45]

Beta blockers slow the rate of discharge of the sinus and ectopic pacemakers and increase the effective refractory period of the atrioventricular node by their beta-adrenergic blocking actions. They also slow both antegrade and retrograde conduction in anomalous pathways.[18] Inasmuch as all beta blockers studied thus far cause an increase in atrioventricular conduction time, advancing AV block is a potential complication when beta blockers are used. Agents with partial agonist activity (intrinsic sympathomimetic activity), such as oxprenolol and pindolol, may provide some protection from the AV conduction impairment induced by beta blockade.[46]

In high doses, beta blockers can induce sinus node dysfunction and lead to sinoatrial block or sinus arrest. These drugs are therefore best avoided in patients with "sick sinus syndrome," a condition that can be exacerbated by beta-adrenergic blockade.[18]

## THERAPEUTIC USES IN CARDIAC ARRHYTHMIAS

Beta-adrenergic blocking drugs have become an important treatment modality for various cardiac arrhythmias (Table 3). Although it has long been acknowledged that beta blockers are more effective in treating supraventricular than ventricular arrhythmias, it has been

**Table 3.** Effects of beta blockers in various arrhythmias

| Arrhythmia | Comment |
|---|---|
| Supraventricular | |
|   Sinus tachycardia | Treat underlying disorder; excellent response to beta blocker, if need to control rate (e.g., ischemia). |
|   Atrial fibrillation | Beta blockers reduce ventricular rate, rarely restore sinus rhythm. May be useful in combination with digoxin. |
|   Atrial flutter | Beta blockers reduce rate, sometimes restore sinus rhythm. |
|   Atrial tachycardia | Effective in slowing ventricular rate, may restore sinus rhythm. Useful in prophylaxis. |
| Ventricular | |
|   PVCs | Variable response to beta blockers, except digitalis-induced, exercise (ischemia)-induced, mitral valve prolapse, or hypertrophic cardiomyopathy. |
|   Ventricular tachycardia | Usually not effective, except in digitalis toxicity or exercise (ischemia)-induced. |
|   Ventricular fibrillation | Electrical defibrillation is treatment of choice. Beta blockers can be used to prevent recurrence in cases of excess digitalis or sympathomimetic amines. Appear to be effective in reducing the incidence of ventricular fibrillation and sudden death after myocardial infarction. |

appreciated only recently that these agents can be quite useful in the treatment of ventricular tachyarrhythmias in the setting of myocardial ischemia.

## Supraventricular Arrhythmias

These arrhythmias have a variable response to beta blockade. Beta blockers are not only therapeutically useful but diagnostically important; by slowing a very rapid heart rate, the drug may permit an accurate ECG diagnosis of an otherwise puzzling arrhythmia.

### Sinus Tachycardia

This arrhythmia usually has an obvious cause (e.g., fever, hyperthyroidism, congestive heart failure), and therapy should be aimed at correction of the underlying condition. However, if the rapid heart rate itself is compromising the patient, for example, causing recurrent angina in a patient with coronary artery disease, then direct intervention with a beta blocker is effective and indicated therapy. Patients with heart failure should not be treated with beta blockers unless they have been placed on diuretic therapy and digitalized, and then only with extreme caution.

### Supraventricular Ectopic Beats

As with sinus tachycardia, specific treatment of these extrasystoles is seldom required, and therapy should be directed to the underlying cause. Although supraventricular ectopic beats are often the precursors to atrial fibrillation (especially in acute myocardial infarction, thyrotoxicosis, and mitral stenosis), there is no evidence that prophylactic administration of beta blockers can prevent the development of atrial fibrillation. Supraventricular ectopic beats related to digitalis toxicity generally respond well to beta blockade. Beta blockers can be useful for those patients in whom supraventricular ectopic activity causes discomforting palpitations.

## Paroxysmal Supraventricular Tachycardia (SVT)

SVTs may be divided into two groups: (1) those related to abnormal conduction (e.g., reciprocating AV nodal tachycardia, and the Wolff-Parkinson-White syndrome, in which there is abnormal conduction through an AV nodal bypass tract), and (2) those caused by ectopic atrial activity, as in digitalis toxicity. Inasmuch as beta blockade delays AV conduction (i.e., increased A–H interval in His bundle electrocardiograms) and prolongs the refractory period of the re-entrant pathways, it is not surprising that many cases of paroxysmal supraventricular tachycardia respond to beta blockers. In acute episodes, vagal maneuvers after beta blockade may effectively terminate an arrhythmia when they may have been previously unsuccessful without beta blockade. Even when beta blockers do not convert an arrhythmia to sinus rhythm, they will often slow the ventricular rate by increasing atrioventricular nodal refractoriness. Additionally, the use of beta-blocking drugs still allows the option of direct current countershock cardioversion (which would be more hazardous if digitalis in high doses was initially used).

## Atrial Flutter

Beta blockade can be used to slow the ventricular rate (by increasing AV block) and may restore sinus rhythm in a large percentage of patients. This is a situation in which beta blockade may be of diagnostic value: given intravenously, beta blockers slow the ventricular response and permit the differentiation of flutter waves, ectopic P waves, or sinus mechanism.

## Atrial Fibrillation

The major action of beta blockers in rapid atrial fibrillation is the reduction in the ventricular response by increasing the refractory period of the AV node. Whereas all beta-blocking drugs have been effective in slowing ventricular rates in patients with atrial fibrillation, they are less effective than quinidine or DC cardioversion in the reversion of atrial fibrillation to sinus rhythm (although this can occur, especially when the atrial fibrillation is of recent onset).

Beta blockers must be used cautiously when atrial fibrillation occurs in the presence of a severely diseased heart that is dependent on high levels of adrenergic tone to avoid myocardial failure. These drugs may be particularly useful in controlling the ventricular rate in situations where this is difficult to achieve with maximally tolerated doses of digitalis (e.g., thyrotoxicosis, hypertrophic cardiomyopathy, mitral stenosis).

Many patients with paroxysmal atrial fibrillation or flutter may have "sick sinus" or "tachy-brady" syndrome, and administration of beta blockers may precipitate severe bradycardic episodes. These patients often require both antiarrhythmic therapy and a pacemaker.

## Ventricular Arrhythmias

Beta-adrenoreceptor blocking drugs can decrease the frequency or abolish ventricular ectopic beats in various conditions. They are particularly useful if these arrhythmias are related to excessive catecholamines (e.g., exercise, halothane anesthesia, pheochromocytoma, exogenous catecholamines), myocardial ischemia, or digitalis excess.

### Premature Ventricular Contractions

The response of these arrhythmias to beta blockade is variable. The best response can be expected in coronary heart disease, particularly when the arrhythmia is secondary to an ischemic event. Because beta blockers are effective in preventing ischemic episodes, arrhythmias generated by these episodes may be prevented.

Beta blockers are also quite effective in controlling the frequency of premature ventricular contractions in hypertrophic cardiomyopathy and in mitral valve prolapse. In these situations, a beta blocker is generally the antiarrhythmic drug of first choice.

## Ventricular Tachycardia

Beta-blocking drugs should not be considered agents of choice in the treatment of acute ventricular tachycardia. Cardioversion or other antiarrhythmic drugs (lidocaine, quinidine, procainamide) should be the initial mode of therapy. Beta-blockers have, however, been shown to be of benefit for prophylaxis against recurrent ventricular tachycardia, particularly if sympathetic stimulation appears to be a precipitating cause. There have been several reported studies showing the prevention of exercise-induced ventricular tachycardia by beta blockers; in many previous cases, there had been a poor response to digitalis or quinidine.[47-49]

## Prevention of Ventricular Fibrillation

Beta-blocking agents can attenuate cardiac stimulation by the sympathetic nervous system, and perhaps reduce the potential for re-entrant ventricular arrhythmias and sudden death.[36,50] Experimental studies have shown that beta blockers raise the ventricular fibrillation threshold in the ischemic myocardium.[36,50] Placebo-controlled clinical trials have shown that beta blockers reduce the number of episodes of ventricular fibrillation and cardiac arrest during the acute phase of myocardial infarction.[51,52] The long-term beta-blocker post–myocardial infarction trials and other clinical studies with beta blockers have demonstrated that there is a significant reduction of complex ventricular arrhythmias.[53-57]

## CLINICAL TRIALS OF BETA-ADRENERGIC BLOCKING DRUGS IN THE PREVENTION OF SUDDEN DEATH

Although no one has demonstrated that suppression of ventricular ectopy reduces sudden cardiac death in human beings, several clinical trials have used beta-adrenergic blocking drugs to assess their efficacy in reducing the incidence of sudden death after myocardial infarction.[53,58-63] However, none of these trials was designed to determine whether changes in sudden death incidence were related to drug efficacy in suppressing ventricular arrhythmias.[36]

Beta-adrenergic blocking drugs have several pharmacologic features that might make them protective against sudden cardiac death. First, beta blockers interfere with the adverse effects of the autonomic nervous system on cardiac electrophysiology, and by this mechanism, could raise the ventricular fibrillation threshold.[13,36,50] Second, some beta blockers have direct intrinsic antiarrhythmic properties[13,27,36] Third, beta blockers can reduce the myocardial workload by their hemodynamic actions, thereby preventing myocardial ischemia and the potential for arrhythmogenesis.[64] More subtle actions of beta blockers include favorable effects on platelet function and myocardial metabolism.[64]

Clinical trials designed to study the effects of beta blockers on survival have focused on two population groups. The first group of studies examined the effects of beta blockers in patients during the hyperacute and early phases of myocardial infarction. These acute-phase studies were directed toward influencing the immediate in-hospital mortality and reducing myocardial infarct size.[65,66] It was postulated that the reduction of myocardial infarction size by beta blockers might favorably affect long-term mortality.[65] However, only one of these early-intervention clinical trials with beta blockers showed statistically significant benefit on survival.[67] Many of these trials actually demonstrated unfavorable effects of beta blockers.[65,68] In the one trial reporting statistically favorable results on survival, it is not known whether the benefit seen with the beta blocker was related to the 90-day oral maintenance regimen, or the early intravenous treatment intervention.[67]

The second group of studies enrolled patients who had survived the early phase of myocardial infarction, and these studies compared survival in those subjects given chronic beta-blocker therapy versus placebo.[69-72] Although prevention of sudden cardiac death was considered a potential beneficial action of beta blockade in these trials, most studies focused on all-cause mortality as the primary endpoint. This may have resulted from the difficulty in defining and establishing sudden cardiac death, and, in part, the importance of all-cause death.

Included in this review are the findings from randomized controlled clinical trials that report on the effects of beta-blocker therapy on the risk of all-cause mortality and sudden cardiac death in patients who had survived an acute myocardial infarction.[53,58-63] Excluded from this review are those trials where sudden cardiac death was not reported,[73,74] and studies that were too small in size to achieve any statistical power.

Study results are presented using the intent-to-treat approach, that is, all randomized patients are accounted for in the group to which they had been assigned. Some of the studies discussed have used other primary statistical analyses, and this explains why the results reported here may differ from those published elsewhere. In the seven trials meeting our review criteria, the beta-blocker intervention was started after patients had stabilized, usually 1 to 3 weeks after infarction, with therapy continued for at least 1 year.[53,58-63] Study design features, including the beta blocker and the dose used, the time when treatment was initiated, and the length of treatment, are shown in Table 4.

## Definition of Sudden Cardiac Death

The primary endpoint in all the trials was death, that is, all-cause mortality. Sudden cardiac death according to various definitions was also an endpoint. In essence, each trial utilized the onset of premonitory symptoms or new symptoms as the starting point for measurement of time. Death occurring within 24 hours of symptom onset constituted the definition in three trials.[58-60] Death occurring within 1 hour of symptoms and excluding only violent deaths, was used in a fourth study.[61] A fifth trial reported all nonviolent deaths both for the 24-hour and 1-hour definition.[53] Another study divided the cardiac deaths known to have taken place within 24 hours into four time segments: first hour, second hour, 1 to 12 hours, and 12 to 24 hours.[62] The seventh report applied the following three definitions: witnessed instantanoues death, death witnessed but preceded by chest pain of less than 1 hour's duration, and patients found dead but seen alive and free of chest pain less than 12 hours earlier.[63] Three trials reported data on the frequency of instantaneous death.[60,61,63]

**Table 4.** Selected design features of long-term beta-blocker trials

| Trial | Patients randomized | Beta blocker | Daily dose (mg) | Entry time* (days) | Mean followup (mo) |
|---|---|---|---|---|---|
| Wilhelmsson et al[58] | 230 | Alprenolol | 400 | 7–21† | 24 |
| Ahlmark et al[59] | 393 | Alprenolol | 400 | 14 | 24 |
| Multicenter International Study[62] | 3053 | Practolol | 400 | 13.2 | 14 |
| Norwegian Multicenter Study[60] | 1884 | Timolol | 20 | 11.5 | 17 |
| BHAT[61] | 3837 | Propranolol | 180–240 | 13.8 | 25 |
| Hansteen et al[63] | 560 | Propranolol | 160 | 4–6 | 12 |
| Julian et al[53] | 1456 | Sotalol | 320 | 8.3 | 12 |

*Entry into study from time of hospitalization for MI.
†From discharge following hospitalization for MI.

**Table 5.** Selected results of long-term beta-blocker trials

| Trial | Patients Randomized | | All-Cause Mortality | | | Definition | Sudden Cardiac Death | | |
|---|---|---|---|---|---|---|---|---|---|
| | Intervention | Control | Intervention (%) | Control (%) | Risk Ratio (I/C) (%) | (hr) | Intervention (%) | Control (%) | Risk Ratio (I/C)(%) |
| Wilhelmsson et al[58] | 114 | 116 | 6.1 | 12.1 | 0.51 | ≤24 | 2.6 | 9.5 | 0.28 |
| Ahlmark et al[59] | 69* | 93* | 7.2 | 11.8 | 0.61 | ≤24 | 1.4 | 9.7 | 0.15 |
| Multicentre International Study[62] | 1533 | 1520 | 6.7 | 8.4 | 0.80 | ≤1 | 2.9† | 4.2† | 0.70 |
| Norwegian Multicenter Study[60] | 945 | 939 | 10.4 | 16.2 | 0.64 | ≤24 | 7.0 | 11.7 | 0.60 |
| BHAT[61] | 1916 | 1921 | 7.2 | 9.8 | 0.74 | ≤1 | 3.3 | 4.6 | 0.72 |
| Hansteen et al[63] | 278 | 282 | 9.0 | 13.1 | 0.69 | ≤1‡ | 4.0 | 8.2 | 0.49 |
| Julian et al[53] | 873 | 583 | 7.3 | 8.9 | 0.82 | ≤24 | 5.5 | 6.5 | 0.84 |
| Total | 5728 | 5454 | 7.7 | 10.7 | 0.72 | | 4.2 | 6.3 | 0.67 |

*Incomplete reporting.
†Sudden cardiac death rates underestimated due to missing information.
‡See text for exact definition.

## Antiarrhythmic Effects of Beta Blockers

Three of the seven trials obtained 24-hour ambulatory electrocardiographic recordings on a subset of their participants both at trial entry and at a subsequent followup visit.[53,60,61] The findings of these three trials are similar. In the subgroup of survivors who entered the trial with frequent ventricular premature beats (VPBs), fewer patients demonstrated this arrhythmia at a later followup visit than in the placebo group.[53,55,57] Among patients with frequent VPBs at entry, many continued to have this arrhythmias at followup, although fewer patients on beta blockers than on placebo.[53,55,57] Although the recorded episodes of ventricular tachycardia were few in all trials at followup, this arrhythmia was less common in patients on beta blockers than on placebo.

## Effect on All-Cause Mortality and Sudden Cardiac Death

All-cause mortality was lower in the beta-blocker-treated group compared with the control group for all seven long-term trials (Table 5). Statistical signficance was reached in three of the trials.[60-62] The relative differences in mortality rates are expressed as risk ratios (intervention group mortality divided by control group mortality), which range from 0.51 to 0.82. When all data are combined, the weighted mean is 0.72, which indicates an overall reduction in all-cause mortality in the trials of 28 percent.

The rates of sudden cardiac deaths are also lower in the beta-blocker group for all seven trials. There seems to be a trend toward a greater overall reduction in sudden cardiac death than in all-cause mortality resulting from beta-blocker treatment (see Table 5). The weighted risk ratios for sudden cardiac death vary between 0.15 and 0.84 with a weighted mean of 0.67, indicating an overall reduction of 33 percent in sudden cardiac deaths. Indeed, if the sudden cardiac deaths are subtracted from all-cause mortality, the remaining death rate is 3.5 percent in the intervention group, and 4.4 percent in control, which represents an intervention/control risk ratio for non-sudden death of 0.80. Thus, while non-sudden deaths are reduced by 20 percent in these trials, the sudden cardiac death rate is reduced to a greater extent.

In the five largest trials, the intervention/control risk ratio for non-sudden death ranged from 0.75 to 1.02.[53,60-63] The two smallest trials had the most favorable risk ratios of intervention to control, that is, 0.51 and 0.61 for all-cause mortality and 0.25 and 0.15 for sudden cardiac death.[58,59] However, these same studies had intervention-to-control risk ratios of 1.4 and 2.8 for non-sudden death. Although it may be argued that this unfavorable difference on non-sudden cardiac death may relate to the specific beta blocker used, a more probable explanation is the potential for chance associated with small patient numbers.

For witnessed instantaneous deaths, an even larger relative benefit from beta-blocker therapy was recorded. The reduction was 59 percent in one study,[60] 46 percent in the second,[63] and 37 percent in the third,[61] corresponding to an average reduction in instantaneous death of 46 percent. For these three trials, the pooled reduction in all-cause mortality was 31 percent, indicating that the relative reduction in instantaneous death is about 50 percent higher than that of all-cause mortality. When, as above, the instantaneous deaths are removed from the all-cause mortality, the pooled reduction in death in the remaining patients becomes 23 percent, and the relative reduction in instantaneous deaths twice as great.

## Conclusions and Clinical Impact

The varied definitions and the difficulty in ascertaining sudden cardiac death have been recognized. When the results of these seven trials involving 11,182 patients are combined, 344 (59 percent) of the 584 deaths in the placebo-treated group are considered sudden.

The results of these long-term beta-blocker trials in survivors of acute myocardial infarction who qualified for treatment demonstrate a clinically and statistically significant reduction in

261

both all-cause mortality and sudden cardiac death of 28 percent and 33 percent respectively. Whether certain beta blockers are more effective than others in improving on this benefit has not been well defined. The two beta blockers approved by the FDA for reducing mortality in infarct survivors (timolol and propranolol) are both nonselective without partial agonism; both drugs have also been shown to favorably affect the risk of sudden cardiac death.[60,61]

Continued efforts are needed to subdivide the population of myocardial infarction survivors into those who will have relatively greater and lower benefits from chronic beta-adrenergic blockade. The prognosis of some patient subgroups may be sufficiently favorable without this prophylactic therapy, so that any improvement on survival with beta blockers may not outweigh the potential side effects, costs, and inconvenience.[75,76] Others believe that all postinfarction patients should be treated even in the low-risk subgroup.[77,78] When treating patients with beta blockers, the length of time following myocardial infarction for which such therapy continues to yield clinical benefit remains undefined. Consensus seems to be that therapy for at least 2 to 3 years is warranted.

Though some details of patient selection may undergo refinement, the role of beta-adrenergic blockers in the management of most survivors of myocardial infarction is now established as a means for decreasing the risk of both sudden and non-sudden cardiac death. Whether or not similar protective benefits on mortality and sudden cardiac death can be achieved in high-risk patients who have not yet had a myocardial infarction remains to be determined.

# REFERENCES

1. AHLQUIST, RP: *A study of the adrenotropic receptors.* Am J Physiol 153:586, 1948.

2. LANDS, AM, ARNOLD, A, MCAULIFF, JP, ET AL: *Differentiation of receptor systems activated by sympathomimetic amines.* Nature 214:597, 1967.

3. DUNLOP, D AND SHANKS, RG: *Selective blockade of adrenoceptive beta-receptors in the heart.* Br J Pharmacol Chemother 32:201, 1968.

4. LEFKOWITZ, RJ: *Selectivity in β-adrenergic response.* Circulation 49:783, 1974.

5. BLACK, JW AND STEPHENSON, JS: *Pharmacology of a new adrenergic β-receptor blocking compound (nethalide).* Lancet 2:311, 1962.

6. FRISHMAN, W: *Clinical pharmacology of the new β-adrenergic blocking drugs: Part 1. Pharmacodynamic and pharmacokinetic properties.* Am Heart J 97:663, 1979.

7. WAAL-MANNING, HJ: *Hypertension: Which β-blocker?* Drugs 12:412, 1976.

8. CONNOLLY, ME, KEUSTING, F, AND DOLLERY, CT: *The clinical pharmacology of β-adrenoreceptor blocking drugs.* Prog Cardiovasc Dis 19:203, 1976.

9. BARRETT, AM AND CULLUM, VA: *The biological properties of the optical isomers of propranolol and their effect on cardiac arrhythmias.* Br J Pharmacol 34:43, 1968.

10. BRUNNER, H, HEADWALL, PR, AND, MAIER, R: *Pharmacologic pro aspects of oxprenolol.* Postgrad Med J (Suppl) 1970, p 5.

11. BASIL, B, JORDAN, R, LOVELESS, AH, ET AL: *β-Adrenoceptor blocking properties and cardioselectivity of M and B 17,803A.* Br J Pharmacol 48:198, 1973.

12. SINGH, BN: *Clinical aspects of the antiarrhythmic action of β-receptor blocking drugs: Part 2. Clinical pharmacology.* NZ Med J 78:529, 1973.

13. SINGH, BN AND JEWITT, DE: *β-Adrenergic receptor drugs in cardiac arrhythmias.* Drugs 7:426, 1974.

14. POWELL, CE AND SLATER, IH: *Blocking of inhibitory adrenergic response.* Circulation 49:783, 1974.

15. OPIE, LH: *Drugs and the heart: β-Blocking agents.* Lancet 1:693, 1980.

16. FRISHMAN, WH AND KOSTIS, J: *The significance of intrinsic sympathomimetic activity in beta-adrenergic blocking drugs.* Cardiovascular Reviews and Reports 30:503, 1982.

17. FRISHMAN, W AND SILVERMAN, R: *Clinical pharmacology of the new β-adrenergic blocking drugs: Part 3: Comparative clinical experience and new therapeutic applications.* Am Heart J 98:119, 1979.

18. FRISHMAN, W AND SILVERMAN, R: *Clinical pharmacology of the new β-adrenergic blocking drugs: Part 2. Physiologic and metabolic effects.* Am Heart J 97:797, 1979.

19. ATTERHOG, JH, DUNER, H, AND PERNOW, B: *Experience with pindolol, a β-receptor blocker in the treatment of hypertension.* Am J Med 60:872, 1976.

20. ARONOW, WS AND UYEYAMA, RR: *Treatment of arrhythmias with pindolol.* Clin Pharmacol Ther 13:15, 1972.

21. KOCH-WESER, J: *Metoprolol.* N Engl J Med 301:698, 1979.

22. LETORA, JJL, MARK, AL, JOHANNSEN, UJ, ET AL: *Selective $\beta_1$-receptor blockade with oral practolol in man.* J Clin Invest 56:719, 1975.

23. FITZGERALD, JD: *Cardioselective $\beta$-adrenergic blockade.* Proc Soc Med 65:761, 1972.

24. FRISHMAN, WH: *Pindolol: A new $\beta$-adrenoceptor antagonist with partial agonist activity.* N Engl J Med 308:940, 1983.

25. FRISHMAN, W AND HALPRIN, S: *Clinical pharmacology of the new beta-adrenergic blocking drugs: Part 7. New horizons in beta-adrenoceptor blockade therapy: Labetalol.* Am Heart J 98:660, 1979.

26. FRISHMAN, WH, STROM, J, KIRTSCHNER, M, ET AL: *Labetalol therapy in patients with systemic hypertension and angina pectoris: Effects of combined alpha and beta-adrenoreceptor blockade.* Am J Cardiol 48:917, 1981.

27. FRISHMAN, W: *$\beta$-Adrenoceptor antagonists: New drugs and new indications.* N Engl J Med 305:500, 1981.

28. JOHNSON, G AND REGARDH, CG: *Clinical pharmacokinetics of $\beta$-adrenoreceptor blocking drugs.* Clin Pharmacokinet 1:233, 1976.

29. FRISHMAN, WH AND TEICHER, M: *Long-acting propranolol.* Cardiovascular Reviews and Reports 4:1100, 1983.

30. FRISHMAN, W: *Nadolol—a new $\beta$-adrenoceptor antagonist.* N Engl J Med 305:678, 1981.

31. FRISHMAN, WH: *Atenolol and timolol—two new systemic $\beta$-adrenoreceptor antagonists.* N Engl J Med 306:1456, 1982.

32. HEEL, RC, BROGDEN, RN, SPEIGHT, TM, ET AL: *Atenolol: A review of its pharmacological properties and therapeutic efficacy in angina pectoris and hypertension.* Drugs 17:425, 1979.

33. HEEL, RC, BROGDEN, RN, PAKES, GE, ET AL: *Nadolol: A review of its pharmacological properties and therapeutic efficacy in hypertension and angina pectoris.* Drugs 20:1, 1980.

34. CRUICKSHANK, JM: *The clinical importance of cardioselectivity and lipophilicity in beta-blockers.* Am Heart J 100:160, 1980.

35. KOCH-WESER, J AND SELLERS, EM: *Binding of drugs to serum albumin.* N Engl J Med 294:311, 526, 1976.

36. PRATT, C AND LICHSTEIN, E: *Ventricular antiarrhythmic effects of beta-adrenergic blocking drugs: A review of mechanism and clinical studies.* J Clin Pharmacol 22:335, 1982.

37. LEVY, JV AND RICHARDS, V: *Inotropic and chronotropic effects of a series of $\beta$-adrenergic blocking drugs: Some structure activity relationships.* Proc Soc Exp Biol Med 122:373, 1966.

38. VAUGHAN WILLIAMS, EM AND PAPP, J: *The effect of oxprenolol on cardiac intracellular potentials in relation to its antiarrhythmic local anesthetic and other properties.* Postgrad Med J 46:22, 1970.

39. FRISHMAN, WH: *$\beta$-Adrenergic blockade in the treatment of coronary artery disease.* In *Clinical Essay on the Heart,* Vol II. McGraw-Hill, New York, 1983.

40. LATOUR, Y, DUMONT, G, BROSSEAU, A, ET AL: *Effects of sotalol in twenty patients with cardiac arrhythmias.* Int J Clin Pharmacol 15:275, 1977.

41. PRAKASH, R, ALLEN, HN, CONDO, F, ET AL: *Clinical evaluation of the antiarrhythmic effects of sotalol.* Am J Cardiol 26:654, 1970.

42. SIMON, A AND BERMAN, E: *Long-term sotalol therapy in patients with arrhythmias.* J Clin Pharmacol 19:547, 1979.

43. BURCKHARDT, D, PFISTERER, M, HOFFMAN, A, ET AL: *Effects of the beta-adrenoceptor blocking agent sotalol on ventricular arrhythmias in patients with chronic ischemic heart disease: A placebo-controlled, double-blind crossover study.* Cardiology 70(Suppl 1):114, 1983.

44. COLTART, DJ, GIBSON, DG, AND SHAND, DG: *Plasma propranolol levels associated with suppression of ventricular ectopic beats.* Br Med J 3:731, 1970.

45. GIBSON, DG: *Pharmacodynamic properties of $\beta$-adrenergic receptor blocking drugs in man.* 7:8, 1974.

46. GIUDICELLI, JF, LHOSTE, F, AND BOSSIER, JR: *$\beta$-Adrenergic blockade and atrioventricular conduction impairment.* Eur J Pharmacol 31:216, 1975.

47. TAYLOR, RR AND HALLIDAY, EJ: *$\beta$-Adrenergic blockade in the treatment of exercise-induced paroxysmal ventricular tachycardia.* Circulation 32:778, 1965.

48. SLOMAN, G AND STANNARD, M: *$\beta$-Adrenergic blockade and cardiac arrhythmias.* 4:508, 1967.

49. GETTES, LS AND SURAWICZ, B: *Long-term prevention of paroxysmal arrhythmias with propranolol therapy.* Am J Med Sci 254:256, 1967.

50. ANDERSON, JL, RODIER, HE, AND GREEN, LS: *Comparative effects of beta-adrenergic blocking drugs on experimental ventricular fibrillation threshold.* Am J Cardiol 51:1196, 1983.

51. RYDÉN, L, ARINIEGO, R, ARNMAN, K, ET AL: *A double-blind trial of metoprolol in acute myocardial infarction: Effects on ventricular tachyarrhythmias.* N Engl J Med 308:614, 1983.

52. YUFUF, S, SLEIGHT, P, AND ROSSI, P: *Reduction in infarct size, arrhythmias, and chest pain by early intravenous beta-blockade in suspected acute myocardial infarction.* Circulation 67(Suppl 1):32, 1983.

53. JULIAN, DG, PRESCOTT, RJ, JACKSON, FS, ET AL: *Controlled trial of sotalol for one year after myocardial infarction.* Lancet 1:1142, 1982.

54. HJALMARSON, Å, HERLITZ, J, HOLMBERG, S, ET AL: *The Goteborg metoprolol study: Effects on mortality and morbidity in acute myocardial infarction.* Circulation 67(Suppl 1):26, 1983.

55. LICHSTEIN, E, MORGANROTH, J, HARRIST, R, ET AL: *Effect of propranolol on ventriuclar arrhythmias: The Beta-Blocker Heart Attack Trial.* Circulation 67(Suppl 1):5, 1983.

56. KOPPES, GM, BECKMANN, CH, AND JONES, FG: *Propranolol therapy for ventricular arrhythmias two months after acute myocardial infarction.* Am J Cardiol 46:322, 1980.

57. VON DER LIPPE, G AND LUND-JOHANSEN, P: *Effect of timolol on late ventricular arrhythmias after myocardial infarction.* Acta Med Scand 651(Suppl):253, 1981.

58. WILHELMSSON, C, VEDIN, JA, WILHELMSEN, L, ET AL: *Reduction of sudden deaths after myocardial infarction by treatment with alprenolol: Preliminary results.* Lancet 2:1157, 1974.

59. AHLMARK, G AND SAETRE, H: *Long-term treatment with beta-blockers after myocardial infarction.* Eur J Clin Pharmacol 10:77, 1976.

60. NORWEGIAN MULTICENTER STUDY GROUP: *Timolol-induced reduction in mortality and reinfarction in patients surviving acute myocardial infarction.* N Engl J Med 304:801, 1981.

61. BETA-BLOCKER HEART ATTACK TRIAL RESEARCH GROUP: *A randomized trial of propranolol in patients with acute myocardial infarction: I. Mortality results.* JAMA 247:1707, 1981.

62. MULTICENTRE INTERNATIONAL STUDY: *Reduction in mortality after myocardial infarction with long-term beta-adrenoreceptor blockade: Supplementary report.* Br Med J 2:419, 1977.

63. HANSTEEN, V, MOINICHEN, E, LORENTSEN, E, ET AL: *One year's treatment with propranolol after myocardial infarction: Preliminary report of Norwegian multicentre trial.* Br Med J 284:155, 1982.

64. FRISHMAN, WH: *Multifactorial actions of β-adrenergic blocking drugs in ischemic heart disease: Current concepts.* Circulation 67(Suppl I):11, 1983.

65. MAY, GS: *A review of acute-phase beta-blocker trials in patients with myocardial infarction.* Circulation 68(Suppl I):21, 1983.

66. MULLER, J, ROBERTS, R, STONE, P, ET AL: *Failure of propranolol administration to limit infarct size in patients with acute myocardial infarction.* Circulation 68(Suppl III):294, 1983.

67. HJALMARSON, Å, ELMFELDT, D, HERLITZ, J, ET AL: *Effect on mortality of metoprolol in acute myocardial infarction.* Lancet 2:823, 1981.

68. WILCOX, RG, ROWLEY, JM, HAMPTON, JR, ET AL: *Randomized placebo-controlled trial comparing oxprenolol with disopyramide phosphate in immediate treatment of suspected myocardial infarction.* Lancet 2:765, 1980.

69. MAY, GS: *A review of long-term beta-blocker trials in survivors of myocardial infarction.* Circulation 68(Suppl I):46, 1983.

70. TAYLOR, SH, SILKE, B, EBBUTT, A, ET AL: *A long-term prevention study with oxprenolol in coronary heart disease.* N Engl J Med 307:1293, 1982.

71. AUSTRALIAN AND SWEDISH PINDOLOL STUDY GROUP: *The effect of pindolol on the two year mortality after complicated myocardial infarction.* Eur Heart J 4:367, 1983.

72. EUROPEAN INFARCTION STUDY GROUP: *European Infarction Study (E.I.S.)—A secondary beta-blocker prevention trial after myocardial infarction.* Circulation 68(Suppl III):294, 1983.

73. BABER, NS, WAINWRIGHT-EVANS, D, HOWITT, G, ET AL: *Multicentre post-infarction trial of propranolol in 49 hospitals in the United Kingdom, Italy and Yugoslavia.* Br Heart J 44:96, 1980.

74. CORONARY PREVENTION RESEARCH GROUP: *An early intervention secondary prevention study with oxprenolol following myocardial infarction.* Eur Heart J 2:389, 1981.

75. CHAMBERLAIN, DA: *Beta-adrenoceptor antagonists after myocardial infarction—where are we now?* Br Heart J 49:105, 1983.

76. GRIGGS, TR, WAGNER, GS, AND GETTES, LS: *Beta-adrenergic blocking agents after myocardial infarction: An undocumented need in patients at lowest risk.* J Am Coll Cardiol 1:1530, 1983.

77. FRISHMAN, WH, FURBERG, CD, AND FRIEDEWALD, WT: *Beta-adrenergic blockade for survivors of acute myocardial infarction.* N Engl J Med 310:830, 1984.

78. FRISHMAN, WH, FURBERG, CD, AND FRIEDEWALD, WT: *The use of beta-adrenergic blocking drugs in patients with myocardial infarction.* Curr Probl Cardiol 9(3):1, 1984.

264

# The Role of Antiarrhythmic Drugs
# in Prevention of Sudden Cardiac Death

*Philip J. Podrid, M.D.*

Sudden cardiac death continues to be a major health problem in the United States. It is the leading cause of mortality, accounting for 400,000 to 600,000 deaths annually.[1] Despite the enormous magnitude of the problem, it has been long ignored by the medical profession. This is largely a result of a prevailing viewpoint that it was the inevitable outcome of far-advanced cardiac pathology. Sudden cardiac death is the most frequent mode of death in patients with coronary artery disease, but it also afflicts those who have other types of heart disease including cardiomyopathy, valvular lesions, and congenital abnormalities. There is a small subset of patients who die suddenly in whom there is no demonstrable structural heart disease and who are considered to have primarily electrical failure.

Although most patients who succumb suddenly have underlying cardiac disease, it is not always extensive or far advanced. The coronary care unit,[2] the mobile coronary units, and large-scale community-based CPR programs[3] have repeatedly shown that the terminal episode can be reversed. Once reversed, it is not likely to recur immediately. This has been found most convincingly in patients who have had a myocardial infarction associated with sudden death. The occurrence of a cardiac arrest during the acute phase does not affect long-term prognosis, and patients may lead normal lives thereafter.

Although sudden death can occur in the setting of an acute myocardial infarction, the majority of out-of-hospital cases of sudden death are not precipitated by coronary thrombosis or myocardial necrosis.[4,5] In most cases, sudden death is the result of primary electrical failure. Unlike a myocardial infarction, this catastrophe occurs instantaneously and without prodromes. It is well established that the underlying rhythm disturbance resulting in sudden cardiac death is ventricular fibrillation[6] (Fig. 1). This terminal arrhythmia is an electrical accident, afflicting the myocardium that is electrically unstable. Such an electrical lesion results from underlying myocardial disease that alters and distorts the electrical properties of the His-Purkinje system and ventricular myocardium. Certain types of ventricular premature beats are the clinical manifestations of this electrical instability.[2,6] Although the presence of this electrophysiologic derangement is a necessary precondition for the occurrence of ventricular fibrillation, it is not sufficient per se to cause sudden death. The electrophysiologic abnormality is continuously present, but ventricular fibrillation is a rare, episodic, and sporadic event that is not likely to immediately recur once terminated. Therefore, there must be a transient "risk factor" that alters the electrical properties of the unstable myocardium and triggers ventricular fibrillation.[1,7] There are a number of such transient factors including electrolyte disorders, pH alteration, coronary spasm, platelet aggregation, drugs, and, most importantly, higher nervous activity. Impulses from the brain, transmitted to the heart via the autonomic nervous system, especially the sympathetic limb, have profound effects on myo-

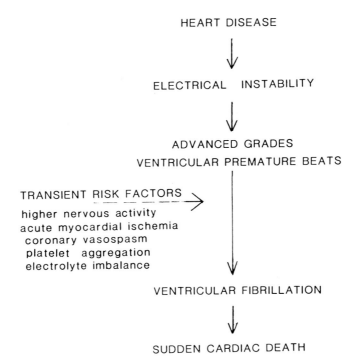

HEART DISEASE

ELECTRICAL INSTABILITY

ADVANCED GRADES
VENTRICULAR PREMATURE BEATS

TRANSIENT RISK FACTORS
higher nervous activity
acute myocardial ischemia
coronary vasospasm
platelet aggregation
electrolyte imbalance

VENTRICULAR FIBRILLATION

SUDDEN CARDIAC DEATH

**Figure 1.** Hypothesis for the occurrence of sudden cardiac death. Heart disease leads to the development of myocardial electrical instability. Ventricular premature beats, especially repetitive forms, are the clinical markers for this instability. Transient risk factors, such as higher nervous activity, can alter the electrical properties of the heart, provoking ventricular fibrillation and sudden cardiac death.

cardial electrophysiologic properties.[8] Changes in autonomic tone have major effects on myocardial vulnerability to ventricular tachyarrhythmias.

## ASSOCIATION OF VENTRICULAR PREMATURE BEATS AND SUDDEN CARDIAC DEATH

The clinical manifestation of myocardial electrical instability is the ventricular premature beat (VPB), which can be readily identified and quantified. A number of studies have shown that there is a direct correlation between VPB frequency and the risk of sudden cardiac death. Hinkle and coworkers[9] monitored 665 asymptomatic men for 6 hours and subdivided them based on the frequency of VPBs. After a 2½-year followup, cardiac mortality in those with more than 10 VPBs per 1000 complexes was almost 12-fold greater compared with those without VPBs. A number of other large scale epidemiologic studies have also demonstrated that the VPB is an independent risk factor for sudden death, especially in persons with coronary artery disease.[10,11] However, in these studies, ECG rhythm strips only were recorded, and thus only a brief period of monitoring data was obtained. More recent studies have extended ambulatory monitoring to periods of up to 24 hours. When these longer periods of monitoring are employed, VPBs can be observed in almost 90 percent of asymptomatic patients as well as those with known coronary artery disease.[12,13] If VPBs are ubiquitous in the population, how then can they be a risk factor?

During the early coronary care unit experience, Lown and Wolf[2] observed that certain types of VPBs were benign, associated with a good prognosis, whereas other forms of ventricular ectopy were serious—often precursors of malignant sustained ventricular tachyar-

**Table 1.** Lown grading system of ventricular premature beats (VPBs)

| Grade | Description |
|---|---|
| 0 | No VPBs |
| 1A | < 30 VPBs/hour and < 1/minute |
| 1B | < 30 VPBs/hour and occasionally > 1/minute |
| 2 | > 30 VPBs/hour |
| 3 | Multiform VPBs |
| 4A | Repetitive VPBs-couplets |
| 4B | Repetitive VPBs-ventricular tachycardia (> 3 sequential) |
| 5 | Early R-on-T VPBs |

rhythmias. On the basis of these observations, they developed a grading system (Table 1). Implicit in the system was that higher grades of VPBs were more serious, associated with greater risk. According to the Lown classification, grades 4 and 5 (the complex VBPs) were particularly hazardous when present in patients with an acute myocardial infarction. A number of studies have confirmed and extended these early observations (Table 2). Kotler and coworkers[14] reported that among 160 patients with a recent myocardial infarction, VPBs increased the incidence of sudden death from 3 to 19 percent during a followup of 30 to 54 months. However, the presence of ventricular tachycardia (VT) further enhanced the risk and was associated with a 60 percent mortality. Vismara and coworkers[15] reported that the frequency of complex arrhythmias in the late hospital phase after a myocardial infarction was significantly greater in those who died during the followup period compared with patients who survived. VanDurme and Pannier[16] reported that repetitive VPBs in patients after myocardial infarction had significant relationship to sudden death. Schulze and coworkers[17] reported that during a 7-month followup of patients after a myocardial infarction, sudden death occurred only among those who had complex arrhythmias and an ejection fraction less than 40 percent. They concluded that the presence of complex arrhythmia was an independent risk factor for differentiating those at greater risk for sudden death. Moss and coworkers[18] followed 978 patients with a definite or probable myocardial infarction for an average of 40 months. In those without VPBs, the sudden death rate was 4 percent. The occurrence of simple VPBs, regardless of frequency, increased the incidence of sudden death to 7 percent, but this was not significant (p = 0.09). The presence of complex VPBs was associated with a sudden death rate of 15 percent. This was significant when compared with the incidence in those who had no VPBs (p < 0.01 or simple VPBs (p = 0.03). When controlling for 10 variables, complex ventricular ectopy was an independent risk factor for sudden cardiac death. An important and decisive study from Ruberman and coworkers[19] of the Health Insurance Plan of New York confirmed the association of complex arrhythmias and

**Table 2.** Ventricular arrhythmias after myocardial infarction

| | | | Sudden death % | |
|---|---|---|---|---|
| Study | N | Duration | No complex VEA | Complex VEA |
| Bigger | 430 | 1 year | 12 | 38 |
| Kotler | 160 | 3 years | 20 | 60 |
| Moss | 978 | 3 years | 4 | 15 |
| Mukhaije | 388 | 14 months | 3 | 16 |
| Rappaport | 139 | 11 months | 6 | 34 |
| Ruberman | 1739 | 5 years | 8 | 25 |

VEA = ventricular ectopic activity.

increased mortality. One hour of sedentary ECG recording was performed on 1739 men, all of whom had a myocardial infarction within 3 months of entry. After a followup of up to 5 years (average 3.5 years) there was a close association between type of VPBs and outcome. The presence of runs of VPBs or early VPBs was associated with a 25 percent incidence of sudden death, contrasted to a 6 percent incidence when no VPBs were present. The occurrence of simple VBPs or any other complex forms increased mortality to 12 percent. The sudden death rate was constant for each year after the baseline evaluation. These authors also evaluated the role of other variables including the presence of congestive heart failure or diuretic use, occurrence of angina, conduction abnormality, ST segment depression, or the duration of heart disease. Regardless of the variable, the presence of complex ventricular arrhythmia increased the risk of sudden death by two- to threefold. Bigger and coworkers[20] found this same association among 430 patients with a myocardial infarction. In their series, the presence of ventricular tachycardia ($\geq$ 3 successive VPBs) increased the risk of death fivefold. Importantly, this association was independent of the rate, frequency, or length of the ventricular tachycardia. Rapaport and Remedios[21] reported that the presence of complex ventricular arrhythmia in patients after myocardial infarction increased the first-year mortality from 6 percent to 34 percent. Finally, Mukhaije and coworkers[22] reported on 325 patients randomized in the multicenter study of infarct size limitation (MILIS) and found that the presence of Lown grades 4A and 4B had the strongest correlation with subsequent sudden death (p = 0.0001).

It can be concluded that in patients with coronary artery disease and recent myocardial infarction, the presence of repetitive arrhythmia constitutes an independent risk factor and places the patient at increased risk for subsequent cardiac mortality, especially sudden death. Similar data in the much larger group of those with coronary artery disease and no prior infarction are as yet lacking. A similar association between complex arrhythmia and sudden death has been observed in patients with congestive cardiomyopathy. In the study by Follansbee and coworkers,[23] 9 of 19 patients with nonsustained ventricular tachycardia on monitoring died suddenly in contrast to only 1 death in the group of 18 patients without this arrhythmia (p < 0.005). As observed in patients with coronary disease, the occurrence of ventricular tachycardia, but not other types of VPBs, was a risk factor.

## DO ANTIARRHYTHMIC DRUGS PREVENT SUDDEN CARDIAC DEATH?

Although there is a clear relationship between the presence of certain types of VPBs and the risk of sudden death, it remains unclear whether suppression of these forms with antiarrhythmic drugs will reduce the incidence of sudden death. In order to answer this question, a population at risk must be identified and studied. The incidence of sudden death in patients with coronary artery disease is approximately 2 to 3 percent a year.[9] Any prospective study involving this population would require several thousand subjects before significance could be established. Patients who have had a myocardial infarction are at increased risk for sudden death during the first year and represent an important group for study.[14,15] There have been a number of such studies in post–myocardial infarction patients using membrane-active antiarrhythmic drugs and beta-adrenergic blocking agents.

## MEMBRANE-ACTIVE DRUGS AFTER MYOCARDIAL INFARCTION

### Lidocaine

Lidocaine was first used in patients admitted to the coronary care units[24] and subsequently has become the most frequently used antiarrhythmic drug for the acute treatment and prevention of ventricular arrhythmias in patients after myocardial infarction. Although the drug is in widespread use, it is unclear whether its prophylactic use has improved survival in the

**Table 3.** Results of randomized trials with lidocaine and its congeners

| Study | Drug | N | Duration of therapy | % Mortality or VF Control | Drug | P |
|-------|------|---|---------------------|---------------------------|------|---|
| Morgensen | Lidocaine | 79 | Days | 11 | 12 | NS |
| Chopra | Lidocaine | 82 | Days | ? | ? | NS |
| Bennett | Lidocaine | 610 | Days | 7 | 16 | NS |
| Lie | Lidocaine | 212 | Days | 10 | 0 | < 0.05 |
| Campbell | Tocainide | 68 | ? | ? | ? | ? |
| Ryden | Tocainide | 112 | 6 months | 8.9 | 8.9 | NS |
| Campbell | Mexiletine | 97 | 48 hours | 3.8 | 2.3 | NS |
| Chamberlain | Mexiletine | 344 | 1 year | 11..6 | 13.2 | NS |
| Hugenholtz | Aprindine | 193 | 1 year | 9.3 | 7.3 | NS |

coronary care unit or whether a reduction in mortality is the result of immediate intervention for termination of serious tachyarrhythmias occuring in the post–myocardial infarction period. There have been a number of studies that have addressed this problem (Table 3). In 1970, Bennett and coworkers[25] compared placebo with intravenous lidocaine in three groups of patients. Group A consisted of 203 patients who received 0.5 mg/min of drug; group B included 203 patients who received 1 mg/min of lidocaine; and 204 patients in group C received placebo. The researchers did not find any significant difference in the occurrence of ventricular premature beats, ventricular tachycardia, or ventricular fibrillation among the three groups. Pitt and coworkers[26] administered lidocaine (2.5 mg/ml) to 108 patients and placebo to 114. The incidence of ventricular arrhythmias was 10 percent in lidocaine-treated patients compared with 30 percent in those not receiving drug (p < 0.01). Although the drug effectively suppressed arrhythmias in those with an uncomplicated myocardial infarction and in patients with hypotension or congestive heart failure, there was no difference in mortality. It is important to note that in this study no loading dose of lidocaine was given and the infusion dose was low, probably subtherapeutic. Moreover, patients in the control group who developed tachyarrhythmias were withdrawn and were treated with lidocaine. From these studies, therefore, the role of lidocaine in preventing sudden death is unclear. In a study by Morgensen,[27] a 75-mg bolus of lidocaine, followed by an infusion of 2 mg/min, was given to 42 patients, and 37 were not treated. Although the frequency of VPBs was not altered, the occurrence of early VPBs and episodes of ventricular tachycardia were significantly reduced by lidocaine (p < 0.05 and p < 0.01 respectively). Mortality, however, was not affected. As with previous studies, patients receiving placebo who developed ventricular tachycardia were treated with 75-mg bolus of lidocaine and were removed from the trial. Chopra and coworkers[28] administered lidocaine or placebo to 82 patients as part of a double-blind trial. A bolus of 50 mg was given initially, followed by an additional 100 mg if arrhythmia persisted. Immediately thereafter, an infusion of lidocaine was instituted at 1 mg/min and increased to 2 mg/min for persistent ventricular arrhythmia. As was reported by other studies, the frequency of ventricular arrhythmia was reduced by lidocaine, but mortality was not affected. Lie and coworkers[29] randomized 212 patients to treatment with lidocaine, 100 mg by bolus followed by 3 mg/min, or placebo. In the 105 patients who received placebo, the incidence of ventricular tachycardia was 6 percent and sudden death occurred in 10 percent. In the lidocaine group, only 2 percent had ventricular tachycardia and there were no episodes of sudden death (p < 0.05).

It can be concluded from these studies that low-dose lidocaine is ineffective for preventing malignant ventricular arrhythmias after MI, whereas there is a significant reduction when higher doses are used. In none of the studies was duration of therapy indicated although it may be assumed that it was limited to several days. Importantly, in some of the reports patients treated with placebo who developed potentially serious arrhythmia were withdrawn and received treatment with lidocaine. Data regarding the frequency of arrhythmia and presence of repetitive or sustained arrhythmia prior to drug therapy are not supplied. It is unclear from these studies whether ventricular tachycardia or fibrillation occurred in those patients with ventricular arrhythmia that persisted despite lidocaine. Nevertheless, it appears that when lidocaine is used in adequate doses, it is effective for preventing malignant ventricular arrhythmia in the immediate post-MI period. Because it is available only for intravenous use, lidocaine has no role in long-term therapy.

## Quinidine

Quinidine, a membrane-stabilizing drug, is an effective oral antiarrhythmic agent and is useful for long-term treatment of arrhythmias. There have been three studies in which this drug has been used in patients after MI (Table 4). Jones and coworkers[30] administered quinidine, 400 mg tid for 72 hours, to 45 patients and placebo to 58 patients. Quinidine significntly reduced the occurrence of clinically important ventricular arrhythmias ($p < 0.05$), especially salvos of ventricular tachycardia ($p < 0.01$). There was a reduction in mortality (8.9 percent versus 10.4 percent), but this decrease was not statistically significant. Holmberg and Bergman[31] used quinidine (600 mg bid) in 49 patients and placebo in 55 patients. Therapy was continued for 15 days and the presence of arrhythmia evaluated by daily auscultation and ECG rhythm strips. These investigators did not find any difference in the occurrence of arrhythmia or death. However, the dosing of drug used was unconventional and perhaps inadequate, while documentation of arrhythmia was crude and inaccurate. In a study by Bloomfield and coworkers,[32] quinidine was given to 27 patients and placebo to 26. The dose of drug was 300 mg q 3h for 3 doses followed by 300 mg q 6h for 5 days. Quinidine significantly reduced the frequency of all ventricular arrhythmias, especially serious ectopy, which the authors defined as $> 5$ VPBs/min, couplets, salvos of ventricular tachycardia, or early VPBs. No episodes of ventricular fibrillation occurred in either group. These authors also reported a 5-day trial of quinidine versus placebo in 23 patients admitted for acute coronary insufficiency without an MI.[33] In the quinidine-treatment group, the frequency of ventricular premature beats and the occurrence of serious ventricular arrhythmias were significantly reduced ($p < 0.001$), but there was no mortality in either group.

Quinidine is an effective antiarrhythmic drug that significantly reduces the frequency of ventricular arrhythmia. However, in the studies reported, the duration of therapy was brief (3 to 15 days), and no conclusions about the long-term efficacy of the drug can be established. The study by Jones and coworkers[30] showed an insignificant reduction in short-term mortal-

**Table 4.** Results of randomized trials with quinidine, procainamide, disopyramide, and phenytoin

| Study | Drug | N | Duration of therapy | % Mortality or VF Control | Drug | P |
|-------|------|---|---------------------|---------------------------|------|---|
| Jones | Quinidine | 103 | 72 hours | 12.4 | 8.9 | NS |
| Holmberg | Quinidine | 104 | 15 days | 7.2 | 10.7 | NS |
| Bloomfield | Quinidine | 53 | 5 days | 0 | 0 | NS |
| Jennings | Disopyramide | 95 | 1 year | 10.2 | 4.3 | NS |
| Zainol | Disopyramide | 60 | 3 weeks | 26.7 | 3.3 | $< 0.05$ |
| Koch Weser | Procainamide | 70 | 2–3 weeks | 6.1 | 0 | $< 0.05$ |
| Kosowsky | Procainamide | 78 | 1 year | 10.3 | 3.7 | $< 0.05$ |
| Collaborative | Phenytoin | 568 | 1 year | 11.0 | 9.4 | NS |
| Peter | Phenytoin | 150 | 2 years | 18 | 24 | NS |

ity, but there was no long-term followup. Therefore, the role of quinidine in preventing sudden death after MI remains unanswered.

## Disopyramide

Disopyramide is a membrane-active drug with electrophysiologic effects similar to those of quinidine. There have been three randomized studies using disopyramide in patients after MI (see Table 4). Jennings and coworkers[34] administered 400 mg of disopyramide daily to 46 patients and placebo to 49. During the 12-month followup, ventricular arrhythmias requiring additional therapy occurred in 42 patients who received placebo, whereas serious arrhythmias were documented in only 21 patients treated with disopyramide (p < 0.005). Death occurred in two patients on disopyramide and in five patients treated with placebo. It is noteworthy that patients who required immediate therapy for ventricular tachycardia, ventricular fibrillation, or frequent, early, or multiformed VPBs were excluded from this study. Zainal and coworkers[35] administered disopyramide to 30 patients with an acute MI admitted to open wards, and 30 patients were given placebo. Compared with placebo, disopyramide therapy resulted in a significant reduction in the number of patients with ventricular tachycardia (5 versus 17 patients, p < 0.01), number experiencing ventricular fibrillation (1 versus 8 patients, p < 0.05), and in total mortality (1 versus 11 patients, p < 0.0025). The authors did not comment, however, about duration of therapy or methods of arrhythmia documentation. Pouleur and coworkers[36] reported no difference in occurrence of serious ventricular arrhythmias among 64 patients treated with disopyramide or placebo. The incidence of sudden death was equivalent, but the number of episodes was small in each group.

The studies with disopyramide provide conflicting data about its role in preventing sudden death. It is unclear whether therapy affords protection, although the study by Zainal and coworkers[35] is suggestive.

## Procainamide

Procainamide is another membrane-stabilizing or local anesthetic agent that has electrophysiologic properties in vitro identical to those of quinidine. It is available for both intravenous and oral use. However, it has a short half-life and must be given every 3 to 4 hours to ensure a constant blood level. Additionally, side effects are frequent and limit long-term use. Koch Weser and coworkers[37] reported on 70 patients with acute myocardial infarctions randomized to therapy with procainamide or placebo (see Table 4). The initial dose of drug was 1000 mg, which was followed by 250 to 300 mg q 3h for an unspecified duration. Procainamide therapy significantly reduced the frequency and severity of ventricular arrhythmias. Over 90 percent of patients receiving placebo had ventricular arrhythmias, 33 percent had ventricular tachycardia, and ventricular fibrillation occurred in 6 percent. In the group receiving procainamide, 62 percent had ventricular arrhythmias but only 8 percent had ventricular tachycardia and there were no episodes of ventricular fibrillation. During the trial, three patients receiving placebo died suddenly, but there were no deaths in those receiving procainamide. Importantly, six patients receiving placebo were removed from study because of serious arrhythmias and each was given procainamide for suppression. Kosowsky and coworkers[38] studied 78 patients randomized to therapy with procainamide or placebo. The dose of drug was 500 mg q 6 to 8h, with treatment continued for 1 year. Early side effects, occurring within the first few weeks, resulted in the discontinuation of procainamide in 9 of 39 patients; and late side effects, after 3 months of therapy, occurred in an additional 14 patients. Nevertheless, the incidence of major ventricular arrhythmias and sudden cardiac death were significantly reduced by procainamide therapy (p < 0.05). Both these studies demonstrate that procainamide is an effective antiarrhythmic agent that reduces sudden cardiac death in the post-infarction period. However, a high frequency of side effects necessitating drug discontinuation is a major problem that limits the usefulness of this agent for long-term therapy and prevention of sudden death.

**Phenytoin**

Phenytoin is primarily an anticonvulsant drug that has antiarrhythmic effects. It has a long half-life and can be given once a day. It also has few side effects, thus making it an attractive agent for long-term trials in patients after myocardial infarction (see Table 4). In 1971, a European collaborative trial using phenytoin was reported.[39] Phenytoin at a dose of 300 to 400 mg daily was given to 283 patients, and placebo (3 or 4 mg of phenytoin) was administered to 285 patients. During the 1-year followup, phenytoin reduced the frequency of symptomatic palpitations and occurrence of VPBs on ECG, but it did not improve survival (91 percent versus 89 percent for placebo, p = NS). In another study by Peter and coworkers,[40] 150 patients were randomized to treatment with phenytoin or placebo. Patients were divided into subgroups based on the presence of mechanical impairment defined as CHF or cardiogenic shock or electrical complications, that is, arrhythmias or conduction abnormalities. For the whole group, there was no significant difference in mortality between drug or placebo therapy (24 percent versus 18 percent) after a 2-year followup. No effect on mortality was observed in any of the subgroups.

Compared with studies using other membrane-active agents, these two trials with phenytoin involved larger numbers of patients followed for a longer period of time, that is, 1 to 2 years. Nevertheless, this drug was ineffective for protecting against death in patients after MI. This finding is consistent with the ineffectiveness of phenytoin for controlling chronic ventricular arrhythmias in adults. Because this agent is of little value and not a first-line antiarrhythmic drug, the negative results of these trials are not surprising and do not provide any further insight into the problem.

**Tocainide**

Although lidocaine is effective for management of acute arrhythmias and prevention of ventricular tachycardia and fibrillation, it can only be given intravenously, thereby precluding long-term therapy. Tocainide, an oral congener of lidocaine, has proven to be effective for long-term therapy of chronic ventricular arrhythmias. Campbell and coworkers[41] randomized 68 patients with a suspected MI to treatment with tocainide or placebo (see Table 3). The drug dosage and duration of therapy were not specified. Tocainide reduced the incidence of ventricular tachycardia, but the authors did not comment about its effect on the occurrence of ventricular fibrillation or mortality. Ryden and coworkers[42] randomized 112 patients to therapy with tocainide or placebo for 6 months. During each visit throughout the entire followup period, patients receiving tocainide had a significant reduction in VPBs and ventricular tachycardia, but there was no significant difference in mortality. However, plasma levels of tocainide were low, suggesting that a suboptimal dose was given. Importantly, tocainide was discontinued in 22 patients because of side effects, compared with 13 patients who were withdrawn from placebo therapy.

Tocainide decreases the frequency of all ventricular arrhythmias including ventricular tachycardia. These results are similar to that observed with the other membrane-active drugs, including intravenous lidocaine. However, during a 6-month followup with oral tocainide, the incidence of sudden death was not reduced. The lack of efficacy may be accounted for by the low blood levels. Additionally, there was a high frequency of side effects, limiting the usefulness of this drug for long-term therapy.

## Mexiletine

Mexiletine, another oral lidocaine congener, is in widespread use in Europe for treatment of ventricular arrhythmias. In a study in post-MI patients, Campbell and coworkers[43] administered mexiletine or placebo for 48 hours to 97 patients (see Table 3). They reported a significant reduction in the frequency of ventricular tachycardia in patients receiving mexiletine compared with placebo (27 versus 200 salvos, $p < 0.005$). Thirty-four patients receiving placebo had serious arrhythmias, defined as ventricular tachycardia, ventricular fibrillation or early VPBs, compared with only seven patients treated with mexiletine ($p < 0.005$). However, the authors did not comment on mortality during this brief study. Chamberlain and coworkers[44] randomized 344 patients to treatment with mexiletine or placebo. Therapy was begun 6 to 14 days after MI and continued for 1 year. Patients with serious arrhythmias that occurred within the 14 days and required antiarrhythmic drug therapy were excluded. As evaluated by ambulatory monitoring, there was no significant difference in the occurrence of ventricular tachycardia, and mortality was the same in the drug and placebo groups (13.2 percent versus 11.6 percent). However, of the 24 patients in the mexiletine group who died, death occurred in 7 after drug was withdrawn because of side effects.

Although mexiletine does not appear to protect against sudden death, definitive conclusions cannot be made. Campbell and associates[43] continued mexiletine therapy for only 48 hours. In the study by Chamberlain,[44] patients who had serious arrhythmias before randomization were excluded. These authors did not observe any difference between the drug and placebo group in the frequency of salvos of ventricular tachycardia as demonstrated on ambulatory monitoring. Mexiletine therapy was therefore continued even if it failed to suppress arrhythmia. It is unclear whether those patients who died had persistent ventricular tachycardia despite therapy. Moreover, 7 of 24 deaths in the mexiletine group occurred after drug was withdrawn because of side effects.

## Aprindine

Aprindine, another oral lidocaine congener, has a long half-life and can be given twice a day. Although infrequent dosing makes it attractive for long-term use, frequent side effects limit its usefulness. The multicenter Rotterdam study[45] randomized 310 patients to aprindine or placebo therapy (see Table 3). After a 1-year followup of 222 patients, abolition of complex arrhythmias, defined as ventricular tachycardia or repetitive or frequent VPBs, occurred in 53 percent receiving aprindine, compared with only 22 percent in the placebo group.[46] However, mortality was equivalent in the two groups.[45]

As observed in studies involving other membrane-active drugs, aprindine is an effective antiarrhythmic agent that abolishes complex arrhythmia in over 50 percent of patients. However, treatment with this drug does not improve survival during the first year after an MI.

## BETA-ADRENERGIC BLOCKING DRUGS AFTER MYOCARDIAL INFARCTION

Since the 1960s, the beta-adrenergic blocking agents have been widely used for therapy of angina, hypertension, and arrhythmias. The physiologic action of these agents is to block the effect of catecholamines on cardiac tissue. It is well established that the sympathetic nervous system and catecholamines have an important role in the genesis of ventricular arrhythmias, especially during myocardial ischemia.[47] Therefore the beta-blocking drugs are of potential benefit in patients with a recent MI (Table 5). Snow and Manc[48] administered 60 mg of propranolol daily to patients for 1 month after MI. They reported a significant decrease in sudden death in the group receiving propranolol. Shortly after this report, a multicenter study involving 195 patients treated with the same dose of propranolol for 28 days failed to show

**Table 5.** Results of randomized trials with beta-blocking drugs

| Study | Drug | N | Duration | % Sudden death Placebo | Drug | P |
|-------|------|---|----------|--------|------|---|
| Snow, Manc | Propranolol | 101 | 28 days | 12.0 | 6.0 | < 0.03 |
| Multicenter | Propranolol | 195 | 28 days | 9.3 | 7.1 | NS |
| Balcon | Propranolol | 114 | 28 days | 10.5 | 12.3 | NS |
| Norris | Propranolol | 454 | 3 weeks | 7.5 | 8.8 | NS |
| BHAT | Propranolol | 3857 | 3 years | 4.6 | 3.3 | < 0.01 |
| Norwegian | Propranolol | 560 | 1 year | 8.2 | 4.0 | 0.038 |
| Wilhelmson | Alprenolol | 230 | 2 years | 9.6 | 2.6 | < 0.05 |
| Ahlmack | Alprenolol | 162 | 1 year | 11.1 | 1.2 | < 0.05 |
| Anderson | Alprenolol | 282 | 1 year | 20.6 | 9.2 | < 0.01* |
| Multicenter | Practolol | 3038 | 1 year | 3.6 | 2.0 | < 0.01 |
| Hjarlmarson | Metoprolol | 1395 | 90 days | 8.9 | 5.7 | 0.03* |
| Norwegian | Timolol | 1884 | 33 months | 13.9 | 7.7 | < 0.001 |
| Julian | Sotalol | 1456 | 1 year | 8.9 | 7.3 | NS |
| Taylor | Oxprenolol | 1103 | 6 years | 9.3 | 8.2 | NS* |

*Total cardiac mortality

any protective effect.[49] Balcon and coworkers[50] randomized 114 patients to treatment with placebo or propranolol (80 mg daily) for 28 days. The incidence of total deaths and sudden cardiac deaths was equivalent in both groups. In a study of 454 patients, Norris and coworkers[51] randomly administered 80 mg of propranolol or placebo for 3 weeks. Patients wtih hypotension, congestive heart failure, heart block, and sinus bradycardia (< 50 beats per min) were excluded from this study. As with other studies, no difference was observed in total mortality or the incidence of sudden cardiac death between the control and drug groups.

Although the initial study with propranolol by Snow and Manc[48] reported that this drug reduced mortality during the first month after an MI, several subsequent studies failed to show any benefit. However, small numbers of patients were involved, small doses of drug were used, and therapy was limited to only 3 to 4 weeks.

In 1982, the Beta Blocker Heart Attack Trial (BHAT) was reported.[52] This multicenter study involved 3857 patients randomized within 5 to 21 days after an MI to therapy with placebo or propranolol (at a daily dose of 160 mg or 240 mg as guided by serum drug level). After an average followup of 25.1 months, propranolol therapy significantly reduced total mortality and sudden cardiac deaths when compared with placebo (7.2 percent versus 9.8 percent and 3.3 percent versus 4.6 percent respectively) (Fig. 2). These findings were supported by a Norwegian multicenter trial involving 560 patients in whom treatment with 100 mg of propranolol was begun 4 to 6 days after an MI.[53] After a 1-year followup, total mortality was reduced compared with placebo (9.0 percent versus 13.1 percent), as was the incidence of sudden deaths (4.0 percent versus 8.2 percent).

Trials with other beta-adrenergic blocking agents have reported similar results. Wilhelmsson and associates[54] reported that compared with placebo, alprenolol significantly reduced the incidence of sudden deaths during a 2-year followup (9.6 percent versus 2.6 percent, p < 0.05). This protective effect occurred primarily in those patients with evidence of significant myocardial damage (defined as the presence of cardiomegaly or atrial arrhythmias). A significant reduction in sudden death in patients receiving alprenolol was also reported by Ahlmack and coworkers.[55] In a study by Andersen and colleagues,[56] alprenolol improved survival only in those patients less than 65 years of age who had a definite or suspected MI.

A multicenter trial with practolol[57] involving 3038 patients followed for 1 year found that the drug significantly reduced total cardiac mortality and sudden death mortality (2.0 percent versus 3.6 percent for placebo, p < 0.01). The major benefit occurred in those patients who

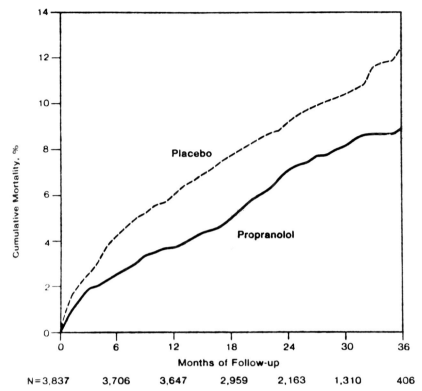

**Figure 2.** Survival results of Beta Blocker Heart Attack Trial (BHAT). A total of 3837 patients were randomized to treatment with propranolol or placebo. After a 3-year followup, there was a significant reduction in mortality in those treated with propranolol. (From Beta Blocker Heart Attack Trial Research Group,[58] with permission.)

sustained an anterior wall infarction. A Norwegian multicenter study[58] involving 1884 patients treated with placebo or timolol reported that the drug reduced the occurrence of sudden death by 44.6 percent (7.7 percent versus 13.9 percent for placebo) after a 33-month followup (Fig. 3). Hjalmarsen and coworkers[59] used intravenous metoprolol during acute myocardial infarction and continued therapy for 3 months with oral drug. Compared with placebo, metoprolol therapy significantly reduced sudden deaths by 34 percent (8.9 percent versus 5.7 percent, p = 0.03).

Although a number of beta-adrenergic blocking agents have a beneficial effect on survival after an MI, not all drugs of this class are effective. Sotalol, which has beta-blocking activity and also prolongs the refractory period by direct action, failed to reduce mortality in a randomized study of 1456 patients.[60] Taylor and coworkers[61] compared oxprenolol with placebo in 1103 patients. Unlike previous beta-blocker drug studies, therapy with drug was begun within 4 months to as long as 7½ years after an MI. For the whole group there was no difference in survival or total cardiac events after a followup extending for as long as 72 months. However, when patients were subgrouped based on the time after MI to entry, important differences were observed. When oxprenolol was begun within 4 months after the MI, there was a significant improvement in survival (95 percent versus 77 percent, p < 0.001). There was no benefit when drug was started 5 to 12 months after an MI, whereas oxprenolol therapy initiated more than 1 year after MI actually reduced survival (79 percent vs 92 percent for placebo, p < 0.002). The protective effect of oxprenolol was therefore limited to the first 4 months of therapy, whereas treatment begun after this time was ineffective. These results are

275

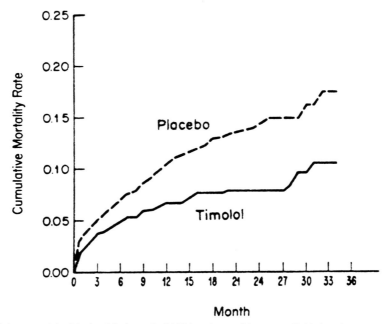

**Figure 3.** Multicenter trial with timolol. A total of 1984 patients with myocardial infarctions were randomized to placebo or timolol therapy. After an average followup of 33 months, there was a significant reduction in mortality in the timolol group. (From Norwegian Multicenter Study Group,[52] with permission.)

consistent with epidemiologic studies that have shown the risk of sudden death to be greatest within the first 6 months after an MI,[15,17] and it is during this period that beta blockers should have their greatest impact. This protection with early usage is also apparent by examination of the survival curves from the BHAT trial[52] as well as the Norwegian timolol[58] and propranolol trials.[53] The major effect of beta-blocking drugs on survival seems to be primarily during the first 6 months of therapy. Thereafter, the survival curves of drug versus placebo become almost parallel.

## METHODOLOGIC PROBLEMS WITH RANDOMIZED DRUG TRIALS

The randomized trials utilizing beta-adrenergic blocker drugs have shown that these agents have beneficial effects on survival, whereas studies with the membrane-active antiarrhythmic drugs have been disappointing. However, many methodologic problems, which plague each of these randomized trials, urge caution in interpretation.

1. With the exception of some of the beta blocker drug trials, small numbers of patients were studied. The endpoints being evaluated were total cardiac mortality or sudden deaths, which are relatively low-frequency events. These endpoints require study of large numbers before any significant differences can be observed.
2. In many of the studies, the duration of therapy was short, often less than 1 month, and therefore inadequate to judge effect of drug on long-term survival.
3. Each trial was double blinded and randomized. All patients entered were treated, without attention to the type or frequency of arrhythmia present before therapy.
4. Effect of the drug on ventricular arrhythmias was not analyzed. Many of the studies do not comment on the method for defining arrhythmia, the type and frequency of

ventricular arrhythmia present, or how the endpoint was documented. In those studies that reported monitoring data, no analysis is provided. There is no certainty that the drug selected was effective for suppressing arrhythmias. None of the trials provide any correlation between survival and the effect of drug on ventricular arrhythmias.

5. Fixed doses of drugs were used, and in many studies the dose employed was subtherapeutic. There was no attention given to blood levels, and drug dosage was not titrated to side effects or effect on arrhythmias.

6. Side effects frequently resulted from therapy with these drugs and caused the withdrawal of patients from study.

7. There are no comments about the addition of other therapies during the trials.

8. Each of the antiarrhythmic drugs has the potential to aggravate arrhythmias. None of the trials dealt with this issue or attempted to establish its occurrence. In our experience, the overall incidence of aggravation of arrhythmia with these drugs is 11 percent.[62] It might be expected that with random use of these agents some patients had an increase in arrhythmias, which could have affected mortality in the drug-treated group.

9. In the beta-blocker trials, many patients eligible for study were excluded. The BHAT study[52] excluded 77 percent of patients admitted with an MI because of contraindications to beta-blocker therapy including bradycardia, congestive heart failure, and asthma; the need for beta-blocker therapy for another indication such as angina, hypertension, or sinus tachycardia; the use of beta blocker at the time of hospital admission; or the potential need for cardiac surgery. The Norwegian propranolol study[53] also excluded 77 percent of patients for the above reasons. Also excluded in this latter trial were those believed to be "good risks" (a term not defined), patients less than 35 years old, and those who required antiarrhythmic therapy. In the timolol study, 48 percent of eligible patients were excluded because of contraindications to the drug including congestive heart failure, bradycardia, hypotension, AV or SA block, VPBs, claudication, renal or hepatic disease, or concurrent illness; other indications for beta blocker therapy; or the need for antiarrhythmic drugs. The metoprolol and sotalol trials also excluded a large number of patients for the same reasons as indicated above. Thus the remaining patients entered into these studies represent a low-risk group, as is evident by the low yearly mortality in the placebo-treated group.

10. Although difficult to define, the effect of other diseases is not evaluated nor is the effect of closer medical supervision and "tender loving care" considered.

These many limitations account, in part, for the disappointing results with the membrane-active drugs. Despite these problems, most of the randomized trials with the beta-blocker drugs showed a significant improvement on survival, although therapy was given to a low-risk group. One of the most important considerations relate to the issue of what arrhythmias need to be suppressed. These many studies did not select patients judged to be at highest risk because of the presence of certain ventricular arrhythmias. In fact, patients with serious arrhythmias were generally excluded from the trials. The previously mentioned studies of patients after an MI have all demonstrated that the risk of sudden death is associated with repetitive forms of ventricular arrhythmias[15-22] It seems logical, therefore, that if survival is to be improved by drug therapy, it must be targeted at suppression of these repetitive forms, rather than empirically administered. Therapy, however, represents a major challenge because there are no guidelines for the selection of an effective drug and no way to predict response. Only 40 to 60 percent of patients will be expected to respond to any one drug; side effects will occur in as many as 50 to 60 percent of patients; and the drug may unpredictably aggravate arrhythmias. In order to establish an effective and well-tolerated program, it is necessary to "tailor" the drug to the individual patient. This goal mandates a systematic and "directed" approach to drug selection.

## SYSTEMATIC APPROACH TO ANTIARRHYTHMIC DRUG THERAPY

Since there are no guidelines to the selection of an effective antiarrhythmic drug, therapy is empiric. The known electrophysiologic properties of the antiarrhythmic agent, the nature of the rhythm disorder, and the underlying heart disease do not provide aid to the effective use of these drugs. Drug selection of appropriate therapy is further complicated by an ever-growing number of antiarrhythmic drugs. Moreover, long-term therapy requires that the drug selected be not only effective but also well tolerated and free of side effects. We have therefore developed a systematic approach for "directed" therapy, which involves a rapid screening of drugs to determine effect on arrhythmia and a short period of therapy to confirm efficacy and safety.[7,63] The following phases of study are involved (Table 6).

PHASE 0. This phase represents a control period for data collection. Upon hospital admission, all antiarrhythmic drugs are discontinued. After at least four half-lives off drug (approximately 24 to 36 hours) patients undergo 48 hours of continuous ambulatory monitoring[12] and a maximal, symptom-limited exercise test on a motorized treadmill.[64] At the completion of these studies, a decision is made regarding the method of drug evaluation. If the patient has high-density and reproducible ventricular arrhythmias, noninvasive evaluation involving repeat ambulatory monitoring and treadmill exercise testing is used to judge drug efficacy. If the arrhythmia is infrequent or not reproducible, invasive electrophysiologic testing is performed.[65]

PHASE 1. Acute drug testing is designed as a method for rapid assessment of effect of the antiarrhythmic drugs on the arrhythmia.[66,67] Each morning the patient is continuously monitored by trendscription for 30 minutes to establish the level of arrhythmia present. A brief period of exercise on a bicycle ergometer is designed to reproduce a level of exercise comparable to what the patient performs during routine daily activities. A 12-lead ECG is obtained, and leads II and $V_2$ or $V_3$ are recorded at 50 mm/sec for measurement of P–R, QRS, and Q–T intervals. At the conclusion of this control period, a large oral dose of drug is administered. The dose is generally one half of the standard daily dose of drug (i.e., quinidine 600

**Table 6.** Systematic approach to arrhythmia management

---

*Phases of Study*

Phase 0. Control period—data collection
    Ambulatory monitoring
    Exercise testing
    Electrophysiologic study (if necessary)

Phase 1. Acute drug testing—rapid screening for drug effect
    Monitoring for 3 hours
    Hourly bicycle ergometry
    Electrophysiologic study

Phase 2. Short-term maintenance—evaluate drug efficacy and patient tolerance
    Ambulatory monitoring
    Exercise
            or
    Electrophysiologic study

Phase 3. Long-term therapy—outpatient management
    Followup every 3–6 months

---

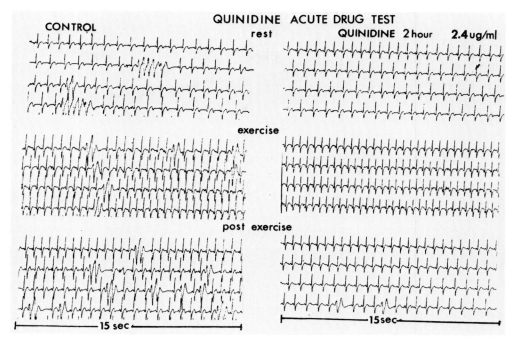

**Figure 4.** Example of an acute drug test with quinidine. During the control period, frequent ventricular ectopy is present at rest, during exercise and in the post-exercise recovery period. Two hours after administration of quinidine (600 mg), arrhythmia is abolished. The quinidine blood level is 2.4 $\mu$g/ml at this time.

mg, procainamide 1500 mg, disopyramide 300 mg). The patient is observed and rhythm continuously recorded by trendscription for 3 hours (Fig. 4). Each hour, blood is obtained for drug level, ECG recorded for intervals, and bicycle ergometry repeated. If the patient is undergoing electrophysiologic testing, this test is performed 2 to 3 hours after drug administration.

PHASE 2. Short-term maintenance follows the completion of a series of acute drug tests. Once effective drugs are identified, therapy with the one or more agents judged to be the best for the patient is initiated and continued for 72 to 96 hours. During this phase, the patient is carefully questioned to elicit any side effects that may limit long-term treatment. Some drugs cannot be tested acutely because several days are required to achieve a therapeutic blood level of drug or active metabolite. The evaluation of these drugs involves only phase 2 testing. At the conclusion of this period of multiple dosing, ambulatory monitoring and treadmill exercise testing (Fig. 5) or electrophysiologic testing (Fig. 6) are repeated.

PHASE 3. This phase involves long-term therapy. If the drug program is judged effective and is tolerated without side effects, the patient is discharged. Followup is done every 3 to 6 months, at which time monitoring and exercise testing are repeated.

A critical issue involves the criteria for judging drug effectiveness. The criteria we have established reflect the substantial evidence that repetitive VPBs impart risk. Therefore, the goal of therapy is the abolition of these forms. When noninvasive techniques are employed, the drug is considered to be effective if the following criteria are met with both monitoring and exercise testing:[7]

1. Total elimination of salvos of ventricular tachycardia.
2. Reduction of $\geq$ 90 percent in the frequency of couplets.
3. Decrease by $\geq$ 50 percent in VPB frequency.

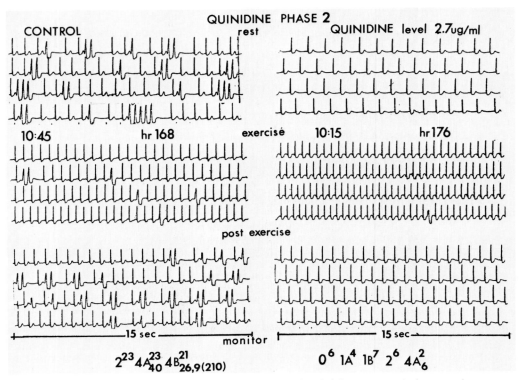

**Figure 5.** Example of phase 2 study with quinidine. During the control period, frequent ventricular ectopy is present at rest, and during and after exercise. Ambulatory monitoring revealed frequent ventricular premature beats (VPBs) for 23 hours (2²³), up to 40 couplets (4A) per hour for 23 hours (4A²³₄₀), and salvos of ventricular tachycardia (4B) for 21 hours (4B²¹). There were as many as 26 salvos per hour with a duration of 9 cycles at a rate of 210 beats per minute. While receiving quinidine (300 mg q 6h), arrhythmia is almost entirely suppressed with exercise. Ambulatory monitoring shows no VPBs for 6 hours (0⁶), infrequent VPBs for 11 hours (1A⁴, 1B⁷), and frequent VPBs for 6 hours (2⁶). Couplets were present for 2 hours with a maximum of 6 per hour (4A²₆).

When invasive electrophysiologic testing is used, the inability to provoke more than two repetitive responses when up to three extrastimuli are added during both sinus rhythm and ventricular pacing constitutes the criterion for drug efficacy.[65]

## Results of "Directed" Therapy

The approach as outlined has been applied to 175 patients who were referred for management of hemodynamically significant arrhythmias including ventricular fibrillation or sustained ventricular tachycardia with syncope. Such patients represent a group who are at highest risk for recurrence, with an annual rate in excess of 30 percent.[68] Noninvasive techniques were employed in the management of 123 patients,[63] whereas 52 patients underwent invasive electrophysiologic studies.[65] Of the patients who had noninvasive studies, 98, or 79.7 percent, were deemed controlled with antiarrhythmic drugs based on the aforementioned criteria. During an average followup to 31.5 months there were six sudden deaths, that is, an annual sudden death rate of 2.3 percent. Twenty-five patients, many of whom were seen in our early experience prior to the availability of newer drugs, were not controlled. Seventeen died suddenly during a followup of 18.8 months, yielding an annual mortality of 43.6 percent (Fig. 7). Fifty-six percent of the patients had left ventricular dysfunction as evaluated by angiography, echocardiography, or radionuclide scanning. The average ejection fraction in this

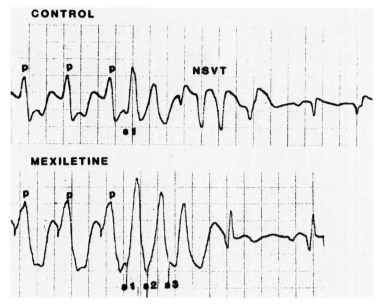

**Figure 6.** Example of phase 2 study employing electrophysiologic techniques. In the control, a single extrastimulus ($S_1$) delivered during a paced (P) rhythm provoked a five-beat salvo of nonsustained ventricular tachycardia (NSVT). During therapy with mexiletine, no arrhythmia was provoked when up to three extrastimuli ($S_1$, $S_2$, $S_3$) were added.

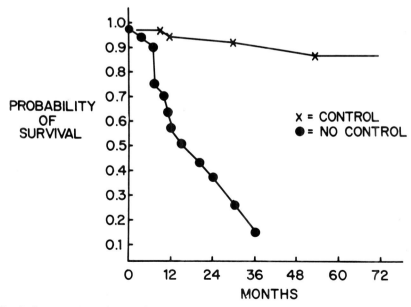

**Figure 7.** Survival among 123 patients undergoing a noninvasive approach to the selection of antiarrhythmic drug therapy. Ninety-eight patients who had salvos of ventricular tachycardia (VT) eliminated by drug therapy were deemed controlled. Annual sudden death rate was 2.3 percent. Despite drug therapy, salvos of VT were still present in 25 patients. Annual sudden death rate in this latter group was 43.6 percent. (From Graboys et al,[63] with permission.)

group was 32 percent. The ability to control arrhythmias was not associated with the presence or extent of left ventricular dysfunction. Those patients with left ventricular dysfunction who were deemed controlled with drugs had a yearly sudden death rate of 3.1 percent, whereas in those with impaired cardiac function not controlled with drugs the annual mortality was 41.5 percent. It may be concluded that when drugs are effective for suppression of repetitive arrhythmias, primarily salvos of ventricular tachycardia, survival is enhanced. This improvement is independent of the state of left ventricular function.

The results of therapy are similar when electrophysiologic testing is used to select an effective drug. Of the 52 patients who had invasive electrophysiologic studies, 45 had provocable arrhythmias. Similar to the results of noninvasive studies, an effective drug program that prevented the provocation of arrhythmias was established in 36 patients (80 percent). After a followup of 21 months only one patient (2.8 percent) had recurrence. Among the nine patients not controlled, five (56 percent) had recurrence. The only difference between patients who had noninvasive studies and those undergoing invasive procedures was the presence of frequent and reproducible spontaneous ventricular arrhythmias. The type and extent of heart disease and the presenting arrhythmias were similar. Regardless of the method of drug selection, it may be concluded that survival is improved when spontaneously occurring or provoked repetitive arrhythmias can be suppressed.

There are several other studies in the literature that confirm that therapy directed at suppression of certain types of ventricular arrhythmias improves survival. Unlike our approach, each of these studies utilized only electrophysiologic testing to guide therapy, regardless of the level of ambient arrhythmias. Ruskin and coworkers[69] reported on 31 patients who survived out-of-hospital sudden death. Twenty-five patients had inducible arrhythmias; antiarrhythmic drugs prevented provocation in 19 (76 percent). None of these 19 patients died suddenly during the 15-month followup period. Six patients still had inducible arrhythmia; three had recurrence of arrhythmias. Horowitz and coworkers[70] reported on 20 patients with inducible ventricular tachycardia during control study. After drug therapy, nine were no longer inducible and only one had recurrence after an average followup of 12.2 months. Of 11 patients in whom drugs were either ineffective or only partially effective, 8 had a recurrence.

The group from Stanford has reported the outcome of antiarrhythmic drug therapy evaluated with electrophysiologic techniques. Their first report involved 21 patients.[71] Twelve of 13 patients controlled by drugs were discharged on the agent deemed effective. There were no recurrences in this group after 8.1 months. In contrast, eight patients were not completely controlled. Five of these patients were discharged on the ineffective drug, and three had recurrences. In a second study involving 55 patients, 13 of 17 patients (76.5 percent) who were still inducible on drug had recurrences after 8.2 months.[71] In contrast, only 4 of 36 patients (11 percent) deemed controlled had recurrences. It should be noted that the criteria for drug efficacy used by these authors differ from those of other groups. They considered a drug to be effective if six or fewer repetitive cycles were induced. In contrast Ruskin, Horowitz, and our group did not consider a drug to be effective if more than two repetitive VPBs were induced. In a much larger group of 239 patients who had electrophysiologic tests, similar results were reported by the Stanford group.[73] Criteria for drug efficacy were the same as in their previous reports. After an average followup of 14.8 months, sudden death occurred in 12 percent of patients without inducible arrhythmias during electrophysiologic testing. In contrast, 31 percent of patients who still had provocable arrhythmias died suddenly. They examined a subgroup of 166 patients who had multiple control studies without drug and in whom ventricular tachycardia was reproducibly provoked. The incidence of sudden death at 2 years was 18 percent in those not inducible after therapy, compared with 41 percent in nonresponders. Although these authors used both medical and surgical approaches for therapy, the important conclusion is that the inability to induce repetitive arrhythmias improved survival. The difference in survival rates between the Stanford group and those of Ruskin and our group reflects, in part, differences in testing protocols, the number of drugs tested, and especially the definition of drug efficacy.

Benditt and coworkers[74] reached similar conclusions. Twenty-one of 23 patients (91 percent) did not have arrhythmias provoked after medical or surgical therapy. Only one patient (5 percent) had sudden death during an 18-month followup. Eight patients did not have inducible arrhythmias or did not undergo testing. Three patients had recurrent sudden deaths within 10 to 19 months.

Despite differences in protocol and criteria of efficacy, the conclusion reached by each study is the same. It seems clear that in patients with a history of sustained ventricular tachyarrhythmia, the suppression by drugs of spontaneously occurring or induced repetitive arrhythmias predicts freedom from recurrent arrhythmias during long-term followup.

## CONCLUSION

The overwhelming evidence suggests that in patients who have had a previous myocardial infarction, the presence of repetitive ventricular arrhythmia increases total cardiac mortality, which is primarily a result of the increase of sudden deaths. Randomized trials of antiarrhythmic agents in patients with a recent myocardial infarction have not shown these drugs to be of benefit. Patients who have survived an episode of out-of-hospital sudden death represent a group who are at highest risk. When antiarrhythmic drug therapy is given empirically to such patients and is not directed at the suppression of complex forms, recurrent sudden death rate is high.[68] Therefore, such empiric therapy is doomed to failure. Selection of an effective and well-tolerated drug requires a systematic approach. Studies in survivors of out-of-hospital sudden death have shown that when therapy is targeted at elimination of repetitive ventricular arrhythmias, recurrent sudden death can be prevented. It is as yet unclear if such "directed therapy" will improve survival in patients after a myocardial infarction. Because the presence of repetitive arrhythmias is what enhances risk, it seems logical that suppression of these forms will significantly reduce the incidence of recurrent sudden deaths. Studies of drug therapy in patients after a myocardial infarction who have complex arrhythmias are necessary to prove this hypothesis. Although drug therapy is effective, there is a need to establish effective methods for noninvasive screening of patients with heart disease to identify those at risk for sudden death. Once identified, there is also a need to develop simple and rapid ways to select an effective drug. In this way, the problem of sudden death can be contained.

## REFERENCES

1. LOWN, B: *Sudden cardiac death: The major challenge confronting contemporary cardiology.* Am J Cardiol 43:313, 1979.

2. LOWN, B AND WOLF, M: *Approaches to sudden death from coronary heart disease.* Circulation 44:130, 1971.

3. COBB, LA, CINN, RD, SAMSON, WE, ET AL: *Prehospital coronary care: The role of rapid response mobile intensive coronary care system.* Circulation 43:11, 1971.

4. REICHENBACK, DD, MOSS, NS, AND MAYER, E: *Pathology of the heart in sudden cardiac death.* Am J Cardiol 39:865, 1977.

5. LONEGRAVE, T AND THOMPSON, P: *The role of acute myocardial infarction in sudden cardiac death—a statistician's nightmare.* Am Heart J 96:711, 1978.

6. LOWN, B AND RUBERMAN, W: *The concept of precoronary care.* Mod Concepts Cardiovasc Dis 39:97, 1970.

7. LOWN, B, PODRID, PJ, DeSILVA, RA, ET AL: *Sudden cardiac death: Management of the patient at risk.* Curr Probl Cardiol 4(12):1, 1980.

8. LOWN, B AND VERRIER, RL: *Neural activity and ventricular fibrillation.* N Engl J Med 294:1165, 1976.

9. HINKLE, LE, CARVER, ST, AND STEVENS, M: *The frequency of asymptomatic disturbances of cardiac rhythm and conduction in middle aged men.* Am J Cardiol 24:629, 1969.

10. The Coronary Drug Project Rearch Group: *Prognostic importance of premature beats following myocardial infarction: Experience in the Coronary Drug Project.* JAMA 223:1116, 1976.

11. Chiang, BN, Perlman, LV, Ostrander, LD, et al: *Relationship of premature systoles to coronary heart disease and sudden death in the Tecumseh epidemiologic study.* Ann Intern Med 70:1159, 1969.

12. Lown, G, Calvert, AC, Armington, R, et al: *Monitoring for serious arrhythmias and high risk of sudden death.* Circulation 51(Suppl III):189, 1975.

13. Calvert, A, Lown, B, and Gorlin, R: *Ventricular premature beats and anatomically defined coronary heart disease.* Am J Cardiol 39:627, 1977.

14. Kotler, M, Tabatznik, B, Mower, MM, et al: *Prognostic significance of ventricular ectopic activity with respect to sudden death in late post infarction period.* Circulation 47:959, 1973.

15. Vismara, LA, Amsterdam, EA, and Mason, DT: *Relation of ventricular arrhythmias in the late phase of acute myocadial infarction to sudden death after hospital discharge.* Am J Med 59:6, 1975.

16. VanDurme, JP and Pannier, RH: *Prognostic significance of ventricular dysrhythmia one year after a myocardial infarction.* Am J Cardiol 37:178, 1976.

17. Schultz, RA, Strauss, HW, and Pitt, B: *Sudden death in the year following myocardial infarction.* Am J Med 62:192, 1977.

18. Moss, AJ, Davis, HT, DeCamilla, J, et al: *Ventricular ectopic beats and their relation to sudden and non-sudden cardiac death after myocardial infarction.* Circulation 60:998, 1979.

19. Ruberman, W, Weinblatt, E, Goldberg, JD, et al: *Ventricular premature complexes and sudden death after myocardial infarction.* Circulation 64:297, 1981.

20. Bigger, JT, Weld, FM, and Rolmitzky, LM: *Prevalence, characteristics and significance of ventricular tachycardia (three or more complexes) detected with ambulatory electrocardiographic recording in the late hospital phase of acute myocardial infarction.* Am J Cardiol 48:815, 1981.

21. Rapaport, E and Remedios, P: *The high risk patient after recovery from myocardial infarction: Recognition and management.* J Am Coll Cardiol 1:391, 1983.

22. Mukhaije, J, Rude, R, Gustafson, N, et al: *Late sudden death following myocardial infarction: Interdependence of risk factors.* J Am Coll Cardiol 1:585, 1983.

23. Follansbee, WP, Michelson, EL, and Morganroth, J: *Nonsustained ventricular tachycardia in ambulatory patients: Characteristics and association with sudden cardiac death.* Ann Intern Med 92:741, 1980.

24. Lown, B and Vassaux, C: *Lidocaine in acute myocardial infarction.* Am Heart J 76:586, 1968.

25. Bennett, MA, Wilner, JM, and Pentecoste, BC: *Controlled trial of lignocaine in prophylaxis of ventricular arrhythmia complicating myocardial infarction.* Lancet 2:909, 1970.

26. Pitt, A, Lipp, H, and Anderson, ST: *Lignocaine given prophylactically to patients with acute myocardial infarction.* Lancet 1:612, 1970.

27. Morgensen, L: *Ventricular tachyarrhythmias and lignocaine prophylaxis in acute myocardial infarction.* Acta Med Scand (Suppl 513):1, 1970.

28. Chopra, MD, Thadane, U, Portal, RW, et al: *Lignocaine therapy for ventricular ectopic activity after acute myocardial infarction: A double blind trial.* Br Med J 3:668, 1971.

29. Lie, KJ, Wellens, HJ, VanChampell, FS, et al: *Lidocaine in the prevention of primary ventricular fibrillation: A double blind randomized study of 212 consecutive patients.* N Engl J Med 291:1324, 1974.

30. Jones, DT, Kostuk, WJ, and Gunton, RW: *Prophylactic quinidine for the prevention of arrhythmias after acute myocardial infarction.* Am J Cardiol 33:655, 1974.

31. Holmberg, S and Bergman, H: *Prophylactic quinidine treatment in myocardial infarction.* Acta Med Scand 181:297, 1967.

32. Bloomfield, SS, Romhilt, DW, Chou, TL, et al: *Quinidine for prophylaxis of arrhythmia in acute myocardial infarction.* N Engl J Med 285:967, 1971.

33. Bloomfield, SS, Romhilt, DW, Chou, TC, et al: *Natural history of cardiac arrhythmias and their prevention with quinidine in patients with acute coronary insufficiency.* Circulation 47:967, 1973.

34. Jennings, G, Jones, MBA, Besterman, EMM, et al: *Oral disopyramide in prophylaxis of arrhythmias following myocardial infarction.* Lancet 1:51, 1976.

35. Zainal, N, Griffiths, JW, Carmichael, DJS, et al: *Oral disopyramide for the prevention of arrhythmias in patients with acute myocardial infarction admitted to open wards.* Lancet 2:887, 1977.

36. Pouleur, H, Chaudin, JM, and Reyns, P: *Effect of disopyramide and aprindine on arrhythmia after acute myocardial infarction.* Eur J Cardiol 5:397, 1977.

37. Koch Weser, J, Klein, SW, Foo-Canto, LL, et al: *Antiarrhythmic prophylaxis with procainamide in acute myocardial infarction.* N Engl J Med 281:1253, 1969.

38. KOSOWSKY, BD, TAYLOR, J, LOWN, B, ET AL: *Long term use of procainamide following acute myocardial infarction.* Circulation 47:1204, 1973.

39. COLLABORATIVE GROUP: *Phenytoin after recovery from myocardial infarction: Controlled trial in 568 patients.* Lancet 1:1055, 1971.

40. PETER, T, ROSS, D, DUFFIELD, A, ET AL: *Effect on survival after myocardial infarction of long term treatment with phenytoin.* Br Heart J 42:1356, 1978.

41. CAMPBELL, RWF, BRYSON, LG, BAILEY, BJ, ET AL: *Oral tocainide in suspected acute myocardial infarction.* Circulation 59(Suppl II):70, 1979.

42. RYDEN, L, ARNMAN, K, CONRADSON, TB, ET AL: *Prophylaxis of ventricular tachyarrhythmias with intravenous and oral tocainide in patients with and recovering from acute myocardial infarction.* Am Heart J 100: 1006, 1980.

43. CAMPBELL, RWF, ACHUFF, SC, POTTAGE, A, ET AL: *Mexiletine in the prophylaxis of ventricular arrhythmias during acute myocardial infarction.* J Cardiovasc Pharmacol 1:43, 1979.

44. CHAMBERLAIN, DR, JULIAN, DG, BOYLE, DM, ET AL: *Oral mexiletine in high risk patients after myocardial infarction.* Lancet 2:1324, 1980.

45. HUGENHOLTZ, PG, HAGEMEIJER, F, LUBSEN, J, ET AL: *One year follow-up in patients with persistent ventricular dysrhythmias after myocardial infarction treated with aprindine or placebo.* In SANDOE, E, JULIAN, DG, AND BELL, JW (EDS): *Management of Ventricular Tachycardia: Role of Mexiletine.* Excerpta Medica, Amsterdam, 1978, pp 572–604.

46. HAGEMEIJER, F, VANDURME, JP, BOGAERT, M, ET AL: *Antiarrhythmic effectiveness of aprindine in patients with ventricular arrhythmias after an acute myocardial infarction.* Circulation 57(Suppl II): 176, 1978.

47. CORBALAN, R, VERRIER, RL, AND LOWN, B: *Psychologic stress and ventricular arrhythmias during myocardial infarction in the conscious dog.* Am J Cardiol 34:692, 1974.

48. SNOW, PJD AND MANC, MD: *Effect of propranolol in myocardial infarction.* Lancet 2:551, 1965.

49. MULTICENTER TRIAL: *Propranolol in acute myocardial infarction.* Lancet 2:1435, 1966.

50. BALCON, R, JEWITT, DE, DAVIES, JPH, ET AL: *A controlled trial of propranolol in acute myocardial infarction.* Lancet 2:917, 1966.

51. NORRIS, RM, LAUGHEY, DE, AND SCOTT, PJ: *Trial of propranolol in acute myocardial infarction.* Br Med J 2:398, 1968.

52. BETA BLOCKER HEART ATTACK TRIAL REARCH GROUP: *A randomized trial of propranolol in patients with acute myocardial infarction: I. Mortality results.* JAMA 247:1707, 1982.

53. HANSTEEN, V, MOINICHIN, E, LORENSTSEN, E, ET AL: *One year's treatment with propranolol after myocardial infarction: Preliminary report of the Norwegian Multicenter Trial.* Br Med J 284:155, 1982.

54. WILHELMSSON, C, WILHEMSSON, L, VEDIN, JA, ET AL: *Reduction of sudden death after myocardial infarction by treatment with alprenolol.* Lancet 2:1157, 1974.

55. AHLMACK, G, SALTRE, H, AND KORSGREN, M: *Reduction of sudden death after myocardial infarction.* Lancet 1:1563, 1974.

56. ANDERSEN, MP, FREDERIKSON, J, JURGENSEN, HG, ET AL: *Effect of alprenolol on mortality among patients with a definite or suspected acute myocardial infarction.* Lancet 2:865, 1974.

57. MULTICENTER INTERNATIONAL STUDY: *Reduction in mortality after myocardial infarction with long term beta adrenoceptor blockade.* Br Med J 2:419, 1977.

58. NORWEGIAN MULTICENTER STUDY GROUP: *Timolol induced reduction in mortality and reinfarction in patients surviving acute myocardial infarction.* N Engl J Med 304:801, 1981.

59. HJALMARSEN, P, HERLITZ, J, MALEK, I, ET AL: *Effect on mortality of metoprolol in acute myocardial infarction.* Lancet 2:823, 1981.

60. JULIAN, DG, JACKSON, FS, PRESCOTT, RJ, ET AL: *Controlled trial of sotalol for one year after myocardial infarction.* Lancet 1:1142, 1982.

61. TAYLOR, SH, SILKE, B, EBBUTT, A, ET AL: *A long term prevention study with oxyprenolol in coronary heart disease.* N Engl J Med 307:1293, 1982.

62. VELEBIT, V, PODRID, PJ, COHEN, B, ET AL; *Aggravation and provocation of ventricular arrhythmias by antiarrhythmic drugs.* Circulation 65:886, 1982.

63. GRABOYS, TB, LOWN, B, PODRID, PJ, ET AL: *Long term survival of patients with malignant ventricular arrhythmias treated with antiarrhythmic drugs.* Am J Cardiol 50:437, 1982.

64. JELINEK, MV AND LOWN, B: *Exercise testing for exposure of cardiac arrhythmia.* Prog Cardiovasc Dis 16:497, 1974.

65. PODRID, PJ, SCHOENBERGER, A, LOWN, B, ET AL: *Use of nonsustained ventricular tachycardia as a guide to antiarrhythmic drug therapy in patients with malignant ventricular arrhythmia.* Am Heart J 105:181, 1983.

66. GAUGHAN, CE, LOWN, B, LANIGAN, J, ET AL: *Acute oral testing for determining antiarrhythmic drug efficacy: I. Quinidine.* Am J Cardiol 38:677, 1976.

67. PODRID, PJ AND LOWN, B: *Selection of an antiarrhythmic drug to protect against ventricular fibrillation. Proceedings of the First US-USSR Symposium on Sudden Death.* Yalta, October 3–5, 1977. DHEW Publication No. (NIH)78-1470, Washington, DC, 1978, pp 259–266.

68. SCHAFFER, WA AND COBB, LA: *Recurrent ventricular fibrillation and modes of death in survivors of out of hospital ventricular fibrillation.* N Engl J Med 293:259.

69. RUSKIN, JN, DIMARCO, J, AND GARAN, H: *Out of hospital cardiac arrest: Electrophysiologic observations and selection of long term antiarrhythmic therapy.* N Engl J Med 303:607, 1980.

70. HOROWITZ, LN, JOSEPHSON, ME, FARSHIDI, A, ET AL: *Recurrent sustained ventricular tachycardia: III. Role of the electrophysiologic study in the selection of antiarrhythmic regimens.* Circulation 58:986, 1978.

71. MASON, J AND WINKLE, R: *Electrode catheter arrhythmia induction in the selection and assessment of antiarrhythmic drug therapy on recurrent ventricular tachycardia.* Circulation 58:971, 1978.

72. MASON, JW AND WINKLE, RA: *Accuracy of the ventricular tachycardia induction study for predicting long term efficacy and inefficacy of antiarrhythmic drugs.* N Engl J Med 303:1073–1077, 1980.

73. SWERDLOW, CD, WINKLE, RA, AND MASON, JW: *Determinants of survival in patients with ventricular tachyarrhythmias.* N Engl J Med 308:1436, 1983.

74. BENDITT, DG, BENSON, IW, KLEIN, GJ, ET AL: *Prevention of sudden cardiac arrest: Role of provocative electropharmacologic testing.* J Am Coll Cardiol 2:418, 1983.

# Mechanisms and Surgical Management of Ventricular Tachyarrhythmias*

*Alden H. Harken, M.D., Lewis Wetstein, M.D.,† and Mark E. Josephson, M.D.‡*

Ventricular tachyarrhythmias are the major cause of morbidity and mortality following infarction. Paradoxically, left ventricular pump failure appears less commonly than electrical disturbances, although ventricular arrhythmias do correlate with the severity of ischemic myocardial damage. Ventricular tachycardia and fibrillation frequently are the initiating arrhythmias leading to sudden cardiac death among patients with ischemic heart disease. The most common substrate for sustained ventricular tachycardia is prior myocardial infarction associated with wall motion abnormalities, specifically akinesis, hypokinesis, or left ventricular aneurysm. Other less common causes of ventricular tachycardia include arrhythmogenic right ventricular dysplasia, idiopathic left ventricular aneurysm, and a variety of miscellaneous diseases. More than 90 percent of patients with ventricular tachycardia associated with coronary artery disease or right ventricular dysplasia can have that rhythm induced and replicated by programmed electrical stimulation. The inducibility of ventricular tachycardia associated with other cardiac disorders or normal hearts is substantially less.

The first surgical approach to the treatment of ventricular arrhythmias associated with coronary artery disease was aneurysmectomy, which was performed initially almost 25 years ago.[1] Since the appearance of this initial report, a variety of surgical procedures have been employed in an attempt to deal with life-threatening arrhythmias, but with limited success.[2] Until electrophysiologic mapping and programmed stimulation had been refined to provide a greater understanding of the basis for this arrhythmia, the most common form of therapy for malignant arrhythmias remained aneurysmectomy with or without coronary artery bypass grafting. The rationale for such surgery was the association of coronary disease, multivessel coronary disease, and aneurysms with ventricular arrhythmias. The success of surgical therapy for these arrhythmias, however, was not uniform and the results are difficult to interpret. The difficulty arises because of a variety of arrhythmias, most of which were not well classified, evaluated, or treated, were included in these early series.[2,3] Furthermore, the methods for treating these patients and for assessing therapy were anecdotal and descriptive. These deficiencies were coupled with the tendency to report successes rather than failure, prohibiting

*Supported in part by grants #HL24278 and #HL22315 from the National Heart, Lung, and Blood Institute, Bethesda, Maryland; grants from the American Heart Association, Southeastern Pennsylvania Chapter, Philadelphia, Pennsylvania; and the Fannie E. Rippel Foundation, Morristown, New Jersey.

†Supported in part by grant G735A from the American Heart Association, Southeastern Pennsylvania Chapter. Recipient of Special Investigatorship Award G735A from the American Heart Association, Southeastern Pennsylvania Chapter.

‡Recipient of Research Career Development Award #HL00361, National Heart, Lung, and Blood Institute, Bethesda, Maryland.

adequate analysis of the effects of aneurysmectomy with or without bypass grafting for the treatment of this disorder. The only data available assessing such surgery in a well-defined group of comparable patients comes from Harken,[4] Mason,[3] and their coworkers, in which sustained ventricular tachycardias inducible by programmed stimulation that were treated by non–electrophysiologically guided surgery had a success rate of 30 to 50 percent. We believed that the reasons for this failure were that the substrate from which the tachycardias originated was at the border of infarction and/or involved the septum, neither of which was addressed by bypass grafting and/or standard aneurysmectomy.

## PATHOLOGIC SUBSTRATE OF VENTRICULAR TACHYCARDIA

Successful surgical intervention requires the resection or isolation of an area of the heart that has been rendered electrophysiologically deranged and thus able to sustain ventricular tachycardia. A better understanding of the electroanatomic milieu essential to sustain malignant ventricular arrhythmias is critical in order to develop appropriate surgical therapy for these arrhythmias. Evidence is accumulating in both animals and patients that myocardial ischemic damage can produce all the pathophysiologic requirements to develop sustained ventricular arrhythmias.

The initial step in the diagnosis of hemodynamically significant cardiac arrhythmias is identification of the origin as supraventricular or ventricular. QRS morphology (width $\geq 0.14$ sec), rate, axis (superior), atrioventricular dissociation, and fusion beats may be helpful in identifying ventricular tachycardia,[5] but these criteria are not absolute. Unequivocal diagnosis depends on intracardiac recording and electrophysiologic testing.

Cardiac arrhythmias are generally ascribed to either automatic or re-entrant mechanisms. Some cardiac cells, including those of the sinus node, certain areas of the atria (e.g., coronary sinus), lower atrioventricular node, and the specialized His-Purkinje system, have the potential to become pacemakers through spontaneous, diastolic depolarization.[6–8] In comparison, the remaining myocardial cells maintain a steady resting potential of approximately $-90$ millivolts until activated. The rate of impulse formation in automatic cells varies and determines which cells will control the rhythm of the heart. Once the automatic cells have depolarized, they stimulate adjacent myocardial cells to depolarize. Usually the sinus node has the highest rate of diastolic depolarization, and therefore it dominates the cardiac rhythm, suppressing potential subsidiary pacemakers.[9,10] Whenever the rate of impulse formation of the sinus node is slower than that of other automatic cells, these latent, subsidiary pacemaker cells will take over and control heart rate.

Several factors can increase or suppress the activity of the normal automatic mechanism, including alterations in autonomic tone, ischemia, hypoxemia, electrolyte fluxes, and drugs. Automatic ventricular tachycardias may occur as the result of increased phase 4 diastolic depolarization, and also they may occur in relation to slow channel–mediated phenomena.[11–14] These tachyarrhythmias are also characteristically associated with hypoxemia,[15] hypokalemia,[16] hypercalcemia,[17,18] increased catecholamines (exogenous or endogenous),[7,19,20] or drugs (typically digitalis).[21,22] Automatic ventricular tachyarrhythmias are common in the early periods following operation and peri–myocardial infarction.[23–26] Onset and termination are often gradual, with an initial warmup and occasional irregularity secondary to exit block from the automatic focus.[27] Automatic ventricular tachycardias may respond to treatment with lidocaine or procainamide, discontinuation of the infusion of sympathomimetic amine, or beta blockade. Phase 4–dependent automatic arrhythmias are neither readily provoked nor terminated by electrophysiologic programmed pacing.

Triggered automaticity is an abnormal rhythm activity that arises during the repolarization phase of a previous impulse rather than arising de novo.[28] This dependency on an initiating stimulus differentiates triggered automaticity from phase 4 automatic activity. The initial spontaneous or triggered impulse is often followed by a train of after-depolarizations that may or may not reach threshold potential, depending upon the amplitude of the after potential or the drive rate, or both. There is a direct relation between the drive rate and the amplitude of the after potential: as the drive rate increases, the amplitude increases. Triggered automaticity cannot always be distinguished from re-entry. However, triggered arrhythmias are more responsive to calcium-channel blocking agents than are most re-entrant ventricular arrhythmias. Although it has been observed experimentally in isolated tissues, the role of triggered activity in human ventricular arrhythmia is unknown.

### Re-entrant Arrhythmias

The vast majority of spontaneous, recurrent, sustained ventricular tachycardias occurring in the setting of chronic ischemic heart disease or previous myocardial infarction are due to re-entrant mechanisms[28,29] Ischemia alters both conduction and refractoriness.[29,30] Thus, during electrical depolarization, an impulse may block in one pathway of a potential re-entrant circuit because of its prolonged refractoriness, and conduct exclusively along the other limb. If conduction is sufficiently slow or the pathway sufficiently circuitous, the impulse may then be able to activate the previously refractory pathway, although retrogradely. After successful retrograde penetration and conduction, the impulse may then re-enter to activate the pathway originally engaged, again antegradely, perpetrating re-entry. Therefore, the electrophysiologic prerequisites for re-entry are unidirectional block, slow conduction over an alternate conduction pathway, and recovery of excitability in the previously refractory pathway.

Although re-entrant ventricular tachyarrhythmias are a recognized sequel to ischemic myocardial damage, only a fraction of afflicted patients appear to be at ongoing risk for malignant, recurrent, sustained ventricular tachyarrhythmias. To devise adequate therapy for these refractory arrhythmias, the electrophysiologic abnormalities predisposing to these arrhythmias must be elucidated.

The origin of these arrhythmias appears to involve peri-ischemic areas of abnormal but viable tissue.[29,30] This boundary between healthy, oxygenated myocardium and muscle that is either infarcted or reversibly or partially damaged may contain the necessary electrophysiologic basis for the initiation and perpetuation of arrhythmia.[31-33] The delineation of a peri-ischemic area has been well demonstrated,[34,35] and it is here that conduction and refractoriness are altered during both acute ischemia and chronic infarction. Adjacent cells in a milieu of interdigitated normal, infarcted and jeopardized, but reversibly damaged myocardium[36] have markedly different refractory periods. A propagated impulse will be blocked in one direction but will conduct in another. In the chronic situation, cells that appear normal and well perfused, but which adjoin ischemic or infarcted tissue, may also behave abnormally, similarly satisfying the conditions for re-entry.[37,38]

In an experimental canine model of heterogeneous infarcts, dogs were highly susceptible to the initiation of ventricular tachyarrhythmias, particularly sustained ventricular tachycardia.[39,40] This susceptibility was most apparent when programmed pacing was done from viable myocardial sites in close proximity to areas of ischemic damage.[40,41] In contrast, dogs with chronic homogeneous infarcts of comparable size were no more susceptible to the initiation of arrhythmia than were noninfarcted and sham-operated control dogs.[42]

The presence of a heterogeneous infarction with multiple interfaces of surviving but altered myocardium interdigitating with both normal and infarcted tissue apparently provides an adequate milieu for re-entrant arrhythmias.[35,43,44] Inasmuch as all tissue may not have been damaged uniformly, adjacent cells may exhibit varying properties of excitability, conduction and refractoriness. Local anatomic and electrophysiologic derangements will dictate whether a conducted impulse is slowed or blocked. This disorganized inhomogeneous pattern of impulse propagation results in the asynchronous activation of adjacent muscle fibers. Neighboring tissue will also recover at significantly disparate times. Finally, as the depressed myocardium recovers, it may be prematurely re-excited or re-entered by impulses from the adjoining muscle, resulting in re-entrant thythm. It is not yet clear what cellular alterations render one animal (or human) susceptible to sustained ventricular tachycardia, while another develops only nonsustained tachycardia or ventricular fibrillation.

In comparison, a homogeneous infarct contains only muscle that is irreversibly damaged. Uniformly viable myocardium is adjacent to the infarct.[33,35,45] Although a border zone abutting the damaged muscle exists, this zone has been demonstrated to be less than 100 microns in width in the normothermic, working heart.[46] Therefore, an impulse that encounters this homogeneous scar will probably be either uniformly propagated or blocked; rarely will the conditions necessary for a sustained re-entrant arrhythmia be satisfied.

Apparently, the geometry of the ischemic area determines both the susceptibility to ventricular tachyarrhythmias induced by pacing and the characteristics of the arrhythmia so initiated. Notably, heterogeneous infarctions are more arrhythmogenic than dense homogeneous infarctions and are also capable of sustaining an impulse along a circuitous pathway, producing ventricular tachycardia.

## INDICATIONS FOR SURGICAL INTERVENTION

Patients advised to undergo surgical ablation of re-entrant ventricular tachyarrhythmia have usually had poor results with conventional medical management. Pharmacologic trials employing programmed electrical stimulation protocols often demonstrate the ineffectiveness of conventional, and sometimes even investigational, antiarrhythmic drugs.[47-50] Unfortunately, invasive electropharmacologic testing can be time consuming (especially with drug-resistant patients—some patients may spend 3 to 4 weeks in the hospital undergoing multiple drug trials); also testing may be stressful and expensive. Moreover, there is a risk of morbidity and, potentially, of mortality. Protocols are being developed to predict the success or failure of medical or surgical approaches using multivariant discriminant analysis of the results of electrophysiologic testing, so that therapeutic regimens likely to fail can be avoided.

Spielman and coworkers[51] evaluated multiple invasive and noninvasive variables in 84 patients studied for sustained ventricular tachycardia to predict the response to serial testing with programmed electrical stimulation (PES). A successful medical result correlated with a patient age of less than 45 years, an ejection fraction of greater than 50 percent, hypokinesis as the only contraction abnormality, or the absence of structural heart disease. Factors associated with drug failure were the induction of ventricular tachycardia with only one extrastimulus, an H–V interval of greater than 60 msec, left ventricular aneurysm, or the presence of Q waves. No single variable adequately predicted the outcome of PES; however, with the use of multivariant discriminant analysis, 20 patients in a prospective series were classified correctly as drug failures, and medical successes were correctly predicted in four of five patients.

Swerdlow and colleagues[52] also used multivariant analysis to predict responses during serial programmed electrical stimulation. Again, no single variable predicted a therapeutic outcome. The absence of structural heart disease, a lower New York Heart Association functional class, fewer coronary arteries stenosed, the absence of left ventricular aneurysm, female sex, and fewer episodes of arrhythmia predicted a higher probability of response to the testing of electrophysiologic drugs.

It is anticipated that further such studies will help determine which patients might benefit from electrophysiologic-pharmacologic testing. Equally important is determining which patients might be spared the expense and morbidity of repeated electrophysiologic studies and possibly be candidates for surgical ablation.

Finally, noninvasive, computerized, surface electrocardiography performed with the use of signal-averaging techniques is also now in a stage of active development and investigation. Preliminary work suggests that patients highly susceptible to recurrent ventricular tachyarrhythmias may be identified by such methods, and perhaps the success or failure of either medical or surgical therapy may be predicted.

## Patient Population

In our first 100 consecutive patients with recurrent sustained ventricular tachycardia refractory to medical therapy who underwent surgery, there were 80 men and 20 women ranging in age from 23 to 74 years. Ninety-four patients had coronary artery disease; 85 also had left ventricular aneurysms. Each of the patients with coronary artery disease had a prior myocardial infarction, and each of the nine patients without aneurysm had an inferior wall myocardial infarction. The cardiac diagnoses in the remaining 6 patients included cardiomyopathy (2 patients—one with obliterative small vessel coronary disease), status of post-repair of tetralogy of Fallot (2 patients), idiopathic left ventricular aneurysm (1 patient), and idiopathic ventricular tachycardia (1 patient). In all but one patient, the tachycardia was replicable by programmed stimulation. In the remaining patient (with idiopathic ventricular tachycardia), the tachycardia could be neither initiated nor terminated by programmed stimulation but was repetitive and incessant and was mapped with catheter recordings using standard procedures.[53-55] Each of the patients had failed to respond to at least two standard antiarrhythmic agents and, in most patients, more than four, including experimental antiarrhythmic agents. Approximately one third of the patients had suffered a cardiac arrest from the ventricular tachycardia.

Catheter endocardial mapping of one or more morphologically distinct ventricular tachycardias was accomplished in all but seven patients. In six of these patients, the tachycardia remained hemodynamically and electrically unstable despite antiarrhythmic agents, and therefore, could not be mapped.

## Intraoperative Electrophysiologic Mapping

Intraoperative mapping was performed after cannulation for cardiopulmonary bypass, as previously described.[54-56] Reference electrograms were recorded from the right and left ventricles. A catheter positioned preoperatively in the right ventricular apex was utilized for programmed stimulation. Three electrocardiographic leads were recorded simultaneously with both reference electrograms and electrograms from a mapping ring electrode (1 to 1.5 mm interelectrode distance) from 54 to 90 preselected epicardial sites from both ventricles during sinus rhythm and ventricular tachycardia. Following completion of the epicardial map of ventricular tachycardia, a left ventricular aneurysm or akinetic area was incised and/or resected. In most patients, the tachycardia continued despite this procedure, and endocardial mapping was undertaken. If the tachycardia stopped following ventriculotomy or resection, it was almost always easily re-initiated by programmed stimulation. Endocardial mapping was performed initially around the cut edge of the aneurysm in a clockwise fashion with 1 cm increasing radii. Typically, 40 to 60 endocardial sites were mapped. In the most recent 20 patients with coronary artery disease, only endocardial mapping was undertaken during ventricular tachycardia owing to accumulated data suggesting that it was endocardium from which the tachycardia originated.

## Results of Intraoperative Mapping

Epicardial mapping was performed during sinus rhythm in the first 90 patients. In 10 of the 84 patients with coronary artery disease, one or more late potentials were recorded during sinus rhythm. In one patient with idiopathic left ventricular aneurysm, late potentials were recorded over the aneurysm. These late potentials occurred 10 to 60 msec following completion of the QRS complex and were usually preceded by a low-amplitude electrogram within the QRS. In all but one instance, the late potential was recorded on or at the border of the ventricular aneurysm. In 5 of the 81 patients with coronary disease, the late potentials bore no relationship to the origin of the tachycardia that arose on the septum. In the remaining 76 patients, the origin of the tachycardia arose on the endocardium of the free wall within 3 cm of the epicardial late potential. Similarly, an epicardial late potential was recorded in proximity to the endocardial origin of the tachycardia in the patient with idiopathic late ventricular aneurysm. Despite this relationship in these six patients, additional tachycardia morphologies were observed to originate at a distant site from the late potential in half of these patients. These data demonstrate that epicardial late potentials are infrequent in the presence of coronary artery disease and that they may not be useful to guide surgery in such patients. These data are in contrast to those of Fontaine[57,58] who always found late potentials in patients with arrhythmogenic right ventricular dysplasia and suggested they identified areas from which the tachycardias arose.

One hundred forty-seven morphologically distinct ventricular tachycardias were induced in the 100 patients intraoperatively. In a patient with automatic ventricular tachycardia, the arrhythmia stopped following anesthesia, and surgery was based on the map obtained in the catheterization laboratory. Fifty-seven patients had more than one morphologically distinct ventricular tachycardia. Although complete epicardial and/or endocardial duration maps were obtained in at least one morphologically distinct tachycardia in most patients, such data were not obtained during each morphologically distinct tachycardia for a variety of reasons, primarily related to inability to initiate all morphologically distinct tachycardias during epicardial and endocardial mapping and/or to a degeneration of the ventricular tachycardia to ventricular fibrillation.

There were 92 tachycardias with right bundle branch block pattern and 55 with left bundle branch block pattern. Epicardial activation during the tachycardia typically began after the onset of the QRS complex except in three patients in whom epicardial activation appeared prior to the onset of the QRS (2 patients), or simultaneously with the onset of the QRS (1 patient). In none of these cases, however, was the epicardial breakthrough the earliest activation recorded. The extent to which epicardial breakthrough followed the onset of the QRS complex was unrelated to the site of origin. In the tachycardias with right bundle branch block morphology, epicardial breakthrough always was on the left ventricle. In those with left bundle branch block morphology, epicardial breakthrough was typically on the right ventricle adjacent to the anterior or inferior interventricular groove (51 patients) or, less commonly, on the left ventricle adjacent to the anterior interventricular groove (5 patients).

Analysis of endocardial activation during ventricular tachycardia revealed that activation from the endocardium was always recorded earlier than that from the epicardium (14 to 85 msec earlier). In all cases, activity preceding the onset of the QRS complex was recorded. In five tachycardias in three patients, continuous activation around the border of an aneurysm was observed. Digital pressure at multiple sites around this pattern of activation could terminate the tachycardia. In approximately half of the patients, electrical activity in systole and diastole could be recorded within a small area of 4 to 6 cm$^2$ either in the same electrogram or in an adjacent electrogram. The significance of these abnormal electrograms has yet to be determined, but we believe they represent terminal components of a re-entrant circuit. Although these findings may represent slowly conducting wavelets unrelated to the re-entrant circuit, termination of the tachycardia by digital pressure at some of these sites and not other areas suggests that our assumption may be right.

Fifty-four patients manifested multiple morphologically distinct tachycardias. In 36 of these patients, earliest activity during two or more of the tachycardias was at the same or adjacent sites. However, in 18 patients, there appeared to be two widely disparate areas of origin. There was no correlation of the site of epicardial breakthrough and the site of earliest recorded endocardial activity when the tachycardias arose on the septum, which was the site

292

of origin in almost two thirds of our patients. When the site of earliest activation was on the endocardium of the free wall of the left ventricle, there was a correlation with epicardial breakthrough in half the patients. In the remaining patients, epicardial breakthrough was still greater than 3 cm from the site of endocardial origin.

In eight patients, intraoperative mappping data either could not be obtained or could not be interpreted, and surgery was based upon the preoperative catheter map. This situation resulted from surgical complications, rapid degeneration of ventricular tachycardia to ventricular fibrillation, inability to determine early from late activation, and one case of automatic tachycardia in which the tachycardia was not present at the time of surgery.

## SURGICAL THERAPY

Because the pathologic basis for the majority of sustained ventricular tachycadias was the sequelae of occlusive disease of the coronary artery, the earliest surgical interventions focused upon the restoration of coronary blood flow. Despite successful anginal control and relief of myocardial ischemia with aortocoronary bypass grafting, simultaneous arrhythmia control was usually not achieved with this procedure.[59,60] Subsequent attempts at revascularization with concomitant resection of ventricular aneurysm also failed to prevent these arrhythmias.[61,62] Apparently, because the origin of the re-entrant focus was often distant from the apparent epicardial border of the aneurysm,[63] so-called blind aneurysmectomy (i.e., without electrophysiologic mapping) was not sufficient to either abolish arrhythmogenic circuits or interrupt the propagation of arrhythmogenic curcuits to the remainder of the ventricles.[64]

### Electrophysiologically Directed Endocardial Excision

On the basis of our intraoperative data demonstrating that (1) aneurysmectomy failed to ablate the arrhythmias and (b) the origin of the tachycardia appeared to be near the endocardium at the border of the infarction and/or aneurysm, we developed the technique of electrophysiologically directed endocardial resection in order to treat this arrhythmia (Fig. 1).[2,56]

In the human, areas of slowed conduction have been identified in the endocardial recordings from patients with ventricular tachycardia.[64] Endocardial electrophysiologic mapping in patients with recurrent ventricular tachycardia has demonstrated the origin of ventricular activation to be near the endocardial edge of the aneurysm or infarction.[65,66] Excision of the endocardium, including the earliest site of activation, has resulted in the control of arrhythmias in patients with disease previously refractory to all medical treatment.[66] Clinical results suggest that the endocardial excision technique is not arrhythmogenic; perhaps the resulting cicatrix in the endocardium behaves as a homogeneous infarct, with propagation of an impulse that encounters this area being either uniformly slowed or blocked.[65–67] Inasmuch as the recognized electrophysiologic substrata of re-entrant arrhythmias are areas of unidirectional block, slow conduction and multiple potential conduction pathways, the procedure for endocardial excision should be successful in abolishing recurrent sustained ventricular tachycardias if (1) the arrhythmia circuit is excised; (2) a critical pathway of conduction is interrupted; or (3) barriers to impulse exits are created.

The Purkinje fibers function as a network of communication that propagates impulses throughout the ventricular myocardium in a rapid but orderly sequence. Stripping the endocardium may interrupt the transmission of impulses; this may suffice for the effective control of arrhythmias. Removal of the endocardium together with the critical Purkinje fiber linkages may be one method of successful endocardial resection.

With this procedure, the endocardium in the region of earliest activity determined by intraoperative mapping and/or catheter mapping was undermined and resected. Typically the excised tissue amounts to 6 to 15 cm$^2$ of tissue from an area occupying 25 to 40 percent of

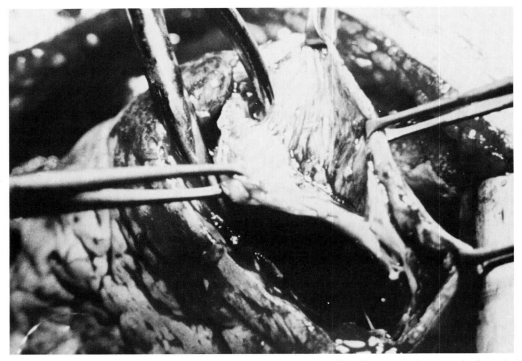

**Figure 1.** Electrophysiologically directed endocardial excision is accomplished by completing a standard surgical aneurysmectomy. The area of earliest activation during ventricular tachycardia is localized electrophysiologically. An endocardial peel is then surgically removed in this area of earliest ventricular activation. Characteristically, this is at the endocardial edge of the aneurysmal border.

the circumference of the aneurysm. All patients have had an endocardial resection at the site of earliest activation. Eighty-five patients have had aneurysmectomies, and our two patients post-repair of tetralogy of Fallot underwent removal of the scar from the prior right ventriculotomy incision. Cryosurgery was added as adjunctive therapy to 13 patients with coronary heart disease in whom the site of earliest activation was at the base of a papillary muscle or intramural and could not be removed by our standard procedure. In our patient with automatic tachycardia, cryothermal injury was directed at the septal aspect of the right ventricular outflow tract underneath the endocardial resection. In two other patients with cardiomyopathy, cryothermia was employed in one case because the tachycardia appeared to arise near the base of the inferior papillary muscle and in another with origin near the base of the anterior papillary muscle. Thus, cryosurgery was utilized when mapping demonstrated early activity below the area resected by the standard endocardial resection or considered unresectable, that is, the papillary muscle. Sixty-one of the 91 patients with coronary artery disease had concomitant coronary bypass grafting, with an average of 1.6 grafts per patient. There were nine operative deaths: seven from pump failure, one from heart failure associated with an intraoperative infarction, and one from disopyramide-induced cardiogenic shock. All but two of the remaining 91 patients underwent electrophysiologic studies 1 to 3 weeks following surgery. The stimulation protocol included single, double, and on occasion triple ventricular extrastimuli from the right and, when necessary, the left ventricle. In addition, 80 patients underwent cardiac catheterization prior to discharge to determine the hemodynamic effects of the surgical procedure. The remaining patients had noninvasive assessment of ventrocular function with echocardiography and MUGA scans.

In 70 patients undergoing electrophysiologic studies, programmed ventricular stimulation was unable to replicate the clinical arrhythmia. In 21 cases, the tachycardia was inducible and/or occurred spontaneously. The induction of tachycardia in these patients was achieved by methods similar to those that induced the arrhythmia prior to surgery. Of note, two of the sustained arrhythmias that were induced were never observed prior to surgery. Serial electrophysiologic drug testing was again performed in each patient with inducible tachycardia. In 13 patients, the tachycardia was no longer inducible following drug therapy, whereas in 8 the tachycardia remained inducible. All patients were sent home on the antiarrhythmic agent or agents that had made the tachycardia noninducible, or on which the tachycardia was inducible but with greater difficulty, and/or which made the tachycardia slower.

Four of the 70 patients with no inducible ventricular tachycardia had recurrences, and 3 of 21 whose tachycardias were inducible after surgery had recurrences. In addition, there were three late sudden deaths in the group that was initially noninducible, one of which was in a patient who had a recurrence of well-tolerated ventricular tachycardia and was placed on quinidine. None of these patients had had a cardiac arrest from tachycardia prior to surgery. Two of the patients who died suddenly had chest pain at the time of cardiac arrest. The remaining patient who died suddenly nearly 3 years postoperatively had had no arrhythmias despite having a well-tolerated ventricular tachycardia (rate 160 beats per min) 15 times in the year prior to surgery. In total, there were 19 late deaths including the three sudden deaths. Of the remaining 16 patients, nine died of heart failure, three died of recurrent myocardial infarction, and one each died of pneumonia, ruptured pulmonary artery, gram-negative sepsis, and ruptured pseudo-infarction in area of recent ischemia. An actuarial survival curve demonstrates almost 60 percent 5-year survival.

Postoperative inducibility and survival appear to be unrelated to the presence or absence of coronary bypass grafts, or the preoperative ejection fraction or left ventricular end-diastolic pressure. Moreover, the results of Holter monitoring were also of no value in predicting inducibility, clinical recurrence, or survival. In fact, most survivors currently have high-grade ectopy. Of note, ejection fractions improved from a mean of 28 percent to a mean of 39 percent and left ventricular end-diastolic pressures decreased from 18 to 15 mm Hg, both of which were statistically significant ($p < 0.05$).[68] There was a high failure rate in those patients requiring adjunctive cryothermia. We believe that this is a result of a subselected population in whom subendocardial resection alone was predicted not to be totally effective and in whom cryothermal ablation was attempted but also failed.

## DISCUSSION

Recurrent sustained ventricular tachyarrhythmias unresponsive to medical therapy were associated with a 1-year mortality of 70 to 85 percent. Patients who are susceptible to these re-entrant arrhythmias usually have a history of previous myocardial infarction or chronic myocardial ischemia. More specifically, these patients demonstrate both anatomic and electrophysiologic derangements. Experimental work suggests that regions of nonuniform damage render the ventricle particularly susceptible to ventricular tachyarrhythmias, and even relatively large areas of homogeneous myocardial ischemic damage may not display the same susceptibility to these arrhythmias. Surgical techniques are being devised to treat patients with ventricular tachyarrhythmias refractory to medical management. These approaches have provided control of arrhythmias in patients whose disease was previously resistant to all medical treatment. The evolving surgical therapies presently employed share either of two physiopathologic consequences that render them successful: the homogeneous ablation of previous heterogeneous myocardial ischemic damage or the delimiting of an arrhythmogenic focus by excluding conduction to surrounding myocardium.

### Advantages and Limitations of Endocardial Resection

The major advantage of electrophysiologically directed endocardial resection is that it is a guided surgical resection that causes no significant hemodynamic impairment and can, in the majority of cases, ablate the arrhythmia.

The technique also allows for the treatment of tachycardias arising on the septum without necessitating septal disarticulation or purposeful creation of a ventricular septal defect. The long-term clinical efficacy and hemodynamic effects of this procedure have been borne out.

The major limitation of the technique is the requirement that each of the observed morphologically distinct tachycardias be induced and mapped at or prior to surgery. Intraoperative mapping cannot always be accomplished, and preoperative catheter endocardial mapping, which permits repeated examination, provides an extremely important tool to localize tachyarrhythmias that may not be induced in the operating room. Although in the vast majority of patients (91 percent), at least one tachycardia can be initiated and mapped in the operating room, this is not always possible and surgical resection must be based on the preoperative catheter map. Thus, the potential inability to accomplish intraoperative endocardial mapping of all morphologic types necessitates preoperative catheter mapping to help guide surgery. Refinement of our mapping techniques has allowed us spatial localization to within approximately 4 cm$^2$.

Another limitation of the technique is the inability to resect the base of the papillary muscles should the tachycardia arise there. Although a limited endocardial resection can be accomplished around the papillary muscle, other techniques, such as cryosurgery, will probably be required to ablate the site of such arrhythmias by creating a homogenous infarction. A similar problem of deep-lying tachycardias within the septum or intramural myocardium also exists. Again, in such cases localization into these deeper areas by intramural mapping may identify cases in which cryothermal injury can create homogeneously infarcted muscle to greater depths than that achieved by endocardial resection, thereby treating the tachycardia successfully. It is clear, therefore, that there must be a large investment of personnel and equipment for this approach or any approach that requries accurate localization of the tachycardia.

### Cryosurgery Alone

Alternatively, an electrophysiologically heterogeneous zone of ischemic injury can be converted into a homogeneous scar by freezing to minus 60°C. This cryosurgical technique permits ablation of the area of activation [69] without disrupting surrounding tissue or myocardial function.[69,70] Moreover, the procedure can be performed without the use of cardiopulmonary bypass in selected patients. The most appealing aspect of this technique is the ability to treat circuits that otherwise would be relatively inaccessible, for example, those in close proximity to papillary muscle or near the mitral annulus, where endocardial excision may not be applicable. At present, there are insufficient reports by which to compare the short-term results or the long-term consequences of cryosurgery with those of excision.

### Encircling Endocardial Ventriculotomy

Encircling endocardial ventriculotomy (EEV) has also been shown to be clinically useful in the surgical management of refractory ventricular tachycardia.[72] This technique was designed to exclude all infarcted and border areas of diseased myocardium from electrical continuity with the remaining normal myocardium.[71,73] EEV is performed thorugh a perpendicular ventricular incision, sparing only the epicardial surface and coronary vessels. The EEV follows the edge of the endocardial extent of the infarction as defined by visual inspection. The resultant near-transmural scar should contain the arrhythmia within its boundaries.

Thus, if ventricular tachycardia were to be initiated, the depolarization wave front issuing from the origin of the tachycardia should not exit into the normal ventricle. Guiraudon, Fontaine, and their colleagues[71,73] reported a successful outcome in 17 of 23 patients who underwent EEV. Two patients (9 percent) died, and 4 of the 21 surviving patients (19 percent) had spontaneous recurrence of ventricular tachycardia postoperatively. Followup observation in this series ranged from 1 to 55 months.

Unfortunately, the hemodynamic consequences of this procedure have been severe.[74-76] Whereas the endocardial excision and cryoablative techniques have demonstrated disruption of re-entrant circuits without destroying functional myocardial integrity, the encircling endocardial ventriculotomy has resulted in significant left ventricular dysfunction owing to decrease in diastolic compliance and to impairment of systolic excursion in the EEV-enclosed regions.[74-77] The overall clinical advantages of this technique have yet to be determined.

## CONCLUSIONS

Postinfarction, recurrent ventricular tachyarrhythmias remain the single most common cause of death in the United States. Recent advances in our understanding of the electroanatomy of these re-entrant ischemic ventricular arrhythmias has provided a foundation for their diagnosis and suggested promising pharmacologic and surgical therapy. Although we have utilized the electrophysiologically guided endocardial excision as the major therapeutic modality, encircling endocardial ventriculotomy and cryosurgery have also been proposed as alternative means to surgically treat arrhythmias. The precise role of these procedures, singly or in combination, in the management of ventricular tachycardia remains to be determined by prospective studies.

## REFERENCES

1. COUCH, OA, JR: *Cardiac aneurysm with ventricular tachycardia and subsequent excision of aneurysm.* Circulation 20:251, 1959.

2. HOROWITZ, LN, HARKEN, AH, JOSEPHSON, ME, ET AL: *Surgical treatment of ventricular arrhythmias in coronary artery disease.* Ann Intern Med 95:88, 1981.

3. MASON, JW, STINSON, EB, AND WINKLE, RA: *Relative efficacy of blind left ventricular aneurysm resection for the treatment of recurrent ventricular tachycardia.* Am J Cardiol 49:241, 1982.

4. HARKEN, AH, HOROWITZ, LN, AND JOSEPHSON, ME: *Comparison of standard aneurysmectomy and aneurysmectomy with directed endocardial resection for the treatment of recurrent sustained ventricular tachycardia.* J Thorac Cardiovasc Surg 80:527, 1980.

5. WELLENS, HJJ, BAR, FWHM, AND LIE, KI: *The value of the electrocardiogram in the differential diagnosis of a tachycardia with a widened QRS complex.* Am J Med 64:27, 1978.

6. BANDURA, JP AND BRODY, DA: *Electronic transmission through blocked canine Purkinje tissue: Role of calcium.* Circulation 52(Suppl II):18, 1975.

7. HOFFMAN, BF AND CRANEFIELD, PF: *Electrophysiology of the Heart.* McGraw-Hill, New York, 1960.

8. HORDOF, AJ, SPOTNITZ, A, MARY-RABINE, L, ET AL *The cellular electrophysiologic effects of digitalis on human atrial fibers.* Circulation 57:223, 1978.

9. WEIDMANN, S: *Heart: Electrophysiology.* Annu Rev Physiol 36:155, 1974.

10. VASSALLE, M: *Generation and conduction of impulses in the heart under physiological and pathological conditions.* Pharmacol Ther B 3:1, 1977.

11. HORDOF, AJ, EDIE, R, MALM, JR, ET AL: *Electrophysiologic properties and response to pharmacologic agents of fibers from diseased atria.* Circulation 54:774, 1976.

12. SINGER, DH, TEN EICK, RE, AND DEBOER, A: *Electrophysical correlates of human atrial tachyarrhythmias.* In DREIFUS, LS AND LIKOFF, W (EDS.): *Cardiac Arrhythmias.* Grune & Stratton, New York, 1973, pp 97–111.

13. SPEAR, JF, HOROWITZ, LN, HODESS, AB, ET AL: *Cellular electrophysiology of human myocardial infarction: I. Abnormalities of cellular activities.* Circulation 59:247, 1979.

14. TALANO, JV, SINGER, DH, LOEB, HS, ET AL: *Intractable ventricular tachyarrhythmias in post-infarction aneurysm: Clinical, electrophysiologic and electropharmacologic studies.* Clin Res 24:242A, 1976.

15. TRAUTWEIN, W: *Membrane currents in cardiac muscle fibers.* Physiol Rev 53:793, 1973.

16. CARMELIET, EE: *Chloride and potassium permeability in cardiac Purkinje fibers.* Bruxelles Presses Academiques Europeennes, Brussels, 1961.

17. FERRIER, GR AND MOE, GK: *Effect of calcium on acetylstrophanthidin-induced transient depolarization in canine Purkinje tissue.* Circ Res 33:508, 1973.

18. WEINGART, R, KASS, RS, AND TSIEN, RW: *Roles of calcium and sodium ions in the transient inward current induced by strophanthidin in cardiac Purkinje fibers.* Biophys J 17:3A, 1977.

19. ARMOUR, JA, HAGEMAN, GR, AND RANDALL, WC: *Arrhythmias induced by local cardiac nerve stimulation.* Am J Physiol 223:1068, 1972.

20. TSIEN, RW: *Effects of epinephrine on the pacemaker potassium current of cardiac Purkinje fibers.* J Gen Physiol 64:293, 1974.

21. DAVIS, LD: *Effect of changes in cycle length on diastolic depolarization produced by ouabain in canine Purkinje fibers.* Circ Res 32:206, 1973.

22. FERRIER, GR, SAUNDERS, JH, AND MENDEZ, CA: *Cellular mechanism for the generation of ventricular arrhythmias by acetylstrophanthidin.* Circ Res 32:600, 1973.

23. FRIEDMAN, PL, STEWART, JF, FENOGLIO, JJ, ET AL: *Survival of subendocardial Purkinje fibers after extensive myocardial infarction in dogs: In vitro and in vivo correlations.* Circ Res 33:597, 1973.

24. HOPE, RR, SCHERLAG, BJ, EL-SHERIF, N, ET AL: *Hierarchy of ventricular pacemakers.* Circ Res 39:883, 1976.

25. HOROWITZ, LN, SPEAR, JF, AND MOORE, EN: *Subendocardial origin of ventricular arrhythmias in 24-hour-old experimental myocardial infarction.* Circulation 53:56, 1975.

26. SPEAR, JF, MICHELSON, EL, SPIELMAN, SR, ET AL: *The origin of ventricular arrhythmias 24 hours following experimental anterior septal coronary artery occlusion.* Circulation 55:844, 1977.

27. FISCH, C, GREENSPAN, K, AND ANDERSON, GJ: *Exit block.* Am J Cardiol 28:402, 1971.

28. WIT, AL AND CRANEFIELD, PF: *Triggered activity in cardiac muscle fibers of the simian mitral valve.* Circ Res 38:85, 1976.

29. SCHERLAG, BJ, EL-SHERIF, N, HOPE, R, ET AL: *Characterization and localization of ventricular arrhythmias resulting from myocardial ischemia and infarction.* Circ Res 35:372, 1974.

30. HAN, J: *Mechanisms of ventricular arrhythmias associated with myocardial infarction.* Am J Cardiol 24:800, 1969.

31. WELLENS, HJJ: *Electrical stimulation of the heart in the study and treatment of tachycardias.* University Park Press, Baltimore, 1971, pp 14–22.

32. BOINEAU, JP AND COX, JL: *Slow ventricular activation in acute myocardial infarction: A source of re-entrant premature ventricular contractions.* Circulation 48:702, 1973.

33. JANSE, MJ, VAN CAPELLE, FJL, MORSINK, H, ET AL: *Flow of "injury" current and patterns of excitation during early ventricular arrhythmias in acute regional myocardial ischemia in isolated porcine and canine hearts; evidence for two different arrhythmogenic mechanisms.* Circ Res 47:151, 1980.

34. SIMSON, MB, HARDEN, W, BARLOW, C, ET AL: *Visualization of the distance between perfusion and anoxia along an ischemic border.* Circulation 60:1151, 1979.

35. WETSTEIN, L, NUSSBAUM, MS, BARLOW, CH, ET AL: *Decrease in acute myocardial ischemia by hyaluronidase in isolated, perfused rabbit hearts.* J Surg Res 30:489, 1981.

36. PHAM, TD, FENOGLIO, JJ, JR, HARKEN, AH, ET AL: *Structural basis for recurrent sustained ventricular tachycardia.* Circulation 64(Suppl):87, 1981.

37. SPEAR, JF, MICHELSON, EL, AND MOORE, EN: *Excitability of cells within a mottled infarct of dogs susceptible to sustained ventricular tachyarrhythmias.* J Am Coll Cardiol 1:1099, 1983.

38. EL-SHERIF, N, SCHERLAG, BJ, LAZZARA, R, ET AL: *Re-entrant ventricular arrhythmias in the late myocardial infarction period: I. Conduction characteristics in the infarction zone.* Circulation 55:686, 1977.

39. MICHELSON, EL, SPEAR, JF, AND MOORE, NE: *Electrophysiological and anatomic correlates of sustained ventricular tachyarrhythmias in a model of chronic myocardial infarction.* Am J Cardiol 45:583, 1980.

40. KARAGUEUZIAN, HS, FENOGLIO, JJ, JR, WEISS, MB, ET AL: *Protracted ventricular tachycardia induced by premature stimulation of the canine heart after coronary artery occlusion and reperfusion.* Circ Res 44:833, 1979.

41. MICHELSON, EL, SPEAR, JF, AND MOORE, EN: *Initiation of sustained ventricular tachyarrhythmias in a canine model of chronic myocardial infarction: Importance of the site of stimulation.* Circulation 63:776, 1981.

42. WETSTEIN, L, MICHELSON, EL, SIMSON, MB, ET AL: *Increased interphase between normoxic and ischemic tissue as the cause for re-entry ventricular tachyarrhythmias.* J Surg Res 32:526, 1982.

43. WETSTEIN, L, MICHELSON, EL, EULER, D, ET AL: *Mechanism and surgical therapy of re-entrant ventricular tachyarrhythmias.* Surg Forum 32:266, 1981.

44. WETSTEIN, L, MICHELSON, EL, SIMSON, MB, ET AL: *Homogeneous ablation of heterogeneous myocardial injury as a method of decreasing ventricular arrhythmogenicity.* Surg Forum 33:288, 1982.

45. WETSTEIN, L, SIMSON, MB, FELDMAN, P, ET AL: *Pharmacologic modification of myocardial ischemia.* Circulation 66:548, 1982.

46. HARKEN, AH, SIMSON, MB, WETSTEIN, L, ET AL: *Early ischemia after complete coronary ligation in the rabbit, dog, pig and monkey.* Am J Physiol 241:H202, 1981.

47. HOROWITZ, LN, JOSEPHSON, ME, FARSHIDI, A, ET AL: *Current sustained ventricular tachycardia: III. Role of the electrophysiologic study in selection of antiarrhythmic regimens.* Circulation 58:986, 1978.

48. MASON, JW AND WINKLE, RA: *Electrode-catheter arrhythmia induction in the selection and assessment of antiarrhythmic drug therapy for recurrent ventricular tachycardia.* Circulation 58:971, 1978.

49. MASON, JW AND WINKLE, RA *Accuracy of the ventricular tachycardia-induction study for predicting long-term efficacy and inefficacy of antiarrhythmic drugs.* N Engl J Med 303:1073, 1980.

50. RUSKIN, JN, DiMARCO, JP, AND GARAN, H: *Out-of-hospital cardiac arrest: Electrophysiologic observations and selection of long-term antiarrhythmic therapy.* N Engl J Med 303:607, 1980.

51. SPIELMAN, SR, SCHWARTZ, JS, McCARTHY, DM, ET AL: *Predictors of the success or failure of medical therapy in patients with chronic recurrent sustained ventricular tachycardia: A discriminant analysis.* J Am Coll Cardiol 1:401, 1983.

52. SWERDLOW, CD, GONG, G, ECHT, DS, ET AL: *Clinical factors predicting successful electrophysiologic-pharmacologic study in patients with ventricular tachycardia.* J Am Coll Cardiol 1:409, 1983.

53. JOSEPHSON, ME, HOROWITZ, LN, FARSHIDI, A, ET AL: *Recurrent sustained ventricular tachycardia: 2. Endocardial mapping.* Circulation 57:440, 1978.

54. JOSEPHSON, ME, HOROWITZ, LN, SPIELMAN, SR, ET AL: *Comparison of endocardial catheter mapping with intraoperative mapping of ventricular tachycardia.* Circulation 61:395, 1980.

55. JOSEPHSON, ME, HOROWITZ, LN, SPIELMAN, SR, ET AL: *The role of catheter mapping in the preoperative evaluation of ventricular tachycardia.* Am J Cardiol 49:207, 1982.

56. HARKEN, AH, JOSEPHSON, ME, AND HOROWITZ, LN: *Surgical endocardial resection for the treatment of malignant ventricular tachycardia.* Ann Surg 190:456, 1979.

57. FONTAINE, G: *Surgical management of ventricular tachycardia unrelated to myocardial ischemia or infarction.* Am J Cardiol 49:397, 1982.

58. FONTAINE, G: *Stimulation studies and epicardial mapping in ventricular tachycardia: Study of mechanisms and selection for surgery.* In KULBERTUS, HE (ED): *Reentrant Arrhythmias: Mechanisms and Treatment.* University Park Press, Baltimore, 1977, pp 334–350.

59. TILKIAN, AG, PFEIFER, JF, BARRY, WH, ET AL: *The effect of coronary bypass surgery on exercise-induced ventricular arrhythmias,* Am Heart J 92:707, 1976.

60. DeSOYZA, N, MURPHY, ML, BISSETT, JK, ET AL: *Ventricular arrhythmia in chronic stable angina pectoris with surgical or medical treatment.* Ann Intern Med 89:10, 1979.

61. TABRY, IF, GEHA, AS, HAMMOND, GL, ET AL: *Effect of surgery on ventricular tachyarrhythmias associated with coronary arterial occlusive disease.* Circulation 58(Suppl):166, 1978.

62. SAMI, M, CHAITMAN, BR, BOURASSA, MG, ET AL: *Long term follow-up of aneurysmectomy for recurrent ventricular tachycardia or fibrillation.* Am Heart J 96:303, 1978.

63. MASON, JW, STINSON, EB, WINKLE, RA, ET AL: *Relative efficacy of blind left ventricular aneurysm resection for the treatment of recurrent ventricular tachycardia.* Am J Cardiol 49:241, 1982.

64. JOSEPHSON, ME, HOROWITZ, LN AND FARSHIDI, A: *Continuous local electrical activity: A mechanism of recurrent ventricular tachycardia* Circulation 57:659, 1978.

65. HOROWITZ, LN, JOSEPHSON, ME, AND HARKEN, AH: *Epicardial and endocardial activation during sustained ventricular tachycardia in man.* Circulation 61:1277, 1980.

66. WITTIG, JH AND BOINEAU, JP: *Surgical treatment of ventricular arrhythmia using epicardial, transmural, and endocardial mapping.* Ann Thorac Surg 20:117, 1975.

67. WETSTEIN, L, MICHELSON, EL, SIMSON, MB, ET AL: *Evaluation of arrhythmogenicity of surgically-induced endocardial vs. ischemic myocardial damage.* J Thorac Cardiovasc Surg (in press).

68. MARTIN, JR, UNTEREKER, WS, HARKEN, AH, ET AL: *Aneurysmectomy and endocardial resection of ventricular tachycardia: Favorable hemodynamic and antiarrhythmic results in patients with global left ventricular dysfunction.* Am Heart J 103:960, 1982.

69. GALLAGHER, JJ, ANDERSON, RA, AND KASELL, J: *Cryoablation of drug-resistant ventricular tachycardia in a patient with a variant of scleroderma.* Circulation 57:190, 1978.

70. KLEIN, GJ, HARRISON, L, AND IDEKER, RF: *Reaction of the myocardium to cryosurgery: Electrophysiology and arrhythmogenic potential.* Circulation 59:364, 1979.

71. GUIRAUDON, G, FONTAINE, G, AND FRANK, R: *La ventriculotomie circulaire d'exlusion; traitement chirurgical des tachycardies ventriculaires compliquant un infarctus du myocarde.* Arch Mal Coeur 71:1255, 1978.

72. GUIRAUDON, G, FONTAINE, G, AND FRANK, R: *Encircling endocardial ventriculotomy: A new surgical treatment for life-threatening ventricular tachycardias resistant to medical treatment following myocardial infarction.* Ann Thorac Surg 26:438, 1978.

73. FONTAINE, G, GUIRAUDON, G, FRANK, R, ET AL: *The surgical management of ventricular tachycardia.* Herz 4:276, 1979.

74. UNGERLEIDER, RM, CALCAGNO, D, WILLIAMS, JM, ET AL: *Encircling endocardial ventriculotomy for refractory ischemic ventricular tachycardia: Effects on regional left ventricular function.* Surg Forum 32:230, 1981.

75. UNGERLEIDER, RM, HOLMAN, WL, STANLEY, TE, III, ET AL: *Encircling endocardial ventriculotomy for refractory ischemic ventricular tachycardia: I. Electrophysiological effects.* J Thorac Cardiovasc Surg 83:840, 1982.

76. UNGERLEIDER, RM, HOLMAN, WL, AND STANLEY, TE, III: *Encircling endocardial ventriculotomy for refractory ischemic ventricular tachycardia: II. Effects on regional myocardial blood flow.* J Thorac Cardiovasc Surg 83:850, 1982.

77. UNGERLEIDER, RM, HOLMAN, WL, AND CALCAGNO, D: *Encircling endocardial ventriculotomy for refractory ischemic ventricular tachycardia: III. Effects on regional left ventricular function.* J Thorac Cardiovasc Surg 83:857, 1982.

# Sudden Death in Infants, Children, and Adolescents

*Victoria L. Vetter, M.D.*

Sudden death is generally considered to be a problem of adults with advanced coronary artery disease. Therefore, the sudden and unexpected death of a young person is considered to be especially tragic. The most common etiologies and the epidemiology of sudden death differ depending on the age of the child. Sudden death in infants will be discussed separately from sudden death in childhood and adolescence.

## SUDDEN INFANT DEATH SYNDROME

The sudden infant death syndrome (SIDS) is defined as the death of an infant that is unexpected by history and in which a thorough postmortem examination fails to demonstrate an adequate cause for death. SIDS is the leading cause of death in the first year of life. Approximately 8000 deaths per year in the United States, or 22 per day, result from this syndrome.[1] The etiology of SIDS and the responsible mechanisms remain the subject of considerable controversy and active research.

The predominant opinion is that few SIDS are caused by a primary cardiac abnormality.[2] The leading hypothesis at present—the apnea hypothesis—states that these infants have an abnormality in the autonomic regulation of cardiovascular or respiratory activity, or both.[3] Protracted apnea may produce secondary changes in cardiac rhythm, predominantly bradycardia.[2]

Numerous pathologic studies have shown subtle abnormalities in these patients; some of these abnormalities involve the heart. Increased smooth muscle has been found in the pulmonary arteries and is believed to be secondary to chronic hypoxia.[4,5] Abnormal thickening of the endocardium has been reported.[6] Abnormal narrowing of the lumen of the sinus node artery has been noted in SIDS infants.[7] Likewise, marked narrowing of the major arterial supply to the AV node has been observed.[8] Changes in the AV node and His bundle that have been found in all neonates have been postulated to play a role in SIDS by producing a degree of electrical cardiac instability.[9-11] This remains a controversial topic.

Abnormal autonomic regulation has been postulated as playing a significant role in SIDS.[2,3] Pathologic evidence that supports this theory includes studies that have shown the central vagal nuclei to be affected.[12] Another study showed a decreased number of small myelinated nerve fibers in the cervical vagus.[13]

Recent clinical studies have suggested that disturbances in autonomic nervous sytem function may be present in babies who experience sudden infant death syndrome.[3,14] One study showed prolonged asystole in response to ocular compression in infants who had had a "near-miss" SIDS episode, suggesting an exaggerated vagal response.[15] Alterations in heart rate and variability of rate have been noted.[3] It has also been postulated that dysfunction of the central mechanism for stabilizing the autonomic response may be an important factor.[16] Further evidence of autonomic nervous system dysfunction has been reported in near-miss infants.[17]

It has been hypothesized that a prolongation of the Q–T interval might be responsible for some of the sudden infant deaths.[18] Early reports that suggested a high percentage of prolonged Q–T intervals in families of SIDS babies[18] have not been substantiated.[19,20] Schwartz has postulated that normal developmental changes in the Q–T interval may predispose the young infant to SIDS.[21]

There are isolated reports of SIDS in patients with the Wolff-Parkinson-White syndrome and other cardiac arrhythmias.[22] However, it seems unlikely that cardiac arrhythmias are responsible for a significant proportion of SIDS.[1] Southall's prospective study found no sudden death in babies who had cardiac arrhythmias on 24-hour electrocardiograms.[23]

Thus, it appears that while the heart may be a factor in some cases of SIDS, a primary cardiac factor cannot be implicated in most cases.

## SUDDEN DEATH IN CHILDREN AND ADOLESCENTS

Fortunately, sudden unexpected death is rare in children. The leading causes of death in childhood include accidental occurrences, malignancies, congenital anomalies, and infectious diseases.[24] Cardiac diseases rank fifth as the cause of death among children 1 to 14 years of age in the United States. Sudden unexpected cardiac death is becoming a significant problem for pediatric cardiologists. Because many of these deaths may be preventable, a discussion of the problem is especially pertinent. The definition of "sudden unexpected (natural) death as death occurring instantaneously or within an estimated 24 hours of the onset of acute symptoms or signs" as used by adult cardiologists will be used for the purposes of this discussion.[25]

As in adult patients, the majority of sudden unexpected deaths in children are of cardiac origin.[26] Other causes include pulmonary problems that produce acute airway obstruction, vascular problems resulting in intracranial or other exsanguinating hemorrhage, and infectious diseases or more chronic diseases including epilepsy and diabetes.

There are few studies of sudden death in children. One recent study from Sweden describes the sudden deaths of 31 children aged 1 to 20 years.[27] Seven were known to have underlying diseases: epilepsy, asthma, diabetes, and cardiomyopathy. Fourteen had been known to have "trivial" disorders of short duration. These disorders included pneumonia, peritonitis, mononucleosis, meningitis, epiglottitis, upper respiratory tract infections, and myocarditis. The remaining 10 individuals died suddenly with no known preceding illnesses. Of these 10 patients, six had cardiac problems: three had myocarditis, one had myocardial fibrosis, one had Wolff-Parkinson-White syndrome and an enlarged heart, and one had coronary artery stenosis with myocardial infarction. Two deaths in this group were related to infectious diseases, one to adrenal failure, and one was unexplained.

The most complete study of sudden unexpected cardiac death in children is the cooperative international study published in 1974 describing 254 cases.[28] Seventy-three percent had no previous surgery and were considered to be medical deaths. Four medical conditions accounted for two thirds of these "medical" deaths. These included congenital aortic stenosis, Eisenmenger's syndrome, cyanotic heart disease with pulmonary stenosis or atresia, and cardiomyopathies. Thirty-three different types of cardiac disease were present, with the diagnosis known or suspected in 95 percent of these patients. Twenty-seven percent of these 254 patients had previous cardiac surgery. The authors stated that approximately one third of these postoperative deaths were presumed to be secondary to arrhythmias. Of 39 sudden-death patients who had open heart surgery, 25 deaths (64 percent) were presumed to be secondary to arrhythmias. The other postoperative sudden deaths occurred in patients who had palliative or closed procedures. The precise circumstances surrounding these deaths were not discussed.

Other lesions associated with sudden unexpected cardiac death in children include congenital coronary artery anomalies,[29,30] atherosclerotic coronary artery disease,[31,32] myocarditis,[33] cardiac tumors,[34,35] mitral valve prolapse,[36,37] aneurysm of aortic cusps with thrombus formation,[38] cardiomyopathies associated with muscular dystrophy and Friedrich's ataxia,[39] obstructive cardiomyopathies,[26,29,40] long Q–T syndromes of Jervell-Lange-Nielson and Romano-Ward,[41,42] aortic rupture or dissection associated with coarctation or Marfan's syndrome,[43] endocardial fibroelastosis and congestive cardiomyopathies,[28] familial conduction system anomalies,[44] and other primary arrhythmias.[45]

The circumstances of sudden death associated with many of the aforementioned cardiac problems will be discussed.

## AORTIC STENOSIS

The incidence of sudden death in children with valvular aortic stenosis has been reported to be approximately 1 percent.[46,47] The patients at highest risk for sudden death appear to be those with severe left ventricular outflow tract obstruction, left ventricular hypertrophy with a strain pattern, syncope, dyspnea, or chest pain.[48,49] Unfortunately, valvulotomy does not obliterate the risk of sudden death inasmuch as sudden death is a common cause of death postoperatively. The postoperative risk has been calculated to be 0.29 percent per annum.[48] The sudden death in patients with aortic stenosis is presumed to be secondary to diminished coronary arterial blood flow. The predisposing factors appear to be left ventricular enlargement, a critical reduction in valve area with a large gradient across the outflow tract, and replacement of the myocardium by fibrosis. In adults, near syncope has been shown to be related to a fall in cardiac output without associated arrhythmias.[50] However, more prolonged syncopal episodes have been shown to be associated with cardiac arrhythmias—specifically, cardiac standstill, ventricular flutter, or ventricular fibrillation.[49] Although children may have less myocardial fibrosis, it seems reasonable to presume that the mechanism of sudden death associated with aortic stenosis would be similar to that encountered in adults. Patients with supravalvar and subvalvar aortic stenosis have also been noted to be at risk for sudden death.

## CARDIOMYOPATHIES

Hypertrophic obstructive cardiomyopathies are frequently mentioned in studies of sudden death in children and account for 9 percent of the sudden deaths in Lambert's series.[28] One study has shown a 31 percent incidence of sudden death in children with idiopathic hypertrophic subaortic stenosis treated medically.[51] Other studies have confirmed a higher incidence of sudden death in children with this lesion as compared with adults.[52,53]

Almot half of the sudden deaths in young athletes reported by Maron had idiopathic hypertrophic subaortic stenosis (IHSS).[29] In most of these cases, cardiac disease was not suspected during life. Many other reports substantiate the presence of IHSS in patients who die during exertion.[26,2840] In many patients, sudden death is the first manifestation of disease. Sudden death in IHSS is associated with youth,[53,55] family history of sudden death,[54] and ventricular arrhythmias on 24-hour electrocardiograms.[53,54] Sudden death occurs more commonly in patients with abnormal electrocardiograms and a moderately to severely thickened ventricular septum.[55] It is disputed whether antecedent syncope increases the risk of sudden death. It is speculated that ventricular arrhythmias are the cause of sudden death.[56–58] In McKenna's study, sudden death in the young patients was unrelated to severe functional limitation, elevated filling pressure, or the presence of a left ventricular outflow tract gradient.[53]

Although surgical myectomy may be effective in relieving obstruction, late postoperative sudden death remains significant—as high as 8 to 11 percent.[60,61] This is a lower incidence than the medically treated patients but remains significant.

In Fiddler's study, young patients treated with propranolol fared better than patients on no treatment.[60] However, other studies have shown that propranolol does not prevent sudden death.[51]

There are reports in the literature of familial or other nonobstructive cardiomyopathies associated with sudden death.[61] Infants and children with endocardial fibroelastosis have also shown a signficant incidence of sudden death.[28,62] The presence of complex or high-grade ventricular arrhythmias in these patients seems to be associated with sudden death.

## MITRAL VALVE PROLAPSE

Sudden cardiac death has been reported in children with mitral valve prolapse,[36] including several reports of sudden death in athletes.[29] This sudden death has been postulated to be secondary to lethal arrhythmias.[63] Although the incidence of sudden death in adults with mitral valve prolapse has been reported to be 1.4 percent,[65] the precise incidence in children and adolescents is not known. Sudden death appears to be associated with the presence of ventricular arrhythmias, previous syncope, and a family history of sudden death.[64,65] Postmortem studies have shown associated involvement of the conduction system that could explain sudden death.[66]

## CORONARY ARTERY ANOMALIES

Coronary artery anomalies may present as sudden death.[67–69] One type of anomaly is anomalous origin of the left main coronary artery from the right sinus of Valsalva. In this condition, the anomalous coronary artery courses between the aorta and pulmonary artery where it may be compressed. These patients are usually asymptomatic and may not be diagnosed until a postmortem examination after a sudden death. These sudden deaths are frequently associated with physical exertion.

Another coronary artery anomaly associated with sudden death is coronary artery isolation by aortic valve adhesion.[70] In addition, ostial stenosis has been associated with sudden death in adolescents.[71] Anomalous origin of the left coronary artery from the pulmonary artery may also predispose to sudden death. Presumably, the mechanism of sudden death is similar in all the patients and is secondary to coronary insufficiency with subsequent ventricular arrhythmias.

Acquired coronary artery lesions may result in sudden death. Of increasing significance are those coronary lesions associated with Kawasaki's disease—the mucocutaneous lymph node syndrome.[72–74] The incidence of sudden death in this syndrome is reported to be approximately 2 percent.[73] Acquired coronary artery disease from progressive systemic sclerosis has been postulated to cause functional coronary artery involvement and sudden death in children.[75]

## ANOMALIES OF AORTA

Sudden death has been reported in patients after repair of coarctation of the aorta.[43,76] Many of these deaths have been shown to be secondary to dissection or rupture of the ascending aorta. Many patients with Marfan's syndrome who have died suddenly have also been shown to have rupture of aortic aneurysms.[28] These patients have also been known to have cardiac arrhythmias.[40] It is not known whether these arrhythmias occur more frequently in those patients with significant mitral valve prolapse.

## MYOCARDITIS

Most series concerning sudden death include cases of acute myocarditis as an importnat etiology. In one study from Canada, 6 percent of the sudden unexpected "natural" deaths were found to have myocarditis.[33] Five percent of the medical deaths in the cooperative study were secondary to myocarditis.[28]

Arrhythmias associated with myocarditis that might result in sudden death include both abnormalities of conduction producing complete heart block and ventricular arrhythmias such as ventricular tachycardia or ventricular fibrillation.

## POSTOPERATIVE CONGENITAL HEART DEFECTS

There is a significant incidence of sudden death in patients who have undergone operative repair of congenital heart defects. The risk of sudden death is greatest in patients who have repair of certain lesions including tetralogy of Fallot (TOF), ventricular septal defect (VSD),[28] complete AV canal (CAVC),[81] and transposition of the great arteries (TGA). Sudden death is stated to occur in 2 to 5 percent of patients with repair of tetralogy of Fallot[77,78] and 2 to 8 percent of patients with repair of transposition of the great arteries.[79,80] Sudden death has also been noted after repair of atrial septal defects (ASD).[28] A recent report noted a 5 percent incidence of sudden death after intracardiac conduit repair of congenital cardiac defects;[82] the deaths were presumed to be secondary to arrhythmias.

In patients with tetralogy of Fallot, sudden death had previously been attributed to conduction disturbances such as right bundle branch block (RBBB) or left anterior hemiblock with presumed progression to complete heart block.[77] However, recent reports are quite suggestive that ventricular arrhythmias may be more important as a cause of sudden death.[83,84] An incidence of sudden death of 30 to 38 percent has been noted in patients with tetralogy of Fallot who have premature ventricular contractions on the resting, stress, or ambulatory electrocardiogram.[78,83,84] Recently, the electrophysiologic study has been used to induce ventricular tachycardia in these patients in an attempt to identify and pretreat those patients at risk for sudden death.[85-88] Those patients with both hemodynamic and electrophysiologic aberrations seem to be at greatest risk for sudden death.[86]

In patients with transposition of the great arteries after a Mustard repair, sudden death has been postulated to be secondary to sick sinus sndrome.[89-91] However, sudden death has been found to be a not-uncommon occurrence in these postoperative patients who also have atrial flutter.[92]

Patients known to have postoperative heart block but who are not treated with pacemakers have a significant incidence of postoperative death of approximately 60 to 80 percent.[93-95] Survival rates are good after pacemaker placement in this group of patients.[95-97]

## PRIMARY PULMONARY HYPERTENSION AND EISENMENGER'S SYNDROME

These two problems represent 17 percent of the sudden deaths in medically treated patients described in the international cooperative sudden death study.[28] Sudden death, presumably from an arrhythmia, is the leading cause of death in these patients.[98]

Sudden death has been reported to occur in 14 to 47 percent of patients with Eisenmenger's syndrome.[99-101] More of these deaths occur in the second decade of life as compared with the first.

Sudden death has been noted frequently in patients with primary pulmonary hypertension.[102] Frequent syncopal episodes in these patients may occur prior to sudden death.[103,104] Death associated with cardiac catheterization in these patients has occurred in association with both bradycardia and ventricular fibrillation.[105]

## CYANOTIC CONGENITAL HEART DISEASE WITH PULMONIC STENOSIS OR PULMONARY ATRESIA

In the cooperative study, 10 percent of the medical sudden deaths occurred in patients with inadequate pulmonary blood flow from pulmonary stenosis or atresia.[28] It has been presumed that these children die from a hypoxic spell. It is possible that severe hypoxia triggers arrhythmias that lead to sudden death. Sudden death also occurred relatively commonly in those patients in the study who had palliative surgery for their cyanotic defects, although the effectiveness of the palliation at the time of death is not discussed.

## EBSTEIN'S ANOMALY

The cooperative study on sudden death indicates that 6 percent of the medical deaths had Ebstein's anomaly of the tricuspid valve.[28] If only patients with Ebstein's anomaly are discussed, it would appear that sudden death occurs in at least 20 percent of these patients over 1 year of age.[106] These patients are known to have a high incidence of cardiac arrhythmias. These include paroxysmal supraventricular arrhythmias, AV nodal re-entry, and supraventricular tachycardia in association with the Wolff-Parkinson-White (WPW) syndrome. Atrial fibrillation and ventricular arrhythmias are also encountered.[107] It has been suggested that these rhythm disturbances are responsible for the high incidence of deaths known to be associated with cardiac catheterization and with surgical repairs.

## CORRECTED TRANSPOSITION OF THE GREAT ARTERIES

Corrected transposition of the great arteries was noted in only one patient in the international study on sudden death.[28] However, reports of patients with corrected transposition do relate a signficant incidence of sudden death.[108-110] Presumably, these sudden deaths are secondary to the arrhythmias known to be associated with corrected transposition, including the Wolff-Parkinson-White syndrome, paroxysmal supraventricular arrrhythmias, and complete heart block.

## ARRHYTHMIAS

Although arrhythmias are uncommon in children, they may be observed in association with congenital heart defects, either preoperatively or postoperatively, in association with acquired cardiac problems, or in normal hearts. The problem of sudden death as associated with specific arrhythmias will be discussed.

### Long Q–T Syndrome

Two hereditary syndromes with prolongation of the Q–T interval have been described in children. These include the syndrome of Jervell and Lange-Nielson associated with congenital deafness[111] and the Romano-Ward syndrome without deafness.[112,113] Asymmetric activation of the sympathetic nervous system is observed in these syndromes. Both are associated with a very high incidence of sudden death, with a mortality of 73 percent in untreated patients. Medical or surgical treatment has markedly lessened the incidence of sudden death but has not abolished it.[114] The sudden death is presumed to be secondary to ventricular arrhythmias.[42]

Sudden death is also associated with prolongation of the Q–T interval secondary to certain drugs such as procainamide, quinidine, and phenothiazines.[26]

## Complete Heart Block

Complete heart block in children may be congenital or acquired. Acquired cases occur in association with specific lesions. For example, patients with corrected transposition of the great arteries have a 30 to 60 percent incidence of developing complete heart block.[108,115] Complete heart block may also be acquired in association with myocarditis or as a postoperative occurrence. It has been reported to occur as late as 14 years postoperatively and is more frequently observed in association with repairs of ventricular septal defects, tetralogy of Fallot, or complete AV canal defects.[116] The current postoperative incidence of complete heart block is less than 1 percent.[94] The incidence of sudden death in postoperative complete heart block without pacemakers is 60 to 80 percent.[93-95]

The incidence of sudden death in congenital complete heart block not treated with a pacemaker is as high as 2 to 3 percent.[117]

## Sick Sinus Syndrome

Sick sinus syndrome is uncommon as a primary arrhythmia in children. It occurs most commonly in association with repair of congenital heart defects such as transposition of the great arteries by the Mustard operation or closure of a sinus venosus atrial septal defect.[118] It is also encountered in acquired heart disease such as myocarditis.[118] Although it is a rare occurrence, severe sinus node dysfunction may present as sudden death in children.[119,120]

## Pre-excitation Syndromes

The Wolff-Parkinson-White syndrome is commonly associated with congenital heart defects, especially Ebstein's malformation of the tricuspid valve and corrected transposition of the great arteries.[121] It may also be encountered in the absence of a congenital heart defect. Sudden death has been noted in children with WPW syndrome. It is presumed to be secondary to ventricular fibrillation induced either by early depolarization of the ventricle from a rapidly conducted premature atrial depolarization or from 1:1 atrioventricular conduction of a rapid supraventricular tachycardia that degenerates to ventricular fibrillation.[121] Digoxin may facilitate conduction in the bypass tract and increase the chances of a life-threatening arrhythmia although this correlation has not been substantiated to date in children. In one study of 11 young patients who had experienced cardiac arrest, two were found to have previously undiagnosed bypass tracts.[122]

## Ventricular Tachycardia

In Benson's study of 11 young patients who had experienced cardiac arrest, ventricular tachycardia could be induced in six patients.[122] Ventricular arrhythmias, especially in the presence of underlying heart disease, appear to increase the risk of sudden death. This is especially true in the presence of mitral valve prolapse, cardiomyopathies, idiopathic hypertrophic subaortic stenosis, and myocarditis.[123] However, sudden death has been reported in the presence of normal hearts when ventricular arrhythmias were present.[124] Familial ventricular arrhythmias associated with sudden death have been reported.[44]

## CONDITIONS OF SUDDEN DEATH

The conditions surrounding sudden death in children differ somewhat from adults. Death is usually instantaneous. Warning syncope occurs in only 16 percent. Most patients are relatively inactive at the time of death, with only a small percentage engaged in active sports.[28]

The cardiac abnormalities most commonly found in athletes or those who die when active include hypertrophic cardiomyopathies, mitral valve prolapse, coronary artery abnormalities, and ruptured aorta.[29,40] Patients with severe aortic stenosis are also at risk for sudden death during strenuous exercise,[26] as are patients with the long Q–T syndrome, myocarditis, cyanotic congenital cardiac defects, and pulmonary hypertension.

## AGE AT DEATH

Certain conditions result in death at younger ages. These include endocardial fibroelastosis and other nonobstructive cardiomyopathies, myocarditis, congenital complete heart block, and cyanotic heart disease with pulmonic stenosis. Patients with aortic stenosis and idiopathic hypertrophic subaortic stenosis tend to experience sudden death at older ages. Overall, more sudden deaths occur during the second decade of life than the first.[28]

## MECHANISMS OF SUDDEN DEATH

The usual mechanism of cardiac sudden death is considered to be an arrhythmia—generally, ventricular fibrillation. Bradycardic cardiac arrest has been documented, especially in young children.[125] In a study on terminal cardiac electrical activity, patients with congenital heart disease were more likely to have ventricular fibrillation as the terminal event.

In children with congenital heart disease, hypoxia and coronary insufficiency have been suggested as mechanisms of sudden death, but ventricular arrhythmias secondary to these factors are most likely reponsible for the deaths.

Hemorrhage associated with ruptured aorta in Marfan's syndrome and hemorrhage associated with ruptured berry aneurysms in children with coarctation of the aorta have been responsible for sudden death in these patients.

Patients with severe congestive heart failure die suddenly, possibly secondary to an arrhythmia induced by low output, hypoxia, and acidosis.

## PREVENTION OF SUDDEN DEATH

It is hoped that identification of high-risk patients with subsequent appropriate intervention and treatment will lead to the prevention of sudden death in children. For example, early or appropriately timed surgical intervention in patients with lesions that produce cyanosis or those lesions prone to develop pulmonary hypertension should be effective in preventing sudden death in these patients.

Treatment of arrhythmias in patients with idiopathic hypertrophic subaortic stenosis or other cardiomyopathies may lower the incidence of sudden death in these patients. The same intervention in patients with mitral valve prolapse should be effective.

Restriction of strenuous physical activity in those patients prone to develop sudden death with activity (IHSS, mitral valve prolapse, long Q–T syndrome) should lower the risk in this group.

With regard to postoperative sudden death, it is hoped that treatment of arrhythmias in postoperative patients after repair of tetralogy of Fallot and transposition of the great arteries will lessen the incidence of sudden death in these patients. Identification of high-risk patients, using the electrophysiologic study, may be helpful.

Pacemaker placement in appropriate patients with congenital or acquired heart block or sick sinus syndrome should prevent sudden death in many of these patients.

Medical treatment of patients with cardiac arrhythmias including ventricular arrhythmias, long Q–T syndrome, or pre-excitation should lower the risks in these groups. Some patients with pre-excitation may benefit from surgical interruption of their bypass tract.

Obviously, a better understanding of the mechanisms of sudden death will allow more appropriate and timely treatment of all of the conditions previously discussed.

## SUMMARY

Sudden death in infants is rarely due to cardiac disease. Sudden death in children and adolescents is usually associated with cardiac disease. The major congenital lesions associated with sudden death are aortic stenosis, cardiomyopathies, idiopathic hypertrophic subaortic stenosis, Eisenmenger's syndrome, and cyanotic congenital defects with pulmonary stenosis or atresia. There is a high incidence of postoperative sudden death, especially associated with repair of tetralogy of Fallot and transposition of the great arteries. Cardiac arrhythmias, including the long Q–T syndrome, sick sinus syndrome, complete heart block, ventricular tachycardia, and pre-excitation are associated with sudden death.

It is hoped that identification of high-risk patients along with appropriate intervention and treatment may significantly lower or prevent sudden death in children.

## REFERENCES

1. *Identification of infants destined to die unexpectedly during infancy: Evaluation of predictive importance of prolonged apnea and disorders of cardiac rhythm or conduction.* Br Med J 286:1092, 1983.

2. VALDÉS-DAPENA, MA: *Sudden infant death syndrome: A review of the medical literature 1974–1979.* Pediatrics 66:597, 1980.

3. SHANNON, DC AND KELLY, DH: *SIDS and near-SIDS.* N Engl J Med 306:959, 1022, 1982.

4. WILLIAMS, A, VAWTER, G, AND REID, L: *Increased muscularity of the pulmonary circulation in victims of sudden infant death.* Pediatrics 63:18, 1979.

5. NAEYE, RL, WHALEN, P, RYSER, M, ET AL: *Cardiac and other abnormalities in the sudden infant death syndrome.* Am J Pathol 82:1, 1976.

6. WILLIAMS, RB AND EMERY, JL: *Endocardial fibrosis in apparently normal hearts.* Histopathology 2:283, 1978.

7. KOZAKEWICH, HPW, McMANUS, BM, AND VAWTER, GF: *The sinus node in sudden infant death syndrome.* Circulation 65:1242, 1982.

8. ANDERSON, KR AND HILL, RW: *Occlusive lesions of cardiac conduction tissue arteries in sudden infant death syndrome.* Pediatrics 69:50, 1982.

9. JAMES, TN: *Sudden death in babies: New observations in the heart.* Am J Cardiol 22:479, 1968.

10. VALDÉS-DAPENA, MA, GREENE, M, BASAVANARD, N, ET AL: *The myocardial conduction system in sudden death in infancy.* N Engl J Med 289:1179, 1973.

11. LIE, JT, ROSENBERG, HS, AND ERICKSON, EE: *Histopathology of the conduction system in the sudden infant death syndrome.* Circulation 53:3, 1976.

12. TAKASHIMA, S, ARMSTRONG, D, BECKER, L, ET AL: *Cerebral hypoperfusion in the sudden infant death syndrome?: Brainstem gliosis and vasculature.* Ann Neurol 4:257, 1978.

13. SACHIS, PN, ARMSTRONG, DL, BECKER, LE, ET AL: *The vagus nerve and sudden infant death syndrome: A morphometric study.* J Pediatr 98:278, 1981.

14. SCHWARTZ, PJ: *Cardiac sympathetic innervation and the sudden infant death syndrome: A possible pathologic link.* Am J Med 60:167, 1967.

15. KAHN, A, RIAZI, J, AND BLUM, D: *Oculocardiac reflex in near miss for sudden infant death syndrome infants.* Pediatrics 71:49, 1983.

16. SALK, L, GRELLONG, BA, AND DIETRICH, J: *Sudden infant death: Normal cardiac habituation and poor autonomic control.* N Engl J Med 291:219, 1974.

17. GUILLEMINAULT, C, ARIAGNO, R, SOUQUET, M, ET AL: *Abnormal polygraphic findings in near-miss sudden infant death.* Lancet 1:1326, 1976.

18. MARON, BJ, CLARK, CE, GOLDSTEIN, RE, ET AL: *Potential role of QT interval prolongation in sudden infant death syndrome.* Circulation 54:423, 1976.

19. KELLY, DH, SHANNON, DC, AND LIBERTHSON, RR: *The role of the QT interval in the SIDS.* Circulation 55:633, 1977.

20. STEINSCHNEIDER, A: *Sudden infant death syndrome and prolongation of the QT interval.* Am J Dis Child 132:688, 1978.

21. SCHWARTZ, PJ, MONTEMERLO, M, AND FACCHINI, M: *The QT interval throughout the first six months of life: A prospective study.* Circulation 66:496, 1982.

22. KEETON BR, SOUTHALL, E, AND RUTTER, N: *Cardiac conduction disorders in six infants with "near-miss" sudden infant deaths.* Br Med J 2:600, 1977.

23. SOUTHALL, DP, RICHARDS, JM, RHODEN, KJ, ET AL: *Prolonged apnea and cardiac arrhythmias in infants discharged from neonatal intensive care units: Failure to predict an increased risk for sudden infant death syndrome.* Pediatrics 70:844, 1982.

24. Monthly Vital Statistics Report 28(13):23, 1980.

25. OGLESBY, P AND SCHATZ, M: Editorial: *On sudden death.* Circulation 43:7, 1971.

26. MANNING, JA: *Sudden unexpected death in children.* Am J Dis Child 131:1201, 1977.

27. MOLANDER, N: *Sudden natural death in later childhood and adolescence.* Arch Dis Child 57:572, 1982.

28. LAMBERT, EC, MENON, VA, WAGNER, HR, ET AL: *Sudden unexpected death from cardiovascular disease in children: A cooperative international study.* Am J Cardiol 34:89, 1974.

29. MARON, BJ, ROBERTS, WC, MCALLISTER, HA, ET AL: *Sudden death in young athletes.* Circulation 62:218, 1980.

30. TSUNG, SH, HUANG, TY, AND CHANG, HH: *Sudden death in young athletes.* Arch Pathol Lab Med 106:168, 1982.

31. BERKHEISER, SW: *Cardiovascular disease in the younger age group.* Aerospace Med 41:1307, 1970.

32. JOHNSON, WD, STRONG, TJ, OALMANN, MC, ET AL: *Sudden death from coronary disease in young men.* Arch Pathol Lab Med 105:227, 1981.

33. WENTWORTH, P, JENTZ, LA, AND CROAL, AE: *Analysis of sudden unexpected death in southern Ontario with emphasis on myocarditis.* Can Med Assoc J 120:676, 1979.

34. JAMES, TN, DEREK, JL, CARSON, DJL, ET AL: *De Subitaneis Mortibus. I. Fibroma compressing the His bundle.* Circulation 48:428, 1973.

35. JOLK, E: *Exercise and cardiac death.* JAMA 218:1707, 1971.

36. ANDERSON, RC: *Idiopathic mitral valve prolapse and sudden death.* Am Heart J 100:941, 1980.

37. COOPER, MJ AND ABINADER, EG: *Family history in assessing the risk for progression of mitral valve prolapse.* Am J Dis Child 135:647, 1981.

38. MANT, AK: *Sudden death due to unusual cardiac pathology.* Forensic Sci 8:7, 1976.

39. JAMES, TN AND MARSHALL, TK: *De Subitaneis Mortibus. XVIII. Persistent fetal dispersion of the atrioventricular node and His bundle within the central fibrous body.* Circulation 53:1026, 1976.

40. LUCKSTEAD, EF: *Sudden death in sports.* Ped Clin North Am 29:1355, 1982.

41. PARK, MK AND GUNTEROTH, WG: *Long Q–T syndrome: A preventable form of sudden death.* J Fam Practice 5:945, 1978.

42. JAMES, TN: *QT prolongation and sudden death.* Mod Concepts Cardiovasc Dis 38:35, 1969.

43. FORFANG, K, ROSTAD, H, SORLAND, S, ET AL: *Late sudden death after surgical correction of coarctation of the aorta.* Acta Med Scand 206:375, 1979.

44. JAMES, TN AND MACLEAN, WAH: *Paroxysmal ventricular arrhythmias and familial sudden death associated with neural lesions in the heart.* Chest 78:24, 1980.

45. JAMES, TN AND PUECH, P: *De Subitaneis Mortibus: X. Type A Wolff-Parkinson-White syndrome.* Circulation 50:1276, 1974.

46. THORNBACH, P AND FOWLER, RS: *Sudden death in children with congenital heart disease.* Presented at the Canadian Pediatric Society Meeting, July 1972.

47. CAMPBELL, M: *The natural history of congenital aortic stenosis.* Br Heart J 30:514, 1968.

48. STEWART, JR, PATON, BC, BLOUNT, SG, JR, ET AL: *Congenital aortic stenosis: Ten to 22 years after valvulotomy.* Arch Surg 113:1248, 1978.

49. SCHWARTZ, LS, GOLDFISCHER, J, SPRAGUE, GJ, ET AL: *Syncope and sudden death in aortic stenosis.* Am J Cardiol 23:647, 1969.

50. FLANN, MD, BRANIFF, BA, KIMBALL, R, ET AL: *Mechanism of effort syncope in aortic stenosis.* Circulation 26:II-109, 1967.

51. MARON, BJ, HENRY, WL, CLARK, CE, ET AL: *Asymmetric septal hypertrophy in childhood.* Circulation 53:9, 1976.

52. MARON, BJ, ROBERTS, WC, AND EPSTEIN, SE: *Sudden death in hypertrophic cardiomyopathy: A profile of 78 patients.* Circulation 65:1388, 1982.

53. MCKENNA, W, DEANFIELD, J, FARUQUI, A, ET AL: *Prognosis in hypertrophic cardiomyopathy: Role of age and clinical, electrocardiographic and hemodynamic features.* Am J Cardiol 47:532, 1981.

54. MARON, BJ, LIPSON, LC, ROBERTS, WC, ET AL: *"Malignant" hypertrophic cardiomyopathy: Identification of a subgroup of families with frequent premature death.* Am J Cardiol 41:1133, 1978.

55. MARON, BJ, ROBERTS, WC, EDWARDS, JE, ET AL: *Sudden death in patients with hypertrophic cardiomyopathy: Characterization of 26 patients without functional limitation.* Am J Cardiol 41:803, 1978.

56. MCKENNA, WJ, ENGLAND, D, DOI, YL, ET AL: *Arrhythmia in hypertrophic cardiomyopathy: I. Influence on prognosis.* Br Heart J 46:168, 1981.

57. MARON, BJ, SAVAGE, DD, WOLFSON, JK, ET AL: *Prognostic significance of 24 hour ambulatory electrocardiographic monitoring in patients with hypertrophic cardiomyopathy: A prospective study.* Am J Cardiol 48:252, 1981.

58. ANDERSON, KP, STINSON, EB, DERBY, GC, ET AL: *Vulnerability of patients with obstructive hypertrophic cardiomyopathy to ventricular arrhythmia induction in the operating room.* Am J Cardiol 51:811, 1983.

59. BEARHS, MM, TAJIK, AJ, SEWARD, JB, ET AL: *Hypertrophic obstructive cardiomyopathy: Ten to 21 year follow-up after partial septal myectomy.* Am J Cardiol 51:1160, 1983.

60. FIDDLER, GI, TAJIK, AJ, WEIDMAN, WH, ET AL: *Idiopathic hypertrophic subaortic stenosis in the young.* Am J Cardiol 42:793, 1978.

61. ROSS, RS, BUCKLEY, BH, HUTCHINS, GM, ET AL: *Idiopathic familial myocardiopathy in three generations: A clinical and pathologic study.* Am Heart J 96:170, 1978.

62. FISHER, JH: *Primary endocardial fibroelastosis: A review of 15 cases.* Can Med Assoc J 87:105, 1962.

63. SWARTZ, MH, TEICHHOLZ, LE, AND DONOSO, E: *Mitral valve prolapse: A review of associated arrhythmias.* Am J Med 62:377, 1977.

64. SHAPPEL, SD, MARSHALL, CE, AND BROWN, RE: *Sudden death and the familial occurrence of mid-systolic click, late systolic murmur syndrome.* Circulation 46:1128, 1973.

65. JERESATY, RM: *Sudden death in the mitral valve prolapse click syndrome.* Am J Cardiol 37:317, 1976.

66. BHARATI, S, BAUERNFEIND, R, MILLER, LB, ET AL: *Sudden death in three teenagers: Conduction system studies.* J Am Coll Cardiol 1:879, 1983.

67. LIBERTHSON, RR, DINSMORE, RE, AND FALLON, JT: *Aberrant coronary artery origin from the aorta.* Circulation 59:748, 1979.

68. CHEITLIN, MD, DECASTRO, CM, AND MCALLISTER, HA: *Sudden death as a complication of anomalous left coronary origin from the anterior sinus of Valsalva: A not so minor congenital anomaly.* Circulation 50:780, 1974.

69. KIMBIRIS, D, ISKANDRIAN, AS, SEGAL, BL, ET AL: *Anomalous aortic origin of coronary arteries.* Circulation 58:606, 1978.

70. KUROSAWA, H, WAGENAAR, SS, AND BECKER, AF: *Sudden death in a youth: A case of quadricuspid aortic valve with isolation of origin of left coronary artery.* Br Heart J 59:748, 1981.

71. KOSKENVUO, K, KARVONEN, MJ, AND RISSANEN, V: *Death from ischemic heart disease in young Finns aged 15 to 24 years.* Am J Cardiol 42:114, 1978.

72. FUJIWARA, H AND HAMASHIMA, Y: *Pathology of the heart in Kawasaki disease.* Pediatrics 61:100, 1978.

73. MORENS, DM, ANDERSON, LJ, AND HURWITZ, ES: *National surveillance of Kawasaki disease.* Pediatrics 65:21, 1980.

74. KATO, H, KOIKE, S, YAMAMOTO, M, ET AL: *Coronary aneurysms in infants and young children with acute febrile mucocutaneous lymph node syndrome.* J Pediatr 86:892, 1975.

75. BUKLEY, BH, KLACSMANN, PG, AND HUTCHINS, GM: *Angina pectoris, myocardial infarction and sudden cardiac death with normal coronary arteries: A clinicopathologic study of 9 patients with progressive systemic sclerosis.* Am Heart J 95:563, 1978.

76. REIFENSTEIN, GH, LEVINE, SA, AND GROSS, RE: *Coarctation of the aorta: A review of 104 autopsied cases of the "adult type", 2 years of age or older.* Am Heart J 33:146, 1947.

77. WOLFF, GS, ROWLAND, TW, AND ELLISON, RC: *Surgically induced right bundle branch block with left anterior hemiblock.* Circulation 46:587, 1972.

78. QUATTLEBAUM, TG, VARGHESE, PJ, NEILL, CA, ET AL: *Sudden death among postoperative patients with tetralogy of Fallot.* Circulation 54:289, 1976.

79. SAALOUKE, MG, RIOS, J, PERRY, LW, ET AL: *Electrophysiologic studies after Mustard's operation for d-transposition of the great vessels.* Am J Cardiol 41:1104, 1978.

80. CHAMPSAUR, GL, SOKOL, DM, TRUSLER, GA, ET AL: *Repair of transposition of the great arteries in 123 pediatric patients.* Circulation 47:1032, 1973.

81. GOLDFADEN, DM, JONES, J, AND MORROW, AG: *Long term results of repair of incomplete persistent atrioventricular canal.* J Thorac Cardiovasc Surg 82:669, 1981.

82. McGOON, DC, DANIELSON, GK, PUGA, FJ, ET AL: *Late results after extracardiac conduit repair for congenital cardial defects.* Am J Cardiol 49:1741, 1982.

83. GILLETTE, PC, YEOMAN, MA, MULLINS, CE, ET AL: *Sudden death after repair of tetralogy of Fallot.* Circulation 56:566, 1977.

84. JAMES, FW, KAPLAN, S, AND CHOU, T: *Unexpected cardiac arrest in patients after surgical correction of tetralogy of Fallot.* Circulation 52:691, 1975.

85. HOROWITZ, LN, VETTER, VL, HARKEN, AH, ET AL: *Electrophysiologic characteristics of sustained ventricular tachycardia occurring after repair of tetralogy of Fallot.* Am J Cardiol 46:446, 1980.

86. GARSON, A, PORTER, C, GILLETTE, PC, ET AL: *Induction of ventricular tachycardia during electrophysiologic study after repair of tetralogy of Fallot.* J Am Coll Cardiol 1:1492, 1983.

87. KUGLER, JD, MOORING, PH, PINSKY, WW, ET AL: *Sustained ventricular tachycardia following repair of tetralogy of Fallot: New electrophysiologic findings.* Am J Cardiol 49:998, 1982.

88. VETTER, VL AND HOROWITZ, LN: *Electrophysiologic results of repair of tetralogy of Fallot.* Am J Cardiol 49:999, 1982.

89. GILLETTE, PC, EL-SAID, GM, SILVARJAN, N, ET AL: *Electrophysiological abnormalities after Mustard operation for transposition of the great arteries.* Br Heart J 36:186, 1974.

90. GILLETTE, PC, KUGLER, JD, GARSON, A, ET AL: *Mechanisms of cardiac arrhythmias after the Mustard operation for transposition of the great arteries.* Am J Cardiol 45:1225, 1980.

91. BHARATI, S, MOLTHAN, ME, VEASY, G, ET AL: *Conduction system in two cases of sudden death two years after the Mustard procedure.* J Thorac Cardiovasc Surg 77:101, 1979.

92. Presented at the Pediatric Dysrhythmia Conference, 55th Scientific Session of the American Heart Association, November 1982.

93. LEVY, MJ, CUELLO, L, TUNA, N, ET AL: *Atrioventricularis communis.* Am J Cardiol 14:587, 1964.

94. LILLEHEI, CW, SELLERS, RD, BONNABEAU, RC, ET AL: *Chronic postsurgical complete heart block.* J Thorac Cardiovasc Surg 46:436, 1963.

95. STANTON, RE, LINDESMITH, GG, AND MEYER, BW: *Pacemaker therapy in children with complete heart block.* Am J Dis Child 129:484, 1975.

96. BENREY, J, GILLETTE, PC, NASRALLAH, AT, ET AL: *Permanent pacemaker implantation in infants, children and adolescents.* Circulation 53:245, 1976.

97. HOFSCHIRE, PJ, NICOLOFF, DM, AND MOLLER, JH: *Postoperative complete heart block in 64 children treated with and without cardiac pacing.* Am J Cardiol 39:559, 1977.

98. GRAHAM, TP, JR: *The Eisenmenger reaction and its management.* In ROBERTS, WC (ED): *Congenital Heart Disease in Adults.* FA Davis, Philadelphia, 1979, pp 531–542.

99. CLARKSON, PM, FRYE, RL, DuSHANE, JW, ET AL: *Prognosis for patients with ventricular septal defect and severe pulmonary vascular obstructive disease.* Circulation 38:129, 1968.

100. YOUNG, D AND MARK, H: *Fate of the patient with Eisenmenger syndrome.* Am J Cardiol 28:658, 1971.

101. WOOD, P: *The Eisenmenger syndrome.* Br Med J 2:701, 1958.

102. PERLOFF, JK: *Primary pulmonary hypertension.* In *The Clinical Recognition of Congenital Heart Disease.* WB Saunders, Philadelphia, 1970, pp 201–204.

103. SLEEPER, JC, ORGAIN, ES, AND McINTOSH, HD: *Primary pulmonary hypertension: Review of clinical features.* Circulation 26:1358, 1962.

104. THILENIUS, OG, NADAS, AS, AND JOCKIN, H: *Primary pulmonary vascular obstruction in children.* Pediatrics 36:75, 1965.

105. KEANE, JF AND FYLER, DC: *Hazards of cardiac catheterisation in children with primary pulmonary vascular obstruction.* Lancet 1:863, 1977.

106. WATSON, H: *Natural history of Ebstein's anomaly of tricuspid valve in childhood and adolescence: An international co-operative study of 505 cases.* Br Heart J 36:417, 1974.

107. BIALOSTOZKY, D, HORWITZ, S, AND ESPINO-VELA, J: *Ebstein's malformation of the tricuspid valve: A review of 65 cases.* Am J Cardiol 29:826, 1972.

108. FRIEDBERG, DZ AND NADAS, AS: *Clinical profile of patients with cogenital corrected transposition of the great vessels.* N Engl J Med 282:1053, 1970.

109. FOSTER, JR, DAMATO, AN, KLINE, LE, ET AL: *Congenitally corrected transposition of the great vessels: Localization of the site of complete atrioventricular block using His bundle electrograms.* Am J Cardiol 38:383, 1976.

110. GILLETTE, PC, BUSCH, U, MULLINS, CE, ET AL: *Electrophysiologic studies in patients with ventricular inversion and "corrected transposition."* Circulation 60:939, 1979.

111. JERVELL, A AND LANGE-NIELSEN, F: *Congenital deaf mutism, functional heart disease with prolongation of Q–T interval and sudden death.* Am Heart J 54:59, 1957.

112. ROMANO, C, GEMME, G, AND PONGIGLIONE, R: *Aritmie cardiache rare dell'eta pediatrica.* La Clinic Paed 45:656, 1963.

113. WARD, OC: *A new familial cardiac syndrome in children.* J Irish Med Assoc 54:103, 1964.

114. SCHWARTZ, PJ, PERITI, M, AND MALLIANI, A: *The long QT syndrome.* Am Heart J 89:378, 1975.

115. WALKER, WJ, COOLEY, DA, MCNAMARA, DG, ET AL: *Corrected transposition of the great vessels, atrioventricular heart block and ventricular septal defect: A clinical triad.* Circulation 17:249, 1958.

116. GODMAN, MJ, ROBERTS, NK, AND IZUKAWA, T: *Late postoperative conduction disturbances after repair of ventricular septal defect and tetralogy of Fallot.* Circulation 49:214, 1974.

117. MICHAELSSON, M AND ENGLE, MA: *Congenital complete heart block: An international study of the natural history.* In ENGLE, MA (ED): *Pediatric Cardiology.* FA Davis, Philadelphia, 1972, pp 85–101.

118. VARGHESE, PJ: *Sinus node disorders.* In ROBERTS, NK AND GELBAND, H (EDS): *Cardiac Arrhythmias in the Neonate, Infant and Child.* Appleton-Century-Crofts, New York, 1977, pp 159–170.

119. JAMES, TN, FROGGATT, P, AND MARSHALL, TK: *Sudden death in young athletes.* Ann Intern Med 67: 1013, 1967.

120. ROLAND, J-M, VARGHESE, PJ, SHEMATEK, J, ET AL: *Sinus node dysfunction in young athletes: A possible cause of sudden death.* Circulation 52(Suppl II):233, 1975.

121. GILLETTE, PC: *The pre-excitation syndromes.* In GILLETTE, PC AND GARSON, A (EDS): *Pediatric Cardiac Dysrhythmias.* Grune & Stratton, New York, 1981, pp 153–176.

122. BENSON, DW, BENDITT, DG, ANDERSON, RW, ET AL: *Cardiac arrest in young, ostensibly healthy patients: Clinical, hemodynamic, and electrophysiologic findings.* Am J Cardiol 52:65, 1983.

123. PEDERSEN, DH, ZIPES, DP, FOSTER, PR, ET AL: *Ventricular tachycardia and ventricular fibrillation in a young population.* Circulation 60:988, 1979.

124. JAMES, TN, MARILLEY, RJ, AND MARRIOTT, HJL: *De Subitaneis Mortibus. XI. Young girl with palpitations.* Circulation 51:743, 1975.

125. WALSH, CK AND KRONGRAD, E: *Terminal cardiac electrical activity in pediatric patients.* Am J Cardiol 51:557, 1983.

# Index

A "t" following a page number indicates a table. A page number in *italics* indicates a figure.

315